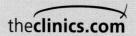

SLEEP MEDICINE CLINICS

Excessive Sleepiness

Guest Editor
CHRISTIAN GUILLEMINAULT, MD

March 2006 • Volume 1 • Number 1

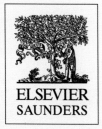

ELSEVIER
SAUNDERS

An imprint of Elsevier, Inc
PHILADELPHIA LONDON TORONTO MONTREAL SYDNEY TOKYO

W.B. SAUNDERS COMPANY
A Division of Elsevier Inc.

1600 John F. Kennedy Boulevard • Suite 1800 • Philadelphia, PA 19103-2899

http://www.sleep.theclinics.com

SLEEP MEDICINE CLINICS Volume 1, Number 1
March 2006 ISSN 1556-407X, ISBN 1-4160-3564-8

Editor: Sarah E. Barth

The ideas and opinions expressed in *Sleep Medicine Clinics* do not necessarily reflect those of the Publisher. The Publisher does not assume any responsibility for any injury and/or damage to persons or property arising out of or related to any use of the material contained in this periodical. The reader is advised to check the appropriate medical literature and the product information currently provided by the manufacturer of each drug to be administered to verify the dosage, the method and duration of administration, or contraindications. It is the responsibility of the treating physician or other health care professional, relying on independent experience and knowledge of the patient, to determine drug dosages and the best treatment for the patient. Mention of any product in this issue should not be construed as endorsement by the contributors, editors, or the Publisher of the product or manufacturers' claims.

Sleep Medicine Clinics (ISSN 1556-407X) is published quarterly by W.B. Saunders Company, 360 Park Avenue South, New York, NY 10010-1710. Months of publication are March, June, September and December. Business and editorial offices: 1600 John F. Kennedy Boulevard, Suite 1800, Philadelphia, PA 19103-2899. Accounting and circulation offices: 6277 Sea Harbor Drive, Orlando, FL 32887-4800. Periodicals postage paid at New York, and additional mailing offices. Subscription prices are $129.00 per year (US individuals), $50.00 (US students), $259.00 (US institutions), $149.00 (Canadian individuals), $85.00 (Canadian and foreign students), $279.00 (Canadian institutions), $149.00 (foreign individuals), and $279.00 (foreign institutions). Foreign air speed delivery is included in all *Clinics* subscription prices. All prices are subject to change without notice. POSTMASTER: Send address changes to *Sleep Medicine Clinics*, Elsevier Periodicals Customer Service, 6277 Sea Harbor Drive, FL 32887-4800. **Customer Service: 1-800-654-2452 (US). From outside of the United States, call 1-407-345-4000. E-mail: hhspcs@wbsaunders.com.**

Reprints: For copies of 100 or more, of articles in this publication, please contact the Commercial Reprints Department, Elsevier Inc., 360 Park Avenue South, New York, New York 10010-1710. Tel.: (212) 633-3813, Fax: (212) 462-1935, e-mail: reprints@elsevier.com.

Printed in the United States of America.

EXCESSIVE SLEEPINESS

CONSULTING EDITOR

TEOFILO LEE-CHIONG, MD
National Jewish Medical and Research Center,
Denver, Colorado

GUEST EDITOR

CHRISTIAN GUILLEMINAULT, MD, BiolD
Professor, Stanford University Sleep Medicine
Program, Stanford, California

CONTRIBUTORS

TORBJÖRN ÅKERSTEDT, PhD
IPM and Karolinska Institutet, Stockholm, Sweden

RICHARD P. ALLEN, PhD
Neurology and Sleep Medicine, John Hopkins
University; Bayview Medical Center,
Baltimore, Maryland

MONICA L. ANDERSEN, PhD
Department of Psychobiology, Universidade
Federal de Sao Paulo, Sao Paulo, Brazil

ISABELLE ARNULF, MD, PhD
Fédération des Pathologies du Sommeil, Hôpital
Pitié-Salpêtrière, Assistance Publique–Hôpitaux
de Paris, Paris, France; and Sleep Disorders
Center, Stanford University School of Medicine,
Stanford, California

CLAUDIO L. BASSETTI, MD
Professor of Neurology and Vice-Chairman,
Department of Neurology, University Hospital
of Zurich, Zurich, Switzerland

MICHEL BILLIARD, MD
Professor of Neurology, Faculté de Médecine,
Hôpital Gui-de-Chauliac, Montpellier, France

SARAH BLUNDEN, PhD
Adjunct Research Fellow, Centre for Sleep
Research, University of South Australia,
Adelaide, Australia

STEPHEN N. BROOKS, MD
Stanford Sleep Disorders Clinic, Stanford, California

RONALD D. CHERVIN, MD, MS
Associate Professor, Department of Neurology,
and Director, Sleep Disorders Center, University
of Michigan, Ann Arbor, Michigan

YVES DAUVILLIERS, MD, PhD
Associate Professor and Director of the
Sleep-Wake Laboratory, Service de Neurologie B,
Hôpital Gui-de-Chauliac; INSERM E0361,
Hôpital La Colombière, Montpellier, France

CHRISTIAN GUILLEMINAULT, MD, BiolD
Professor, Stanford University Sleep Medicine
Program, Stanford, California

TIMOTHY F. HOBAN, MD
Associate Professor, Departments of Pediatrics
and Neurology; Director, Pediatric Sleep
Medicine Program, University of Michigan,
Ann Arbor, Michigan

YU-SHU HUANG, MD, PhD
Departments of Child Psychiatry and Sleep
Medicine, Chang Gung Memorial Hospital,
Taipei, Taiwan; and Sleep Disorders Center,
Stanford University School of Medicine,
Stanford, California

ALEX IRANZO, MD
Neurology Service, Hospital Clínic de Barcelona and Institut D'Investigació Biomèdiques August Pi i Sunyer (IDIBAPS), Barcelona, Spain

CLETE A. KUSHIDA, MD, PhD
Stanford Sleep Disorders Clinic, Stanford University Center of Excellence for Sleep Disorders, Stanford, California

SCOTT M. LEIBOWITZ, MD
Stanford Sleep Disorders Clinic, Stanford University Center of Excellence for Sleep Disorders, Stanford, California

MARIA-CECILIA LOPES, MD
Stanford Sleep Disorders Clinic, Stanford University Center of Excellence for Sleep Disorders, Stanford, California; and Department of Psychobiology, Universidade Federal de Sao Paulo, Sao Paulo, Brazil

SEIJI NISHINO, MD, PhD
Associate Professor of Psychiatry and Behavioral Sciences, Director, Sleep and Circadian Neurobiology Laboratory, Associate Director, Center for Narcolepsy, Stanford University School of Medicine, Palo Alto, California

MAURICE M. OHAYON, MD, DSc, PhD
Associate Professor and Director, Stanford Sleep Epidemiology, School of Medicine, Stanford University, Palo Alto, California

KANNAN RAMAR, MD
Fellow in Sleep Medicine, Stanford University Sleep Medicine Program, Stanford, California

MICHAEL H. SILBER, MB, ChB
Professor of Neurology, Sleep Disorders Center and Department of Neurology, Mayo Clinic College of Medicine, Rochester, Minnesota

PHILIPP VALKO
Resident of Neurology, University Hospital of Zurich, Zurich, Switzerland

EXCESSIVE SLEEPINESS

Volume 1 • Number 1 • March 2006

Contents

Pathologic sleepiness is a fundamental symptom of sleep disorders. Mechanisms include increased sleep debt, circadian dysrhythmias, and decreased wakefulness drive. A detailed clinical history from the patient and observers, aided by quantitative sleepiness scales, is essential. Polysomnography and the Multiple Sleep Latency Test are the investigations most often required to reach a diagnosis. Other tests, such as the maintenance of wakefulness test, may be helpful in selected situations.

Excessive daytime sleepiness (EDS) has not been as extensively studied in the general population as insomnia. This article reviews more than 20 epidemiologic studies performed in different parts of the world. EDS has been defined in various ways, making comparisons between the studies hazardous. EDS was not gender-related in most of the studies. Evolution with age has given conflicting results. It has been associated with sleep-disordered breathing, mental disorders, and physical illness. Studies that used similar methodologies suggest that cultural differences might be involved in the observed differences in prevalence. From these studies, however, it seems that a uniform operational definition of EDS is still missing, jeopardizing the interpretation of the findings.

Circadian rhythm sleep disorders are caused by a mismatch between the sleep-wake pattern and circadian phase. Sleep at the circadian high is impaired, while alertness is reduced during wakefulness. This article explores the various circadian rhythm sleep

Sleep Deprivation and Sleepiness Caused by Sleep Loss 31

Scott M. Leibowitz, Maria-Cecilia Lopes, Monica L. Andersen, and Clete A. Kushida

Sleep deprivation and sleep loss are pervasive in modern society, largely stemming from societal demands of increased productivity. This increased productivity does not come without a cost to basic physiologic processes that have been explored by animal and human sleep deprivation research over the last century. These studies have provided some understanding of the molecular and neurochemical ramifications of sleep loss, and the circadian and homeostatic processes involved with sleep-wake mechanisms. Clinicians have several tools to assess daytime sleepiness as a consequence of sleep loss, and often this sleep loss is related to sleep and medical conditions. A better understanding of the causes and consequences of sleep loss can lead to recognition and curtailment of voluntary sleep deprivation and management of disorders that result in sleep loss.

Narcolepsy 47

Seiji Nishino

Narcolepsy is characterized by excessive daytime sleepiness, cataplexy, and other dissociated manifestations of rapid eye movement sleep. The major pathophysiology of human narcolepsy has recently been revealed by the extension of discoveries of narcolepsy genes in animal models. This directly led to the development of new diagnostic tests. The disease is currently treated with amphetamine-like compounds and modafinil for excessive daytime sleepiness and anticataplectics for cataplexy. Clinical, pharmacologic, pathophysiologic aspects of narcolepsy and future directions are discussed.

Excessive Daytime Sleepiness and Obstructive Sleep Apnea Syndrome 63

Kannan Ramar and Christian Guilleminault

Daytime sleepiness is a major symptom of obstructive sleep apnea syndrome and presents great public health concern. The underlying mechanisms are poorly understood. Poor correlation often exists between subjective and objective test measures, but new analytic methods have given hope for better results. Further study and validation of these methods, and development of alternative subjective and objective tests for sleepiness, will facilitate the clinical assessment of excessive daytime sleepiness. Compliance with the primary treatment must be maintained during provision of supplemental medication to sustain healthy outcomes.

Chronic Hypersomnia 79

Yves Dauvilliers and Michel Billiard

Although considerable progress has been made in understanding hypersomnia, the pathophysiology of idiopathic hypersomnia (IH) is still totally unknown. This article details the concept of IH with long sleep time and without long sleep time, and reports the main differential diagnosis. Also explored is hypersomnia caused by medical conditions, hypersomnia following infection, and nonorganic hypersomnia. There is a definite need further to develop sleep laboratory investigations to assess the correct diagnosis. Studies at the genetic and biologic levels are also needed to further the understanding of the pathophysiology of IH and to develop specific treatment.

The Kleine-Levin Syndrome

Yu-Shu Huang and Isabelle Arnulf

> The essential clinical criterion of Kleine-Levin syndrome (KLS) is recurrent episodes of hypersomnia. Patients have to experience at least one of the following symptoms during the episodes: (1) cognitive disturbances, (2) megaphagia, (3) hypersexuality, (4) irritability or odd behavior. Recent imaging studies have shown involvement of the thalamus, and raise the question of persistent hypoperfusion in some brain areas during the asymptomatic period. There is no clear etiology for the syndrome, although some more frequent HLA genotypes suggest a possible auto-immune mediation of the disease. No treatment as been shown systematically to improve KLS despite many trials with drugs. No therapeutic recommendation can be made today.

Sleepiness in Children

Sarah Blunden, Timothy F. Hoban, and Ronald D. Chervin

> Sleepiness is a common often underdiagnosed problem in children. Causes lie in both intrinsic and extrinsic sleep disorders of either a primary or secondary nature. Daytime sequelae of sleepiness in children include neuropsychologic and psychosocial deficits.

Neuromuscular Disorders and Sleepiness

Stephen N. Brooks

> Excessive daytime sleepiness (EDS) is a common symptom among patients with neuromuscular disease and may have a significant negative impact on the health and well-being of these individuals. Sleep-disordered breathing is often the most important cause of EDS in these patients. Additional causes of EDS in patients with neuromuscular disease may include nocturnal sleep disruption from pain, secretions, limited mobility or abnormal movements, central nervous system involvement as part of the primary disorder, or even medications used to treat the neuromuscular disease. With awareness of the problem, appropriate evaluation can lead to effective treatment of EDS in most of these cases.

Parkinson's Disease and Sleepiness

Alex Iranzo

> Sleepiness in Parkinson's disease is a common and complex phenomenon that may lead to automobile accidents and social problems because of excessive daytime somnolence and events of sudden-onset sleep. Sleepiness in Parkinson's disease is multifactorial. The main contributing factors are the intrinsic pathology of the disease itself and the sedative effects of dopaminergic agents used in its treatment.

Poststroke Hypersomnia

Claudio L. Bassetti and Philipp Valko

> Hypersomnia, defined as excessive sleepiness or sleep-like behavior, can reflect insufficient arousal following disruption of the arousal systems or increased production of sleep. Poststroke hypersomnia affects about 20% of patients with stroke. Severe and persistent hypersomnia is suggestive of a bilateral paramedian thalamic or mesencephalic stroke and large hemispheric strokes with mass effect. Poststroke hypersomnia can be documented by actigraphy, whereas the correlation with wake and sleep EEG is relatively poor. Persistent poststroke hypersomnia can occasionally be improved with stimulants or dopaminergic drugs.

Richard P. Allen

It has been assumed that periodic leg movements in sleep and the frequent arousals associated with them cause clinically significant insomnia and daytime sleepiness, but studies do not support this relationship. Restless legs syndrome (RLS) is associated with decreased sleep efficiency and short sleep times. RLS studies have consistently failed to find presence of the daytime sleepiness expected for the short sleep time. Some of the other effects of chronic sleep deprivation have been shown clinically and one recent report documented the expected cognitive impairment of frontal lobe function. RLS patients seem to have some altered arousal increasing alertness and overcoming sleepiness despite profound sleep loss.

FORTHCOMING ISSUES

June 2006

Sleep in the Elderly
Sonia Ancoli-Israel, PhD, *Guest Editor*

September 2006

Insomnia
Thomas Roth, PhD, *Guest Editor*

December 2006

Sleep Disordered Breathing
Max Hirschkovitz, MD, *Guest Editor*

ELSEVIER SAUNDERS

SLEEP
MEDICINE
CLINICS

Sleep Med Clin 1 (2006) xi

Foreword
Excessive Sleepiness

Teofilo Lee-Chiong, MD
National Jewish Medical and Research Center
1400 Jackson Street, Room J232
Denver, CO 80206, USA

E-mail address:
lee-chiongt@njc.org

In the highly tumultuous decade of the 1910s, the year 1912 was rather uneventful.

The war in Europe was to start in 2 years. The ocean liner RMS Titanic struck an iceberg on its maiden voyage and sank. It would be another 16 years before Fleming would discover penicillin and 17 more until the Black Thursday collapse of the stock market ushered in the Great Depression. In the midst of all these historic events, 1912 stood alone in its relative obscurity.

It was, nonetheless, in this transitory year of 1912 that the *Clinics of North America* began, with the publication of its *Surgical Clinics.*

A physician reading the *Clinics* that year knew close to nothing about sleep, certainly very little about insomnia, and not much, if at all, about circadian rhythmicity. Snoring was merely an "indelicate" subject, and psychiatrists everywhere were attempting to unravel the mysteries of dreaming even as they tried to comprehend the meaning of its fantasies. The dangers of sleep apnea had yet to be described.

Since then, the *Clinics* has expanded to include 60 titles, each with a worldwide distribution. The *Sleep Medicine Clinics* is the latest addition to this series.

This premiere issue on excessive sleepiness will be followed by issues on sleep in the elderly, insomnia, and sleep apnea in this initial year of the *Sleep Medicine Clinics.* Future issues will feature pediatric and adolescent sleep, sleep among women, parasomnias, circadian rhythms, forensic sleep medicine, cardiovascular disorders, endocrine diseases, and much more.

It will take another 94 years before the *Sleep Medicine Clinics* becomes as seasoned and revered as its surgical counterpart. We expect to have covered the breadth and width of sleep medicine several times over by then.

Welcome to the *Sleep Medicine Clinics.*

doi:10.1016/j.jsmc.2006.01.001

SLEEP
MEDICINE
CLINICS

Sleep Med Clin 1 (2006) xiii–xiv

Preface
Excessive Sleepiness

Christian Guilleminault, MD, BiolD
Kannan Ramar, MD
Stanford University Sleep Medicine Program
401 Quarry Road, Suite 3301
Stanford, CA 94305, USA

E-mail address:
cguil@stanford.edu

Daytime sleepiness is a state that may be ignored for many years by affected subjects. Subjective scales have been developed for assessment of daytime sleepiness, but the controversies regarding their efficacy are many. Subjects with obstructive sleep apnea of similar apnea–hypopnea index may have an Epworth sleepiness scale (ESS) score that can be as low as 5 and as high as 15. Correlation between subjective scales and polysomnographic tests exploring daytime sleepiness are also often poor. Subjects with an ESS score of 6 have shown a mean sleep latency of 6 minutes as measured with the multiple sleep latency test (MSLT) and 8 minutes as measured with the maintenance of wakefulness test (MWT). Alternatively, subjects with an ESS score of 13 have shown a mean sleep latency of 14 minutes (by way of MSLT) and of 15 minutes (by way of MWT). Individuals may deny sleepiness but report "fatigue" or "tiredness" when they wake up that increases with time during the day. Many attempts have been made at defining sleepiness, and various tests have been used to measure attention and performance in sleepy patients with limited success.

Investigation of sleep deprivation or sleep restriction has shown that important variability exists in the way subjects respond to these challenges. In one of our studies with 7 days of sleep restriction to 4 hours per night, important individual differences in performance, subjective alertness scales, and polysomnographic tests were already evident by day 2. These differences persisted until the end of the experimental condition despite the fact that the flattening of the leptin secretion curve associated with sleep restriction and the increase in food intake were similar in all subjects [1]. We are far from understanding the biological basis of these individual differences. Our study on sleep restriction in young adults also showed dissociation between subjects in the decrements noted in different tests used over time; some were present in all subjects and some were present only in a subgroup of normal individuals. Additionally, the severity of the impairment, related to similar sleep restriction or deprivation, judged with specific performance tests or the MWT varied from mild to severe.

Clearly, we do not possess "the test" that can appropriately evaluate impairment due to daytime sleepiness, and we cannot effectively determine all impairments related to sleepiness in a given subject at all hours of the day. It is also difficult to properly assess the personal and societal risks that may arise when an individual is coping with sleep restriction, abnormal schedules, or a sleep-disturbing illness or mechanisms to maintain alertness. Finally, genetic and environmental factors, as always in medicine, may interact to produce excessive daytime sleepiness (EDS).

doi:10.1016/j.jsmc.2006.01.002

Complaints of EDS exist, however, and its effects are clearly pronounced in everyday events such as decreased social/cognitive function and motor vehicle accidents. Epidemiologic studies have shown a very wide range of response to this matter. In the United States, many different methodologies have been applied to the study of EDS, making it difficult to compare studies; the reported prevalences vary from 0.3% to 16.3%. The Cardiovascular Health Study [2] found a 20% prevalence of participants being "usually sleepy in the daytime" in a sample of 4578 adults aged 65 and older. In Europe, the prevalence varied from 5% to 16% in adults aged 20 years and older. In addition, most investigations of the prevalence of EDS have been performed on Caucasians, and we lack information on the prevalence of the complaint in other ethnicities.

The notion that sleep restriction, shift work hours, and poor sleep hygiene—characteristics often linked with industrialization—are associated with EDS is recognized by many. Additionally, the fact that syndromes such as narcolepsy are associated with EDS—and that the symptoms can be a major element in the pathology of EDS—is well acknowledged. Systematic investigation of narcolepsy–cataplexy has lead to the discovery of the hypocretin/orexin system in the brain, and recognition of the importance of this system in the maintenance of alertness. However, we are still far from having a good grasp of the different neuronal systems involved in maintenance of normal alertness and the brain circuits associated and activated with EDS. Von Economo, studying encephalitica lethargica [3], identified brain regions critical for the maintenance of alertness, and since then many have tried to use the anatomic-pathology approach to investigate the problem. We have more tools at our disposal, but many points remain unclear. Recently, EDS was investigated in a large cohort study, the Honolulu-Asia Aging study cohort, and an increased risk of subsequent development of Parkinson disease was shown in men with EDS [4].

This issue of the *Sleep Medicine Clinics* covers many avenues, from evaluation of the sleepy patient to the many possible factors behind a complaint of EDS. Can we use the understanding of neurologic disorders to paint a clearer picture of EDS? What can we offer to subjects who complain of EDS? What is behind intermittent but recurrent hypersomnia? What are the risks associated with EDS in children and in adults? We are still far from finding responses to all these questions, but advances have been made during the past few years. These advances are outlined in this issue, as are the many remaining unanswered questions that our field needs to tackle.

References

[1] Guilleminault C, Powell NB, Martinez S, et al. Preliminary observations on the effect of sleep time in a sleep restriction paradigm. Sleep Med 2003;3:177–84.

[2] Whitney CW, Enright PL, Newman AB, et al. Correlates of daytime sleepiness in 4578 elderly persons: the Cardiovascular Health Study. Sleep 1998;21:27–36.

[3] Von Economo C. Encephalitis lethargica: its sequelae and treament. Oxford (UK): Oxford University Press; 1931.

[4] Abbott RD, Ross GW, White LR, et al. Excessive daytime sleepiness and subsequent development of Parkinson disease. Neurology 2005;65:1442–6.

SLEEP
MEDICINE
CLINICS

Sleep Med Clin 1 (2006) 1–7

The Investigation of Sleepiness

Michael H. Silber, MB, ChB

- ■ Clinical approach
- ■ Sleepiness scales
- ■ Polysomnography
- ■ The Multiple Sleep Latency Test
- ■ Maintenance of Wakefulness Test
- ■ Performance testing
- ■ Other tests
- ■ References

Abnormal sleepiness is one of the primary symptoms of sleep disorders. Sleepiness is a normal physiologic phenomenon, however, and only becomes excessive when it occurs in situations when individuals can be reasonably expected to be awake and alert [1]. The degree of sleepiness depends on interplay between two factors: the time in the circadian cycle (process C), and the length of time from the last sleep period (process S) [2]. In subjects with normal circadian rhythmicity, sleepiness is maximal between 2 and 6 AM with a second minor peak 12 hours earlier in the afternoon. This rhythm is modified by the degree of accumulated sleep debt, a process that results in a homeostatic drive to induce sleep. Sleepiness is counterbalanced by alerting mechanisms, modulated predominantly by monoaminergic neuronal systems, such as dopaminergic and histaminergic pathways. The cluster of hypocretin (orexin) secreting neurons in the hypothalamus may be the master controller modulating monoaminergic systems, with projections from these neurons being widely distributed to the brainstem, diencephalon, and basal forebrain [3].

Sleepiness can be conceptualized as having two components: the subjective perception of the need to sleep, and the ability to transition from a state of wakefulness to a state of sleep [4]. The perception of the need to sleep is usually accompanied by objective manifestations, such as yawning, loss of neck extensor tone, pupillary constriction, ptosis,

and a decreased attention span. The ability to fall asleep can be measured objectively using electroencephalographic activity and this forms the basis for the Multiple Sleep Latency Test (MSLT). The two components of sleepiness may dissociate; some patients with pathologic sleepiness have little or no warning of sleep onset, whereas patients with restless legs syndrome or psychophysiologic insomnia may have an intense desire to fall asleep but be unable to do so.

Excessive sleepiness may be caused by factors that disrupt circadian rhythmicity, increase sleep debt by either voluntary curtailment of sleep time or fragmentation of sleep, or decrease the drive toward alertness [Box 1] [4]. Disorders of circadian rhythmicity include intrinsic disorders, such as delayed sleep phase syndrome, and extrinsic causes, such as the effects of shift work. Insufficient sleep syndrome, perhaps the commonest cause of excessive sleepiness, is caused by voluntary sleep curtailment. Fragmentation of sleep by diseases, such as obstructive sleep apnea syndrome, or environmental factors, such as exposure to a bed partner's snoring [5], reduce the restorative value of sleep and increase sleep debt. Narcolepsy, in association with cataplexy, is caused by reduced activity of the wakefulness system secondary to decreased hypocretin production. Histamine receptor antagonists reduce alertness, as do benzodiazepine receptor agonists, such as benzodiazepines, barbiturates, and alcohol.

Sleep Disorders Center and Department of Neurology, Mayo Clinic College of Medicine, 200 1st Street, Rochester, MN 55905, USA
E-mail address: msilber@mayo.edu

doi:10.1016/j.jsmc.2005.11.005

The exact mechanisms by which other drugs cause sleepiness are often uncertain. Similarly, the pathophysiology of some intrinsic disorders of hypersomnolence, such as idiopathic hypersomnia, remains obscure.

Tiredness is not always synonymous with sleepiness. The term "fatigue" is used in sleep medicine to refer to a feeling of exhaustion with an inability to perform physical activities at the level one might expect. It is often associated with mental fatigue characterized by poor concentration and memory. Patients with fatigue generally do not complain of falling asleep inappropriately and their symptoms are usually not caused by a primary sleep disorder. Causes include chronic medical conditions, such as infections, malignancies, autoimmune disorders, and endocrinopathies; neurologic disorders, such as myasthenia gravis, Parkinson's disease, and multiple sclerosis; and psychiatric disorders, such as depression, somatoform disorders, and personality disorders. A subgroup of patients with chronic tiredness have chronic fatigue syndrome.

Clinical approach

The elucidation of excessive sleepiness commences with a careful history from the patient, supplemented by collateral history from a bed partner when available. First, a detailed account of a typical night's sleep is elicited, including bedtime, time asleep, wakenings during the night, and morning rise time. Reasons for periods of wakefulness while in bed should be determined, such as physical complaints, environmental factors, or an active mind. A patient's sleep patterns may vary with work shifts and days off work, and these differences should be noted. A change in sleep patterns at the onset of sleepiness may be relevant. Next, the occurrence of specific respiratory and motor symptoms during sleep should be explored. A history of snoring, waking with a choking sensation in the throat, or apnea observed by the bed partner are strong indicators to consider sleep apnea syndrome. A history of restless legs at night or observed periodic limb movements during sleep may be helpful.

The nature of the patient's complaint of sleepiness should be fully explored, with fatigue differentiated from sleepiness. The degree of somnolence experienced under varying circumstances should be ascertained, such as working at a computer, watching television, sitting in a theater, or talking with a single person. Special emphasis should be paid to sleepiness driving, including drifting of the car off the road or across the center line. The presence of cataplexy, the sudden bilateral loss of muscle strength caused by emotion, is very specific for a diagnosis of narcolepsy. The occurrence of hypnagogic hallucinations and sleep paralysis is less specific, because these phenomena may be seen in a variety of sleep disorders and in normal persons [6,7]. A detailed psychosocial history is essential, including occupations, social relationships, psychiatric disorders, stressors, and substance use. Past medical history and family history of sleep disorders may be revealing.

The goals of history taking in the sleepy patient are to determine if extrinsic environmental factors are responsible for the patient's symptoms, and to obtain clues to the presence of one or more disorders causing somnolence. Insufficient sleep syndrome, sleepiness caused by drugs or medications, and environmental sleep disorder can usually be diagnosed, especially if collateral history is available. With these conditions, further investigations are generally not required. If the history results in suspicion of disorders, such as obstructive sleep apnea syndrome or narcolepsy, or if there are no indicators to the underlying diagnosis, then further testing is needed, including polysomnography and MSLT.

Sleepiness scales

Sleepiness scales are standardized questions designed to quantitate subjective sleepiness. They have the advantage of being easy and cheap to administer and to reflect the patient's own opinion on the severity of the symptoms; however, they do not measure any objective parameter of sleepiness. They are used to supplement the history and to follow the effects of treatment.

The most commonly used scale is the Epworth Sleepiness Scale, developed in 1991 [8]. This scale poses eight situations, such as sitting and reading, or sitting in a car while stopped for a few minutes in traffic. Patients are asked to rate their chance of dozing in each situation on a scale of 0 to 3, with zero indicating no chance of dozing and 3 a high chance of dozing. The possible total score is 24. The normal upper limit, derived from two studies of 72 and 182 normal subjects, is generally considered to be 10 to 11 points [9,10]. The Epworth Sleepiness Scale has acceptable test-retest reliability [11]. The score has been shown to correlate with the intensity of psychologic symptoms [12] and is consistently higher in women than men [13]. There is surprisingly poor correlation with MSLT results [14,15]. This does not necessarily indicate that the Epworth Sleepiness Scale has low validity but rather that it may be measuring a different component of sleepiness. The scale is useful clinically as an adjunct to the history, and a supplement to the MSLT, especially when mean latencies fall between 5 and 10 minutes (see later). It can also be used to judge quantitative changes in sleepiness following therapy.

An older scale, used since 1972, is the Stanford Sleepiness Scale [16]. This scale measures sleepiness at a specific time and is often administered just before the trials of MSLT to assess whether the patient's perception is in keeping with the objective results. It consists of eight options, each comprising a series of descriptors of increasing drowsiness, such as "relaxed," "awake," "not at full alertness," or "let down." Visual analog scales have also been used to assess sleepiness, and these may be especially helpful in monitoring the intensity and duration of the effect of stimulants administered at different times of the day [4].

Polysomnography

Polysomnography, the fundamental investigation in sleep medicine, consists of the simultaneous recording of multiple physiologic parameters during sleep. The minimum signals recorded are electroencephalography, electro-oculography, submental and anterior tibial surface electromyography, electrocardiography, measures of airflow and thoraco-abdominal expansion, and oxyhemoglobin saturation. Sleep is scored into different stages according to standard criteria [17] and a summary of the frequency of respiratory disturbances and periodic limb movements is prepared.

Polysomnography is vital in the investigation of the sleepy patient. First, it is the method whereby the spectrum of sleep-disordered breathing, including obstructive and central sleep apnea syndromes, is diagnosed. Polysomnography is also necessary for the diagnosis of periodic limb movement disorder. Second, polysomnography is required the night before a MSLT, as discussed later.

The Multiple Sleep Latency Test

The MSLT is the most frequent objective test of sleepiness used in clinical practice. First described in 1977 [18], it remains widely used despite concerns regarding its ability to distinguish accurately normal and pathologic sleepiness. It is essential to understand the limitations of the test and the preconditions that need to be fulfilled for its results to be meaningful. When used correctly as one element in the comprehensive assessment of a sleepy patient, however, it remains a powerful diagnostic tool. In broad outline, the MSLT consists of four or five nap opportunities at 2-hour intervals during the course of the day. The mean time from lights out to sleep onset is calculated and the presence of any rapid eye movement (REM) sleep on the naps is noted. The first attempt to standardize the MSLT was made in 1986 [19], with revised guidelines formulated by a panel of experts using the RAND-UCLA appropriateness method published by the American Academy of Sleep Medicine in 2005 [20]. Face validity for the MSLT as a measure of the ability to stay awake is provided by studies demonstrating its correlation with prior sleep deprivation [21], subjective measurements of sleepiness [22], and the effect of drugs known to be sedating [23]. Intrarater reliability is 0.87 [24], interrater reliability 0.85 to 0.9 [24,25], and test-retest reliability in normal subjects 0.97 [26].

Preparation for the MSLT includes discontinuation of all psychotropic medications that can cause sleepiness or suppress REM sleep 2 weeks before the date of the test (6 weeks for fluoxetine) [20]. This includes antidepressants, stimulants, hypnotics, tranquillizers, and narcotics. Although often inconvenient for the patient, this can generally be achieved with careful planning, sometimes delaying the test to a time when the patient can take time off from work and refrain from driving. In situations when it is clinically unacceptable to discontinue medications, such as active major depression or epilepsy, it is better not to perform the test at all at that time than to obtain uninterpretable results. In those circumstances, diagnoses should be made based on all other information available and clinical judgment. Discontinuing medications too close to the date of the test can result in REM sleep rebound during the naps and may result in an incorrect diagnosis of narcolepsy. A urine drug screen should be performed on the morning of the test to rule out continued medication use or concealed drug abuse. Caffeinated beverages are not permitted during the test and should ideally be kept to a minimum for several days before the study. Smoking should not occur at least 30 minutes before each test.

The MSLT is sensitive to prior sleep time. The first studies of the test were performed in subjects who had undergone voluntary sleep deprivation [18,27] and demonstrated significant correlations between sleep latency and degree of sleep loss. Extending the time in bed to 10 hours a night for 2 weeks in 23 subjects who had reported spending 6 to 9 hours sleeping a night resulted in a change in the MSLT mean sleep latency from 6.5 to 11.5 minutes [28], confirming an earlier similar study [29]. In contrast, a retrospective analysis of the effects of prior sleep time on the MSLT was performed using normal controls in 10 studies with sleep time the previous night greater than 435 minutes compared with seven studies with sleep time the previous night less than 425 minutes [1]. The former group had significantly shorter mean MSLT latencies than the latter group. It is hard to reconcile this paradoxical result with the data associating shorter MSLT mean latencies with increasing sleep deprivation. Published guidelines suggest a minimum sleep time the night before the test of 6 hours [20]. It is required that polysomnography be performed the night before, both to measure sleep time accurately and to rule out sleep-disordered breathing as a cause for sleepiness. Sleep logs should be obtained for 1 week before the study to assess sleep-wake schedules and some sleep centers routinely use wrist actigraphy to obtain a more objective measure of sleep and wakefulness. Many sleep specialists regard the minimum suggested sleep time of 6 hours the night before the MSLT as too short and strive to achieve at least 7 hours sleep a night for a week before the study, especially on the night before the test.

The MSLT is sensitive to alerting factors, such as physical activity [30], ambient temperature, light, and noise. The nap opportunities should take place in a dark, quiet room with the patient lying comfortably in bed [20]. Exercise and exposure to bright sunlight should not be permitted between naps and all stimulating mental activity should cease 15 minutes before each test. A light breakfast and lunch should be provided at least an hour before the first and third nap opportunities. The first test should take place 1.5 to 3 hours after waking from the night's sleep and then about every 2 hours thereafter. Although five nap opportunities are recommended, a shorter four-nap test can be performed unless sleep-onset REM sleep has occurred on one of the first four naps.

At the start of each nap opportunity, biocalibrations should be performed and the patient should then be asked to lie quietly in a comfortable position with eyes closed and try to fall asleep [20]. Sleep latency is defined as the time from lights out to the first epoch of any stage of sleep (more than 15 seconds sleep in a 30-second epoch). If no sleep is obtained, the test is terminated 20 minutes after lights out and the latency is recorded as 20 minutes. If sleep occurs, then the test should continue for 15 minutes from sleep onset, including any subsequent wakefulness epochs. The mean sleep latency is calculated for the four or five naps. REM sleep latency is defined as the time from sleep onset to the first epoch of REM sleep, irrespective of any intervening epochs of wakefulness. A sleep-onset REM period (SOREMP) occurs if REM sleep commences within 15 minutes of sleep onset. The number of SOREMPs is counted.

The interpretation of the MSLT mean sleep latency is controversial. The original studies of 14 control subjects showed mean latencies of 10.7 minutes compared with 3 minutes in a group of 27 narcoleptic patients [31]. Despite standard deviations of more than 5 minutes in the control group, the authors suggested a "preliminary guideline" of less than 5 minutes indicating pathologic sleepiness. The subsequent 1986 guidelines established a "generally accepted rule of thumb," with mean latencies of less than 5 minutes indicating definite excessive daytime sleepiness, latencies greater than 10 minutes indicating normal alertness, and latencies in the range of 5 to 10 minutes falling in a "diagnostic gray area" of uncertain significance [19]. Very few subsequent studies of normative data have been published; the largest with 176 subjects reported a mean latency 11.1 minutes in younger and 12.5 minutes in older subjects, but standard deviations were not given [32]. An analysis of combined data from normal control subjects in 27 studies using the MSLT has been reported [1]. The mean latency was 10.4 ± 4.3 minutes for studies with four naps and 11.6 ± 5.2 minutes for studies with five naps. In none of the studies, however, was the primary outcome the development of MSLT norms. The total sleep time the preceding night was not always recorded and deviations from the standard

MSLT protocol often occurred, especially with reference to the definition of sleep onset. Other studies have shown that the mean MSLT sleep latency is also sensitive to age [32], with longer latencies being recorded from preadolescent children [33].

With these imperfect data, the MSLT should be interpreted in clinical practice as one of a number of pieces of important diagnostic information. Mean latencies should be regarded as representing a continuum of sleepiness, with lower values indicating greater sleepiness than higher values. Although some ostensibly normal research subjects may have mean latencies below 5 minutes, values in this range generally indicates pathologic sleepiness caused by disease or insufficient sleep. The closer the mean latency approaches 10 minutes, the more overlap there is with a normal population, but some patients with pathologic sleepiness fall into the 5- to 10-minute range. Clinical judgment, supplemented by quantitative sleepiness scales, should be used to supplement the MSLT in this group. Mean latencies of 10 and above fall within the statistically normal range and indicate sleepiness that is not significantly greater than a control population.

The presence of SOREMPs on two or more naps is generally considered abnormal. This finding is the characteristic neurophysiologic marker for narcolepsy, but is not entirely sensitive or specific. Pooling of data from eight studies showed a sensitivity of 0.78 and a specificity of 0.93 for the diagnosis of narcolepsy [20]. SOREMPs are also seen in 7% of patients with obstructive sleep apnea syndrome [34] and this finding emphasizes the importance of ruling out obstructive sleep apnea by polysomnography the night before an MSLT. Obstructive sleep apnea and narcolepsy may coexist, but the latter should only be diagnosed with an MSLT following at least several weeks of confirmed effective therapy for sleep-disordered breathing. SOREMPS may also be caused by withdrawal of REM-suppressant medication, sleep deprivation, sleep-wake schedule disorders, and occasionally major depression. Precise attention to the correct preparation of patients for the test results in exclusion of most of these confounding causes. In addition to SOREMPS, patients with narcolepsy generally have very short mean sleep latencies on the MSLT, with pooled data from different studies revealing a value of 3.1 ± 2.9 minutes [1]. The International Classification of Sleep Disorders, 2nd edition [35], suggests a mean latency of 8 or less minutes as one of the criteria for the diagnosis of narcolepsy. Data on the use of the MSLT in the diagnosis of idiopathic hypersomnia are less clear, because most studies require a short MSLT mean sleep latency as a diagnostic criterion for the disorder [35].

Maintenance of Wakefulness Test

The Maintenance of Wakefulness Test (MWT), a variant of the MSLT, tests the ability to remain awake rather than the drive to fall asleep. It is not used as a test of sleepiness but rather to measure the effectiveness of therapy. An objective measure of therapeutic response may be useful when public safety is at risk, such as when patients with treated sleep disorders wish to drive school busses or fly airplanes. Indeed, the United States Federal Aviation Administration mandates the test before pilots treated for obstructive sleep apnea syndrome are allowed to resume flying [20]. The MWT may also be useful in the assessment of patients who still describe sleepiness despite high doses of stimulant medication to differentiate between the development of drug tolerance and fatigue from an unrelated problem [20]. The MWT has been used as an end point in large studies of modafinil in the treatment of narcolepsy and has been shown to be sensitive to stimulant effect [36,37].

There are several differences between the MSLT and the MWT. The MWT may be more susceptible to motivational factors than the MSLT. The MWT attempts to assess alertness in real-life situations, so a preceding sleep log or polysomnogram is usually not necessary [20]. Drug therapy should not be changed before the study. The patient should be seated in bed with back and head supported by a bed rest (bolster pillow) in such a way that the neck is comfortable. Careful attention should be paid to ambient light; a 7.5-W night light placed 1 ft off the floor and 3 feet lateral to the patient's head should be the only illumination in the room. At the start of each trial, the patient should be asked to sit still and remain awake as long as possible but extraordinary measures, such as singing or slapping the face, are not permitted. Each trial is terminated after three epochs of stage 1 non-REM sleep or one epoch of any other stage. If no sleep occurs, the trial is stopped after 40 minutes. Sleep latency is defined in the same manner as in the MSLT and mean sleep latency are calculated.

In contrast to the MSLT, a multicenter normative study of 64 subjects aged 30 to 70 years has been performed [38]. The mean sleep time by polysomnography the night before the study was 417 ± 63 minutes. Mean MWT latencies did not correlate with the total sleep time, suggesting that sleep deprivation may not have affected the results. A truncated distribution of mean latencies was noted with subjects remaining awake for 40 minutes in over 75% of the trials. The mean latency was 32.6 ± 9.9 minutes. The choice of a reasonable mean sleep latency to indicate acceptable alertness is fraught with difficulties. The MWT is a laboratory test and the results may not correlate with the ability to remain awake while driving a bus or flying an airplane. The 5th percentile (approximately 11 minutes) is probably an inappropriately low cutpoint, because it implies that some patients with ostensibly normal mean sleep latencies may be less alert than about 90% of the normal population. Conversely, requiring patients to remain awake for 40 minutes on all four trials implies a standard of alertness achieved by less than half the normal population, imposing a higher standard to be met by the sick than the healthy. Mean sleep latency at the 15th percentile (approximately 22.5 minutes) has been suggested as an arbitrary lower limit of acceptable alertness [4], but this value has not been validated; it might be equally reasonable to use the 25th, 50th, or 75th percentiles. Physicians must use clinical judgment in interpreting the results in a particular patient, taking into account the illness, its treatment, and the activities for which the patient needs to be alert.

Performance testing

Performance tests have been developed to assess alertness using psychophysiologic rather than electrophysiologic measures. These include the psychomotor vigilance test in which motor responses to sounds of varying intensities in a quiet environment are assessed [39], and driving simulation tasks in which a subject has to respond to road emergencies interspersed between long periods of monotonous steering [40]. These tests may, at least in theory, provide a more realistic measure of alertness in real life than the MSLT. Although frequently used in research, they have not been widely used in the clinical assessment of the sleepy patient.

Other tests

Although metabolic disturbances, such as hypothyroidism or hepatic failure, may result in fatigue, they rarely give rise to sleepiness, unless severe enough to cause an encephalopathy. If the distinction between fatigue and sleepiness is clinically unclear, however, it is reasonable to check thyroid, adrenocortical, hepatic, and renal function.

HLA DQB1*0602 is found in about 90% of patients with narcolepsy with cataplexy and in 35% to 56% of patients with narcolepsy without cataplexy [41,42]. It also occurs in about 20% of the normal population [43], however, and has low specificity and predictive value for the diagnosis of narcolepsy. There is little role for its use in routine clinical practice. Cerebrospinal hypocretin-1 (orexin-A) concentration is low or zero (≤110 pg/mL) in about 90% of patients with nar-

colepsy with cataplexy [44]. It is normal, however, in more than 80% of patients with narcolepsy without cataplexy and in most cases of idiopathic hypersomnia [44,45]. It is only useful as a diagnostic tool if cataplexy if present. The test is currently used only as a research technique, but soon may become more widely available. Possible future indications for its use include confirming a diagnosis of narcolepsy in patients with sleepiness and cataplexy who cannot undergo a meaningful MSLT because of the presence of concomitant disorders, such as obstructive sleep apnea syndrome, or the use of medications interfering with the interpretation of the test.

References

[1] Arand D, Bonnet M, Hurwitz T, et al. The clinical use of the MSLT and the MWT: review by the MSLT and MWT Task Force of the Standards of Practice Committee of the American Academy of Sleep Medicine. Sleep 2005;28:123–44.

[2] Borbely AA, Achermann P. Sleep homeostasis and models of sleep regulation. In: Kryger MH, Roth T, Dement WC, editors. Principles and practice of sleep medicine. 4th edition. Philadelphia: Elsevier Saunders; 2005. p. 405–17.

[3] Mignot E. Sleep, sleep disorders and hypocretin (orexin). Sleep Med 2004;5(Suppl 1):S2–8.

[4] Silber MH, Krahn LE, Morgenthaler TI. Sleep medicine in clinical practice. London: Taylor and Francis; 2004.

[5] Beninati W, Harris C, Herold DL, et al. The effect of snoring and obstructive sleep apnea on the sleep quality of bed partners. Mayo Clin Proc 1999;74:955–8.

[6] Ohayon MM, Priest RG, Caulet M, et al. Hypnagogic and hypnopompic hallucinations: pathological phenomena? Br J Psychiatry 1996;169:459–67.

[7] Ohayon MM, Zulley J, Guillaminault C, et al. Prevalence and pathologic associations of sleep paralysis in the general population. Neurology 1999;52:1194–200.

[8] Johns MW. A new method for measuring daytime sleepiness: the Epworth sleepiness scale. Sleep 1991;14:540–5.

[9] Johns MW, Hocking B. Daytime sleepiness and sleep habits of Australian workers. Sleep 1997;20:844–9.

[10] Parkes JD, Chen SY, Clift SJ, et al. The clinical diagnosis of the narcoleptic syndrome. J Sleep Res 1998;7:41–52.

[11] Johns MW. Sleepiness in different situations measured by the Epworth sleepiness scale. Sleep 1994;17:703–10.

[12] Olson LG, Cole MF, Ambrogetti A. Correlations among Epworth Sleepiness Scale scores, Multiple Sleep Latency Tests and psychological symptoms. J Sleep Res 1998;7:248–53.

[13] Chervin RD. Sleepiness, fatigue, tiredness, and

lack of energy in obstructive sleep apnea syndrome. Chest 2000;118:372–9.

[14] Chervin RD, Aldrich MS. The Epworth Sleepiness Scale may not reflect objective measures of sleepiness or sleep apnea. Neurology 1999;52:125–31.

[15] Benbadis S, Mascha E, Perry MC, et al. Association between the Epworth Sleepiness Scale and the Multiple Sleep Latency Test in a clinical population. Ann Intern Med 1999;130:289–92.

[16] Hoddes E, Zarcone V, Smythe H, et al. Quantification of sleepiness: a new approach. Psychophysiology 1973;10:431–6.

[17] Rechtschaffen A, Kales A. A manual of standardized terminology, techniques, and scoring system for sleep stages of human subjects. Bethesda: National Institute of Neurological Disease and Blindness; 1968.

[18] Carskadon MA, Dement WC. Sleep tendency: an objective measure of sleep loss. Sleep Res 1977;6:200.

[19] Carskadon MA, Dement WC, Mitler MM, et al. Guidelines for the multiple sleep latency test (MSLT): a standard measure of sleepiness. Sleep 1986;9:519–24.

[20] American Academy of Sleep Medicine. Practice parameters for clinical use of the Multiple Sleep Latency Test and the Maintenance of Wakefulness Test. Sleep 2005;28:113–21.

[21] Rosenthal L, Roehrs TA, Rosen A, et al. Level of sleepiness and total sleep time following various time in bed conditions. Sleep 1993;16:226–32.

[22] Carskadon MA, Dement WC. The Multiple Sleep Latency Test: what does it measure? Sleep 1982;5(Suppl 2):S67–72.

[23] Bliwise D, Seidel W, Karacan I, et al. Daytime sleepiness as a criterion in hypnotic medication trials: comparison of triazolam and flurazepam. Sleep 1983;6:156–63.

[24] Drake CL, Rice MF, Roehrs TA, et al. Scoring reliability of the Multiple Sleep Latency Test in a clinical population. Sleep 2000;23:911–3.

[25] Benbadis SR, Qu Y, Perry MC, et al. Interrater reliability of the Multiple Sleep Latency Test. Electroencephalogr Clin Neurophysiol 1995;95:302–4.

[26] Zwyghuizen-Doorenbos A, Roehrs T, Schaefer M, et al. Test-retest reliability of the MSLT. Sleep 1988;11:562–5.

[27] Carskadon MA, Dement WC. Effects of total sleep loss on sleep tendency. Percept Mot Skills 1979;48:495–506.

[28] Roehrs T, Shore E, Papineau K, et al. A two-week sleep extension in sleepy normals. Sleep 1996;19:576–82.

[29] Carskadon MA, Dement WC. Nocturnal determinants of daytime sleepiness. Sleep 1982;5(Suppl 2):S73–81.

[30] Bonnet MH, Arand DL. Sleepiness as measured by modified multiple sleep latency testing as a function of preceding activity. Sleep 1998;21:477–83.

[31] Richardson GS, Carskadon MA, Flagg W, et al. Excessive daytime sleepiness in man: multiple sleep latency measurement in narcoleptic and control subjects. Electroencephalogr Clin Neurophysiol 1978;45:621–7.

[32] Levine B, Roehrs T, Zorick F, et al. Daytime sleepiness in young adults. Sleep 1988;11:39–46.

[33] Carskadon MA. The second decade. In: Guilleminault C, editor. Sleeping and waking disorders: indications and techniques. Menlo Park: Addison-Wesley; 1982. p. 99–125.

[34] Aldrich MS, Chervin RD, Malow BA. Value of the Multiple Sleep Latency Test (MSLT) for the diagnosis of narcolepsy. Sleep 1997;20:620–9.

[35] American Academy of Sleep Medicine. The international classification of sleep disorders: diagnostic and coding manual. 2nd edition. Westchester (IL): American Academy of Sleep Medicine; 2005.

[36] US Modafinil in Narcolepsy Multicenter Group. Randomized trial of modafinil for the treatment of pathological somnolence in narcolepsy. Ann Neurol 1998;43:88–97.

[37] US Modafinil in Narcolepsy Multicenter Group. Randomized trial of modafinil as a treatment for excessive daytime somnolence in narcolepsy. Neurology 2000;54:1166–75.

[38] Doghramji K, Mitler MM, Sangal RB, et al. A normative study of the Maintenance of Wakefulness Test (MWT). Electroencephalogr Clin Neurophysiol 1997;103:554–62.

[39] Van Dongen HPA, Maislin G, Mullington JM, et al. The cumulative cost of additional wakefulness: dose-response effects on neurobehavioral functions and sleep physiology from chronic sleep restriction and sleep deprivation. Sleep 2003;26:117–26.

[40] Findley LJ, Suratt PM, Dinges DF. Time-on-task decrements in "steer clear" performance of patients with sleep apnea and narcolepsy. Sleep 1999;22:804–9.

[41] Mignot E, Hayduk R, Black J, et al. HLA DQB1*0602 is associated with cataplexy in 509 narcoleptic patients. Sleep 1997;20:1012–20.

[42] Rogers AE, Meehan J, Guillaminault C, et al. HLA DR15 (DR2) and DQB1*0602 typing studies in 188 narcoleptic patients with cataplexy. Neurology 1997;48:1550–6.

[43] Fernandez-Vina M, Gao X, Morales M, et al. Alleles at four HLA class II loci determined by oligonucleotide hybridization and their associations in five ethnic groups. Immunogenetics 1991;34:299–312.

[44] Ripley B, Overeem S, Fujiki N, et al. CSF hypocretin/orexin levels in narcolepsy and other neurological conditions. Neurology 2001;57:2253–8.

[45] Krahn LE, Pankratz VS, Oliver L, et al. Hypocretin (orexin) levels in cerebrospinal fluid of patients with narcolepsy: relationship to cataplexy and HLA DQB1*0602 status. Sleep 2002;25:733–6.

SLEEP
MEDICINE
CLINICS

Sleep Med Clin 1 (2006) 9–16

Epidemiology of Excessive Daytime Sleepiness

Maurice M. Ohayon, MD, DSc, PhD

- How excessive daytime sleepiness is assessed in the general population
- Prevalence of excessive daytime sleepiness
  North America
  South America
  Europe
- Excessive daytime sleepiness and cognitive deficits

- Excessive daytime sleepiness and mortality
- Factors associated with excessive daytime sleepiness
- Summary
- References

Falling asleep occasionally while watching television or after a copious meal may be normal. But daytime sleepiness becomes excessive when sleep episodes repeat during the day. These episodes are more likely to occur during monotonous activities but they can also occur unexpectedly (eg, during a meeting, in public transportation, or during a conversation with other people).

Excessive daytime sleepiness has received less attention than insomnia from epidemiologists. The lack of a clear definition of the symptom and the complexity of the concept are partly responsible. In addition, contrary to insomnia, excessive daytime sleepiness is not a diagnosis; it can be a symptom or a consequence of a sleep disorder, a physical illness, or a mental disorder. Consequently, studying prevalence, incidence, and risk factors for excessive daytime sleepiness bears little impact on the development of new treatments for this symptom. Considering, however, that excessive daytime sleepiness is a disabling symptom that adversely affects the quality of life of individuals in various areas of functioning, and that it is a good indicator of the presence of health problems, it

certainly deserves more extensive studying in the general population.

How excessive daytime sleepiness is assessed in the general population

Epidemiologic studies on daytime sleepiness can be divided into two main categories: those measuring hypersomnia symptoms and those assessing excessive daytime sleepiness. The main problem encountered in the study of excessive daytime sleepiness is the lack of uniformity in the definition of excessive daytime sleepiness. The earliest studies were mostly focused on hypersomnia symptoms, such as getting too much sleep or napping. In the studies of the past decade, daytime sleepiness has referred to sleep propensity in situations of diminished attention. The terms "hypersomnia" and "excessive daytime sleepiness" are often used interchangeably, however, and excessive daytime sleepiness is defined differently across surveys. As seen in Table 1, definitions of excessive daytime sleepiness are different from one study to another [1–22]. The time frame (eg, past week, past month, past year) fre-

This work was supported by an educational grant from Cephalon, Inc.
Stanford Sleep Epidemiology, School of Medicine, Stanford University, 3430 West Bayshore Road, Palo Alto, CA 94303, USA
E-mail address: mohayon@stanford.edu

doi:10.1016/j.jsmc.2005.11.004

Table 1: Prevalence of excessive sleepiness in the general population

Authors	N	Age	Sample selection	Type of interview	Description	Prevalence (%) (M/F)
Karacan et al [18] Alachua county, Florida, USA, 1976	1645	≥18	Random sample	Household	Hypersomnia	0.3
Bixler et al [1] Los Angeles, USA, 1979	1006	≥18	Random stratified sample	Household	Sleep too much	4.2
Klink and Quan [3] Tucson, USA, 1987	2187	≥18	Random stratified sample	Self-administered questionnaire	Falling asleep during the day	12.3/11.7
Ford and Kamerow [2] Baltimore, Durham, Los Angeles, USA, 1989	7954	≥18	Household probability sample	Household	Sleep too much lasting 2 wk or more, and professional consultation, sleep-enhancing medication intake, or interferes a lot with daily life	2.8/3.5
Hays et al [4] North Carolina, USA, 1996	3962	≥65	Random sample	Household	Frequent feeling of sleepiness during the day or evening that requires taking a nap	25.2
Enright et al [5] Forsyth, Sacramento, Washington, Pittsburgh counties, USA, 1996	5201	≥65	Random sample of the Health Care Finance Administration Medicare eligibility lists	Self-administered questionnaire plus clinical examination	Usually sleepy in the daytime	17/15
Foley et al [6] Island of Oahu, Hawaii, USA, 2001	2346 men	71–93	Cohort of the Honolulu Heart Program	Face-to-face clinical interviews	Usually sleepy in the daytime	7.7
Rockwood et al [7] Canada, 2001	1659	65–99	National representative sample	Screening questionnaire and clinical interview	Tendency to sleep all day	3.9
Téllez-Lòpez et al [8] Monterrey, Mexico, 1995	1000	≥18	Not specified	Household	Getting too much sleep Strong need to sleep during the day	9.5 21.5
Hara et al [9] Bambui, Brazil, 2004	1066	≥18	Random sample	Household	Presence of sleepiness during the previous month, ≥3d/wk	16.8
Lugaresi et al [19] San Marino, Italy, 1983	5713	≥3	Representative sample	Household	Sleepiness independent of meal times	8.7
Gislason et al [10] Uppsala, Sweden, 1987	3201 men	30–69	Random sample	Postal questionnaire	Moderate daytime sleepiness Severe daytime sleepiness	16.7 5.7
Liljenberg et al [20] Gävleborg and Kopparberg counties, Sweden, 1988	3557	30–65	Random sample	Postal questionnaire	Daytime sleepiness often or very often	5.2/5.5

Study	N	Age	Sampling	Data collection	Definition	Prevalence (%)
Martikainen et al [12] Tampere, Finland, 1992	1190	36–50	Random stratified sample	Postal questionnaire	Consider themselves more clearly tired than others, or Daily experience of desire to sleep during normal activities, or Feel tired every day	9.8
Janson et al [11] Reykjavik, Iceland Uppsala and Göteborg, Sweden, Antwerp, Belgium, 1995	2202	20–45	Two phases: (1) random sample of the gen. pop. (2) random sample of the phase 1 responders	(1) Postal questionnaire (2) Structured interview plus self-administered questionnaire	Daytime sleepiness ≥3 d/wk	11–21
Hublin et al [13] Finland, 1996	11,354	33–60	Twin cohort	Postal questionnaire	Daytime sleepiness every or almost every day	6.7/11
Asplund [21] Västerbotten and Norrbotten, Sweden, 1996	6143	≥65	None	Postal questionnaire	Often sleepy during the day Often naps in daytime	32/23.2 29.4/14.4
Ohayon et al [14] United Kingdom, 1997	4972	≥15	Two stages: random stratified sample plus household probability sample	Telephone	Feel sleepy during the day A lot or greatly, ≥1 mo Moderately, ≥1 mo	4.4/6.6 21.5/17.9
Nugent et al [15] Northern Island, 2001	2364 men	≥18	Random sample from the 1989 Electoral Register	Postal questionnaire	Moderate daytime sleepiness (fall asleep when relaxing and sudden attacks of sleep or has to pull off the road while driving) Severe daytime sleepiness (fall asleep against their will)	8 11.8
Ohayon et al [16] Germany, 2002	4115	≥15	Two stages: random stratified sample plus household probability sample	Telephone	Tendency to fall easily asleep during the day ≥3 d/wk Periods of sudden and irresistible sleep ≥3 d/wk Feeling sleepy during the day A lot or extremely Moderately	7.8 9 3.2 13
Ohayon et al [16] Italy, 2002	3970	≥15	Two stages: random stratified sample plus household probability sample	Telephone	Tendency to fall easily asleep during the day ≥3 d/wk Periods of sudden and irresistible sleep ≥3 d/wk Feeling sleepy during the day A lot or extremely Moderately	0.8 1.6 1.5 4.5

(continued on next page)

Table 1: *(continued)*

Authors	N	Age	Sample selection	Type of interview	Description	Prevalence (%) (M/F)
Ohayon et al [16] Portugal, 2002	1858	≥18	Two stages: random stratified sample plus household probability sample	Telephone	Tendency to fall easily asleep during the day ≥3 d/wk	1.1
					Periods of sudden and irresistible sleep ≥3 d/wk	1.6
					Feeling sleepy during the day	
					A lot or extremely	2
					Moderately	4.3
Ohayon et al [16] Spain, 2002	4065	≥15	Two stages: random stratified sample plus household probability sample	Telephone	Tendency to fall easily asleep during the day ≥3 d/wk	0.8
					Periods of sudden and irresistible sleep ≥3 d/wk	0.4
					Feeling sleepy during the day	
					A lot or extremely	2
					Moderately	3.5
Ohayon and Vechierrini [17] France, 2002	1026	60–101	Two stages: random stratified sample plus household probability sample	Telephone	Tendency to fall easily asleep during the day ≥1 d/wk	5.3
					Feeling sleepy during the day	
					A lot or extremely	5.2
					Moderately	6
Takegami et al [22] Hokkaido region, Japan 2005	4412	≥20	Random sample	Questionnaire distributed at home	Epworth Sleepiness Scale	9.6/8.8

quency, severity, and duration are inconsistently assessed. The evaluation of the symptom is mostly limited to a single question. Consequently, the variance in results across studies does not make it possible to reach any definite conclusions in the matter.

Prevalence of excessive daytime sleepiness

North America

Four United States studies that investigated hypersomnia reported rates varying from 0.3% to 16.3%. Bixler and coworkers [1] simply mentioned that they assessed hypersomnia and reported a prevalence of 4.2%. In the Ford and Kamerow study [2], participants were asked whether they had gone 2 weeks or more in which they slept too much (hypersomnia). This yielded a 6-month prevalence of hypersomnia of 3.2%. Using the same definition, Breslau et al [23] found a lifetime prevalence of hypersomnia of 16.3% in their young adult sample (21–30 years of age). Klink and Quan [3] examined how many participants fell asleep during the day and found an overall prevalence of 12%.

Four studies were performed on elderly samples in the United States. Hays and coworkers [4] reported a 25.2% prevalence of elderly subjects with a frequent feeling of sleepiness during the day or evening that required taking a nap. Another study using 5201 subjects 65 years and older [5] reported a prevalence of 17% of men and 15% of women being "usually sleepy in the daytime." Using the same definition, Foley and coworkers [6] obtained a prevalence of 7.7% in a sample of 2346 Japanese-American men, whereas the Cardiovascular Health Study [24] found a 20% prevalence of participants being "usually sleepy in the daytime" in a sample of 4578 adults aged 65 and older. A Canadian study [7] using a national sample of 1659 elderly obtained a prevalence of 3.9% of subjects who had a tendency to sleep all day.

South America

Three general-population studies in South America assessed excessive daytime sleepiness. The first one, a Mexican study [8], reported a prevalence of 9.5% of the sample who claimed to get too much sleep, and 21.5% of the sample who reported experiencing a strong need to sleep during the day. A Brazilian community study [25] used the Epworth Sleepiness Scale to measure excessive daytime sleepiness in a sample of 408 adults from Campo Grande city. They found a prevalence of 18.9%. Another Brazilian study performed in Bambui [9] with 1066 subjects observed a prevalence of 16.8%

of subjects with daytime sleepiness in the past month occurring at least 3 days per week.

Europe

In Europe, the Swedish study by Gislason and coworkers [10] yielded a prevalence rate of 16.7% for moderate daytime sleepiness and of 5.7% for severe daytime sleepiness in their male sample. Janson and coworkers [11] found a prevalence of daytime sleepiness occurring at least 1 day per week of about 40%; daily daytime sleepiness was observed in about 5% of their young adult sample (20–44 years of age) drawn from three countries. Martikainen and coworkers [12], who used a more restrictive definition of excessive daytime sleepiness, found that 9.8% of their 1190 Finnish respondents aged 36 to 50 years reported being "clearly more tired than others," experiencing a "daily desire to sleep in the course of normal activities," or feeling "very tired daily." Hublin and coworkers [13] found a prevalence of daytime sleepiness occurring daily or almost daily of 9% in their Finnish twin cohort. Ohayon and coworkers [14] assessed daytime sleepiness on a severity scale in their United Kingdom sample of 4972 subjects. Severe daytime sleepiness was observed in 5.5% of their sample, and moderate daytime sleepiness in 15.2%. A Northern Irish community study [15] involving 2364 subjects aged between 18 and 91 years reported a prevalence of 19.8% of moderate or severe excessive daytime sleepiness.

A study in five European countries [16] measured excessive daytime sleepiness using three definitions: (1) a tendency to fall easily asleep during the day occurring at least 3 days per week; (2) periods of sudden and irresistible sleep occurring at least 3 days per week, and (3) feeling sleepy during the day. They observed an important variability between the countries: subjects of the United Kingdom and Germany reported more frequent daytime sleepiness than the three South European countries (Italy, Spain, and Portugal) on all three items. Furthermore, there were small correlations between the questions: about 15% of the subjects reported positive answers on at least two of the questions. This observation clearly indicates the multidimensionality of excessive daytime sleepiness and also that current epidemiologic studies have assessed only a part of it.

Excessive daytime sleepiness and cognitive deficits

Two epidemiologic studies have linked excessive daytime sleepiness to cognitive deficits. In a study involving 2346 Japanese-American men aged between 71 and 93 years, Foley and coworkers [6] found that men who reported excessive daytime sleepiness at baseline were twice as likely to be diagnosed with dementia 3 years later than those without daytime sleepiness. In another study involving 1026 subjects aged 60 years or older, Ohayon and Vechierrini [17] found that after controlling for age, gender, physical activity, occupation, organic diseases, use of sleep or anxiety medication, sleep duration, and psychologic well-being, subjects with excessive daytime sleepiness were twice as likely to have attention-concentration deficits, difficulties in orientation, and memory problems than did the others.

Excessive daytime sleepiness and mortality

Some general population studies have investigated the mortality risks associated with excessive daytime sleepiness. The study of Hays et al [4] assessed mortality risks in a sample of 3962 elderly individuals (65 years and older). In that study, excessive daytime sleepiness was defined by the presence of naps during the daytime. They found that individuals who reported napping most of the time had a mortality risk of 1.73. Another study [7] found a small increased mortality risk (1.89) from daytime sleepiness in their elderly sample. This risk was nonsignificant, however, when they adjusted the model for age, depression, cognitive deficits, and illness.

Factors associated with excessive daytime sleepiness

Unlike insomnia symptoms, excessive daytime sleepiness is generally not gender-related. Whether its prevalence increases or decreases with age is not clear, because both trends have been observed [3,10,15,16]. Excessive daytime sleepiness can be caused by various factors, such as poor sleep hygiene [13,14], work conditions [14], and psychotropic medication use [13–15]. Excessive daytime sleepiness has been found to be associated also with sleep-disordered breathing [14,16–18]; psychiatric disorders, especially depression [2,4,13–15,23]; and physical illnesses [11,14,15].

Summary

From these epidemiologic studies, it is clear that a uniform operational definition of excessive daytime sleepiness is still missing. None of these epidemiologic studies used a standardized questionnaire to assess daytime sleepiness. Although many surveys have been undertaken on the topic, differences in definition and the variance in results do not make it possible to reach any definite conclusions.

The causes and consequences of excessive sleepiness are rarely presented as a whole. The prevalence of transient or seasonal patterns of excessive daytime sleepiness is unknown. Hypersomnia is an associated symptom in depressive disorders in the DSM-IV classification. No epidemiologic study has investigated such a relationship, however, even though mental disorders are present in about 10% of sleepy individuals who consult in sleep disorders clinics and about 10% to 75% of depressed patients complain of hypersomnia. Few polysomnographic studies have been performed with patients having a mood disorder in relationship to hypersomnia or excessive daytime sleepiness. The Multiple Sleep Latency Test did not reveal abnormalities in the daytime sleep latency [26]. Several clinical studies have also pointed out the high occurrence of subjective excessive daytime sleepiness in association with mental disorders, organic disorders, or both. This high comorbidity may hide a more complex problem based on the definition of excessive daytime sleepiness.

At this point, only one test exists that measures excessive daytime sleepiness objectively and scientifically: the Multiple Sleep Latency Test, which is considered the gold standard. This test, however, must be administered in a sleep laboratory, limiting its uses in epidemiologic studies unless a subsample is invited to perform this test in a sleep laboratory. Consequently, it is very highly desirable that a self-administered questionnaire be developed to assess excessive daytime sleepiness. If it is done, however, it should be kept in mind that one passes from an objective measure to a subjective measure of excessive daytime sleepiness. One of the most commonly used self-administered sleepiness scales is the Epworth scale [27,28]. Unfortunately, studies that measured the agreement between this scale and the Multiple Sleep Latency Test revealed a poor agreement between them [28,29].

Few of the epidemiologic studies have reported results by ethnic group, or indicated the ethnic makeup of their sample. In fact, there have been almost no data published on ethnocultural differences in excessive daytime sleepiness in the United States or elsewhere [16,30]. Some investigators have interpreted data from the Human Relations Area Files as indicating that certain aspects of sleep, such as daytime napping, may occur more in some cultural groups [31], but epidemiologic data on such cross-cultural differences actually are quite rare. A recent study of college students in Mexico City found no support for the "siesta culture" concept, characterized by a strong tendency for daytime naps and daytime sleepiness [32]. More similarities than differences were noted between the sample from Mexico and samples from other countries on sleep patterns.

There are yet several areas that need to be clarified regarding excessive daytime sleepiness in the general population. First, an operational definition needs to be developed so that it can be used in general population studies. Once the agreement is made on the definition of excessive daytime sleepiness and the criteria necessary to conclude to its presence, several questions still remain. How can one differentiate daytime sleepiness from fatigue? To what extent do these two concepts overlap? Is daytime sleepiness always a cause of fatigue, or can daytime sleepiness occur without fatigue? To what extent can subjective daytime sleepiness assessment be compared with objective daytime sleepiness assessment? How can one distinguish between the different causes of excessive daytime sleepiness?

References

[1] Bixler EO, Kales A, Soldatos CR, et al. Prevalence of sleep disorders in the Los Angeles metropolitan area. Am J Psychiatry 1979;136:1257–62.

[2] Ford DE, Kamerow DB. Epidemiologic study of sleep disturbances and psychiatric disorders: an opportunity for prevention? JAMA 1989;262:1479–84.

[3] Klink M, Quan SF. Prevalence of reported sleep disturbances in a general adult population and their relationship to obstructive airways diseases. Chest 1987;91:540–6.

[4] Hays JC, Blazer DG, Foley DJ. Risk of napping: excessive daytime sleepiness and mortality in an older community population. J Am Geriatr Soc 1996;44:693–8.

[5] Enright PL, Newman AB, Wahl PW, et al. Prevalence and correlates of snoring and observed apneas in 5,201 older adults. Sleep 1996;19:531–8.

[6] Foley D, Monjan A, Masaki K, et al. Daytime sleepiness is associated with 3-year incident dementia and cognitive decline in older Japanese-American men. J Am Geriatr Soc 2001;49:1628–32.

[7] Rockwood K, Davis HS, Merry HR, et al. Sleep disturbances and mortality: results from the Canadian Study of Health and Aging. J Am Geriatr Soc 2001;49:639–41.

[8] Téllez-Lòpez A, Sánchez EG, Torres FG, et al. Hábitos y trastornos del dormir en residentes del área metropolitana de Monterrey. Salud Mental 1995;18:14–22.

[9] Hara C, Lopes Rocha F, Lima-Costa MF. Prevalence of excessive daytime sleepiness and associated factors in a Brazilian community: the Bambui study. Sleep Med 2004;5:31–6.

[10] Gislason T, Almqvist M, Erikson G, et al. Prevalence of sleep apnea syndrome among Swedish men: an epidemiological study. J Clin Epidemiol 1988;41:571–6.

[11] Janson C, Gislason T, De Backer W, et al. Daytime sleepiness, snoring and gastro-oesophageal reflux amongst young adults in three European countries. J Intern Med 1995;237:277–85.

[12] Martikainen K, Hasan J, Urponen H, et al. Daytime sleepiness: a risk factor in community life. Acta Neurol Scand 1992;86:337–41.

[13] Hublin C, Kaprio J, Partinen M, et al. Daytime sleepiness in an adult Finnish population. J Intern Med 1996;239:417–23.

[14] Ohayon MM, Caulet M, Philip P, et al. How sleep and mental disorders are related to complaints of daytime sleepiness. Arch Intern Med 1997;157:2645–52.

[15] Nugent AM, Gleadhill I, McCrum E, et al. Sleep complaints and risk factors for excessive daytime sleepiness in adult males in Northern Ireland. J Sleep Res 2001;10:69–74.

[16] Ohayon MM, Priest RG, Zulley J, et al. Prevalence of narcolepsy symptomatology and diagnosis in the European general population. Neurology 2002;58:1826–33.

[17] Ohayon MM, Vechierrini MF. Daytime sleepiness is an independent predictive factor for cognitive impairment in the elderly population. Arch Intern Med 2002;162:201–8.

[18] Karacan I, Thornby JI, Anch M, et al. Prevalence of sleep disturbance in a primarily urban Florida county. Soc Sci Med 1976;10:239–44.

[19] Lugaresi E, Cirignotta F, Zucconi M, et al. Good and poor sleepers: an epidemiological survey of the San Marino population. In: Guilleminault C, Lugaresi E, editors. Sleep/wake disorders: natural history, epidemiology, and long-term evolution. New York: Raven Press; 1983. p. 1–12.

[20] Liljenberg B, Almqvist M, Hetta J, et al. The prevalence of insomnia: the importance of operationally defined criteria. Ann Clin Res 1988;20:393–8.

[21] Asplund R. Daytime sleepiness and napping amongst the elderly in relation to somatic health and medical treatment. J Intern Med 1996;239:261–7.

[22] Takegami M, Sokejima S, Yamazaki S, et al. An estimation of the prevalence of excessive daytime sleepiness based on age and sex distribution of Epworth sleepiness scale scores: a population based survey. Nippon Koshu Eisei Zasshi 2005;52:137–45 [in Japanese].

[23] Breslau N, Roth T, Rosenthal L, et al. Sleep disturbance and psychiatric disorders: a longitudinal epidemiological study of young adults. Biol Psychiatry 1996;39:411–8.

[24] Whitney CW, Enright PL, Newman AB, et al. Correlates of daytime sleepiness in 4578 elderly persons: the Cardiovascular Health Study. Sleep 1998;21:27–36.

[25] Souza JC, Magna LA, Reimao R. Excessive daytime sleepiness in Campo Grande general population, Brazil. Arq Neuropsiquiatr 2002;60:558–62.

[26] Nofzinger EA, Thase ME, Reynolds III CF, et al.

Hypersomnia in bipolar depression: a comparison with narcolepsy using the Multiple Sleep Latency Test. Am J Psychiatry 1991;148:1177–81.

[27] Johns MW. A new method for measuring daytime sleepiness: the Epworth sleepiness scale. Sleep 1991;14:540–5.

[28] Johns MW. Sleepiness in different situations measured by the Epworth Sleepiness Scale. Sleep 1994;17:703–10.

[29] Olson LG, Cole MF, Ambrogetti A. Correlations among Epworth sleepiness scale scores, multiple sleep latency tests and psychological symptoms. J Sleep Res 1998;7:248–53.

[30] Morin CM, Edinger JD. Sleep disorders: evaluation and diagnosis. In: Turner SM, Hersen M, editors. Adult psychopathology and diagnosis. 3rd edition. New York: John Wiley & Sons; 1997. p. 483–507.

[31] Webb WB, Dinges DF. Cultural perspectives on napping and the siesta. In: Dinges DF, Broughton RJ, editors. Sleep and alertness: chronobiological, behavioral and medical aspects of napping. New York: Raven Press; 1989. p. 247–65.

[32] Valencia-Flores M, Castano VA, Campos RM, et al. The siesta culture concept is not supported by the sleep habits of urban Mexican students. J Sleep Res 1998;7:21–9.

ELSEVIER
SAUNDERS

SLEEP
MEDICINE
CLINICS

Sleep Med Clin 1 (2006) 17–30

Sleepiness and Circadian Rhythm Sleep Disorders

Torbjörn Åkerstedt, PhD

- Shift work sleep disorder
- *Physiologic alertness*
- *Subjective alertness*
- *Performance and accidents at work*
- *Sleep*
- Jet lag

- Delayed sleep phase syndrome
- Advanced sleep phase syndrome
- Non–24-hour sleep-wake syndrome
- Irregular sleep-wake syndrome
- References

Sleepiness is heavily regulated by homeostatic influences, mainly related to sleep loss and time awake. The circadian system exerts a powerful influence, directly through its regulation of metabolism, and indirectly through its interference with or promotion of sleep, depending on circadian phase. This circadian influence is at the core of the circadian rhythm sleep disorders. Essentially, the problem derives from a mismatch between the circadian system and the sleep-wake pattern of the individual.

The central oscillator is situated in the suprachiasmatic nuclei of the hypothalamus [1]. It is a self-sustained oscillator and drives much of human physiology in an approximately 24-hour cycle. Core components of the circadian pacemaker work on the basis of feedback loops of gene expression and repression. The Period (Per) gene family is a central component in the molecular machinery that generates circadian rhythms [2]. The Per family provides negative autofeedback on its own expression. Per transcripts and PER proteins oscillate with period lengths correlated to the observed period (tau) [3]. Phosphorylation targets PER for degradation, imposing a rate-limiting step on the amount of PER protein available for dimerization and subsequent nuclear translocation. CLOCK, the protein product of the circadian gene *Clock*, acts as a positive regulator of both Per2 and Per3 and a mutation in this gene in mice is associated with lengthening of endogenous circadian period (tau) [4].

It receives input for light and other stimuli that synchronize the pacemaker to the environmental light-dark cycle, so called "zeitgebers," which entrain (influence the clock through the light-dark changes of the normal environment). Essentially, light before the circadian trough phase delays the biologic clock (1–2 hours) and light after the trough phase advances the clock [5].

The influence of the circadian system on sleep was demonstrated in month-long isolation studies in which individuals could live according to their own preferred sleep-wake schedule. This led in some individuals to an estimate of the circadian rhythm having a period of around 25 hours [6] and the finding that some individuals desynchronized, that is showed different period lengths for the "day" of their sleep-wake rhythm and that of the rhythm of metabolism (rectal temperature) [7]. The present estimate of the period length with control for light, however, is 24.1 hours [8].

It was later shown that whenever the sleep-wake rhythm placed sleep around the acrophase (circa-

IPM and Karolinska Institutet, Box 230, Stockholm 17177, Sweden
E-mail address: torbjorn.akerstedt@ipm.ki.se

doi:10.1016/j.jsmc.2005.11.009
sleep.theclinics.com

dian maximum) of rectal temperature, sleep was shortened, and when sleep was placed around the circadian trough (or low), sleep was promoted [9]. The previous studies were performed under conditions of long-term (around a month) isolation from all zeitgebers, but the same circadian dependence has also been demonstrated in individuals who are entrained and merely isolated for 36 hours [10]. The latter essentially showed that as bedtime was delayed to 3:00 AM, 7:00 AM, or 11:00 AM, sleep duration was gradually shortened, down to 4.5 hours. Then sleep started to increase with further displacement so that a bedtime at 7:00 PM yielded 10.5 hours of sleep (note that prior wake duration also increased from the 20 hours at 3:00 AM to 36 hours at 7:00 PM).

Sleepiness ratings were part of most of the studies cited and the results essentially show self-rated sleepiness to follow the circadian rhythm of rectal temperature, with a slight delay [11] and with a strong dependence on circadian phase and homeostatic influences (duration of time awake or sleep loss). The same influences combine also to regulate sleep content (sleep stages) [12].

The experimental studies clearly demonstrate that misalignment between the sleep-wake pattern and the circadian physiology lead to suboptimal sleep and wakefulness and that optimal entrainment serves to stabilize alertness on an optimal (high level) during the daylight hours [13]. Misalignment is the mechanism of circadian rhythm disorders. Displacing the sleep-wake pattern, like in shift work or travel across time zones, affects sleep and alertness negatively. Similarly, if the circadian system is shifted in relation to the societal requirements of a work-sleep pattern, a similar negative effect ensues. This may involve having a delayed sleep phase (being an extreme evening type), that is a circadian system that runs late in relation to the ideal sleep-wake pattern. The case is the opposite with advanced sleep phase. There is also the possibility of a circadian system that runs with a different period than the expected sleep-wake rhythm. All result in disturbed sleep and in sleepiness.

This article reviews sleepiness in relation to the major types of circadian misalignment. It starts with shift work sleep disorder, because it may be the most prevalent type of circadian rhythm sleep disorder. It is also the disorder in which most data on sleepiness are available. The second type is jet lag, where also considerable data on sleepiness exist. The other diagnostic groups, delayed sleep phase, non–24-hour sleep disorder, advanced sleep phase disorder, and irregular sleep pattern, offer very limited systematic data on sleepiness and conclusions have to be made through inference.

Shift work sleep disorder

Large proportions of the population have work schedules that interfere with night sleep and it is well established that this causes disturbed sleep and sleepiness [14]. The effects are for the most part transient (limited mainly to night shifts), however, and shift work sleep disorder has not received much clinical attention despite the fact that the severity of the sleep impairment in shift and night work is as great as that in traditional insomnia and seems to affect three fourths of those who work shifts or at night [15]. The *Diagnostic and Statistical Manual of Mental Disorders-IV* [16] defines shift work sleep disorder as "report of difficulty falling asleep, staying asleep, or non-restorative sleep for at least one month" and it must be associated with "a work period that occurs during the habitual sleep phase." There are also required effects on impairment of wakefulness. In the recent version of International Classification of Sleep Disorders [17] excessive sleepiness is included. Note that normal night sleep and normal daytime alertness should be present when the individual is not working nights. See also Reid and Zee [18] for a recent review of shift work sleep disorder as a circadian rhythm sleep disorder.

Virtually no data on sleepiness are available on this diagnostic category, mainly because the diagnosis has been used rather seldom. In one recent attempt to estimate the prevalence of shift work sleep disorder the authors arrived at 10% of a population of shift workers [19]. Insomnia was defined according to [17] difficulties falling asleep, staying asleep, or nonrestorative sleep for at least 1 month. Shift work sleep disorder was defined according to the International Classification of Sleep Disorders [17] as the symptoms previously discussed (including excessive sleepiness) occurring "sometimes" or "often" and with a severity of at least 6 on a 1 to 10 scale. The Epworth Sleepiness Scale level for excessive sleepiness was 13 (usually 10). The prevalence of excessive sleepiness in this study was 24.7% in night workers, 20.3% in rotating workers, and 15.5% in day workers. Using the established cutoff at 10, the values were 44.8%, 35.8%, and 32.7%, respectively. Those shift workers suffering from insomnia or excessive sleepiness also showed a higher prevalence of ulcers, depression, sleepiness-related accidents, missed work days, and missed family or social events than those without sleep or sleepiness problems. These differences were not seen in day workers. In another study of 400 shift workers it was found that the proportion with a very negative attitude to work hours constituted 8% and were mainly characterized by marked sleepiness and sleep complaints [20].

There is a large number of studies of effects of shift work on sleep and sleepiness in normal samples of shift workers. This is the basis on which it is possible to build a coherent picture of sleepiness (and sleep) in relation to shift work. Most of the data derive from self-ratings of sleepiness and this is from where most of the data on effects of particular shift system characteristics derive. Physiologic sleepiness has been measured frequently enough to give a picture of what a night shift per se may cause in terms of sleepiness.

Physiologic alertness

Physiologic measures give strong support to the notion of night shift sleepiness. In an electroencephalogram (EEG) study of night workers at work (train drivers) it was found that one quarter showed pronounced increases in alpha (8–12 Hz) and theta (4–8 Hz) activity, and slow eye movements toward the early morning, but these were absent during day driving [21]. The correlations with ratings of sleepiness were quite high ($r = .74$). In some instances obvious performance lapses, such as driving against a red light, occurred during bursts of slow eye movements and of alpha-theta activity. The pattern is very similar in truck drivers during long-haul (8–10 h) drives [22,23], and similar results have been demonstrated for air crews during long-haul flights [24].

In process operators there was found not only sleepiness-related increases in alpha and theta activity, but also full-fledged sleep during the night shift (but not during other shifts) [25]. Such incidents of sleep proper occurred in approximately one quarter of the subjects. Usually they occurred during the second half of the night shift and never in connection with any other shift. Importantly, sleep on the job was not condoned by the company, nor was there any official awareness that sleep would or could occur during work hours. Interestingly, the subjects were unaware of having slept, but were aware of sleepiness. Furthermore, hospital interns on call showed "attentional failures" (defined as sleep intrusions in the EEG) particularly during early morning work [26]. This was reduced when continuous on-call duty across days was broken up to permit relatively normal amounts of sleep each day.

Increased alpha and theta activity have also been demonstrated in truck drivers driving a truck simulator at night [27], in power station operators during a night shift [28], or in shift workers driving a simulator home after a normal night shift [29]. All also showed large increases in subjective sleepiness and the driving simulator studies showed impaired performance in the form of increased variation in lateral position.

With respect to the Multiple Sleep Latency Test, which is the standard clinical polysomnographic measure of sleepiness, only data from post–night shift bedtimes exist in field studies [23,25,30–33]. Essentially they indicate short (<5 minute) latencies, attesting to excessive sleepiness according to clinical criteria [34]. The reason for the lack of field studies with this method is probably the difficulty of getting workers off from work to perform the 20 minute Multiple Sleep Latency Test several times during a night shift; finding a suitable quite place to make the measurements; and getting workers to wear electrodes (for fast hook-up to the polysomnograph) while working. There have been, however, a large number of simulated night shift studies showing short latencies, but the controlled and soporific laboratory situation is not likely to be representative of a real life situation, at least not with respect to absolute levels of sleepiness. Even in the training simulator for a power station, which is very similar to the work task, the rated night shift sleepiness was significantly higher than that in at the real workplace [28]. The explanation during debriefing was that the normal social interaction and physical activity did not occur in the simulator.

It should also be emphasized that the types of EEG changes previously described in the shift workers have also been demonstrated in laboratory studies [21,35–38]. The latter study demonstrated that the closest correlation with sleepiness was obtained for the 5- to 9-Hz range. The EEG changes are also closely related to performance lapses and errors [39–44]. High levels of alpha and or theta power density indicate impaired performance; the severely sleepy individual is not functioning and perceives major difficulties keeping his or her eyes open and is aware of "fighting sleep" (level 8–9 on the Karolinska Sleepiness Scale) [35,43]. Slow eye movements or long eye closures are sensitive indicators of sleepiness [21,35,41,45–49]. Incidentally, the amount of alpha power density is usually a direct function of the eye closure duration (long blinks), whereas much of the EEG delta power activity seems to be caused by eye-blink artifacts [50].

Even though physiologic indicators clearly show sleepiness during night work the effects are not as dramatic as one expects from subjective reports. The reason may be that many individuals start counteracting sleepiness when they start feeling the symptoms. This probably prevents sleepiness from appearing in many physiologic indicators, because EEG and electro-oculugram signs of sleepiness only occur at higher levels of sleepiness when the individual is "fighting sleep" and has reached maximum level of sleepiness [35]. Physiologic changes may occur only when no countermeasures are applied.

Subjective alertness

With respect to the prevalence of perceived sleepiness there is a wealth of questionnaire studies suggesting that most shift workers experience sleepiness in connection with night shift work, whereas day work is associated with no, or marginal, sleepiness [51–54]. The studies by Verhaegen and coworkers [53] and Paley and Tepas [54] are somewhat unusual in that they had an experimental design and showed that reported fatigue increased on entering and decreased on leaving shift work. In many studies most shift workers admit to having experienced involuntary sleep on the night shift, whereas this is rare on day-oriented shifts [55,56]. Between 10% and 20% report falling asleep during night work. The popular Epworth scale has not been used very frequently in relation to shift work but one recent study showed values of 9.2 in night workers, 8.6 in rotating shift workers, and 8 in day workers [19]. The differences are small, however, and the Epworth scale [57] in its present form may not be ideal for studying shift work because the questions often refer to activities that are difficult to relate to nighttime work.

If one wants to obtain a detailed impression of subjective sleepiness in shift work one needs to obtain repeated measurements during the different shifts and days off and several times during each shift and during leisure time. When this has been done, the results indicate moderate to high sleepiness during the night shift and no sleepiness at all during the day shifts [58–60]. Two of the present author's studies are used next to illustrate subjective sleepiness in shift work. These studies are presented here because the same self-rating scale of sleepiness is used throughout and therefore, it is possible to make comparisons. The scale is the Karolinska Sleepiness Scale, which ranges from 1 to 9, with 1, very alert; 3, rather alert; 5, nether alert nor sleepy; 7, sleepy but no difficulty remaining awake; and 9, very sleepy (fighting sleep, an effort to remain awake) [35].

The first study [Fig. 1] shows subjective sleepiness in 60 workers in the paper industry working an extremely rapidly rotating shift system with very short rest between the shifts [20]. The schedule started with a night shift (2100–0600 hours), followed by 8 hours off; an afternoon shift (1400–2100 hours), 8 hours off; and a morning shift (0600–1400 hours). This triad was followed by 56 hours off and included two normal night

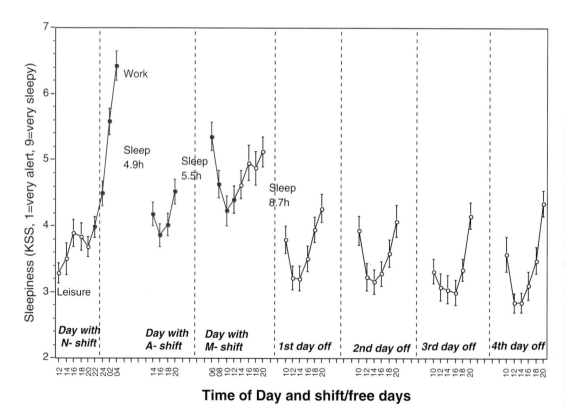

Fig. 1. Subjective sleepiness (Karolinska Sleepiness Scale) in rapidly rotating shift workers (mean ± se). Filled points (*gray*) indicate sleepiness during work hours.

sleeps. The triad pattern was repeated seven times and the cycle ended with 8 days off. Fig. 1 shows the last triad, together with the first 2 days off. Sleepiness rose to high levels during the first night shift (6.5); fell to intermediate levels during the afternoon shift (after 5.4 hours of sleep); and reached high levels again during the morning shift (after an additional 4.5 hours of sleep). Sleepiness was back to normal levels (mostly <4) on the first recovery day. The morning shift effect usually seems to be similar to midnight shift levels but is present throughout the entire shift [58,61].

The second illustration [Fig. 2] concerns adjustment to night work under rather special circumstances. Adjustment to night shifts normally does not occur because shifts alternate and because of the exposure to daylight when returning home from the night shift, which counteracts the expected delay of the circadian clock [62]. When light is not interfering, however (eg, when night workers are provided with strong sunglasses for the morning commute home) adjustment occurs [62]. This may also be seen in situations when no daylight is present. Fig. 2 shows the results from seven workers on an oil production platform in the North Sea [63]. They worked 14 consecutive days between 1900 and 0700 hours. These were followed by 3 weeks off. The workers were not exposed to outdoor light because the platform was a self-contained workplace in which all aspects of life take took place indoors. Fig. 2 shows the sleepiness pattern across the working days and the first 6 days off. Sleepiness reached extremely high levels during the first days, but the pattern gradually changed. In about the middle, the pattern and levels become similar to day work patterns, although at a level of intermediate sleepiness. On return home the pattern was strongly changed again and sleepiness levels remained high for 4 to 5 days. In fact, daytime levels never seem to reach normal day life levels. Because the study did not

include further weeks off it is unclear whether recovery may have proceeded further.

The sleep data during the night work period showed that the bedtime gradually changed from 0800 hours to close to 1100 hours. Similarly, the time of awakening changed from 1700 hours to 1800 hours, yielding a sleep length of just below 8 hours. During the days off a midnight bedtime was adopted throughout, but the time of awakening changed from 0600 hours to 0800 hours on Day 6. Taken together, the results suggest that the circadian system adjusted strongly to night work, although not perfectly, and that the readjustment back to reasonably normal levels took around 6 days. Indeed, it is possible that even some days more would have been required to reach full recovery.

The effect of shift work on sleepiness is obviously profound, but an important question is whether it is related to the ability to function. This seems to be the case in most studies [64,65] even if it has been suggested that the relation may be rather moderate [66,67]. Yang and coworkers [68] have shown that if the self-rating is performed after a minute of sitting quietly with closed eyes the correlation is increased. In most studies self-ratings are performed without any control of the situation leading up to the rating, whereas performance tests are performed under controlled conditions and with a task load that may unmask sleepiness.

Performance and accidents at work

As may be expected from the effects of shift work on sleepiness, performance and safety also are affected [69]. Road transport is the area where the link between safety and night work sleepiness is most pronounced. Harris [70] and Hamelin [71] and others [72,73] convincingly demonstrated that single vehicle truck accidents have the greatest probability of occurring at night (early morning). Furthermore, the US National Transportation Safety Board found that 30% to 40% of all United States truck accidents are fatigue related (and grossly underestimated in conventional reports). The latter investigation was extended to search for the immediate causes of fatigue-induced accidents [74]. It was found that the most important factor was the amount of sleep obtained during the proceeding 24 hours and split-sleep patterns, whereas the length of time driven seemed to play a minor role. The National Transportation Safety Board also found that the Exxon Valdez accident in 1989 was caused by fatigue, as a result of reduced sleep and extended work hours [75]. The extent of fatal, fatigue-related accidents is considered to lie around 30% [76]. This is compared with approximately the same level of incidence in the air-traffic sector,

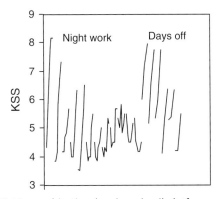

Fig. 2. Mean subjective sleepiness in oil platform workers on 12 night shifts and 6 days off (*dashed lines*).

whereas equivalent accidents at sea are estimated at slightly below 20%.

In industry a classic study is that of Bjerner and coworkers [77] who showed that errors in meter readings over a period of 20 years in a gas works had a pronounced peak on the night shift. There was also a secondary peak during the afternoon. Similarly, Brown [78] demonstrated that telephone operators connected calls considerably slower at night. Wojtczak-Jaroszowa and Pawlowska-Skyga [79] found that the speed of spinning threads in a textile mill went down during the night. From conventional industrial operations less data are available [80,81] but indicate that overall accidents tend to occur, not surprisingly, when activity is at its peak. But these values do not take account of exposure. Most other studies show a night shift dominance [82–84], but not all.

Most other studies of performance have used laboratory-type tests and demonstrated, for example, reduced reaction time or poorer mental arithmetic on the night shift [60] or reaction time performance [85]; for a review see Folkard [86]. A number of laboratory studies have been performed either simulating night shift work or extending performance testing to the night hours for other reasons. All have found that most types of tasks that require sustained attention, including vigilance performance, reaction time performance, or throughput in cognitive tasks, all result in a marked reduction of capacity during the late night hours [87,88]. The performance decrement during simulated night work has been compared with the effects of blood alcohol levels of 0.08% [89].

It is also believed that the (nighttime) nuclear plant meltdown at Chernobyl was caused by human error related to work scheduling [90]. Similar observations have been made for the Three Mile Island reactor accident and the near miss incidents at the David Beese reactor in Ohio and at the Rancho Seco reactor in California. These are all anecdotal, however, and very little other data seem available. The most carefully executed study, from car manufacturing, seems to indicate a moderate increase (30%–50%) in accident risk on the night shift [91]. Åkerstedt and coworkers [92] showed that fatal occupational accidents were higher in shift workers in a prospective study of shift workers (controlling for physical work load, stress, and other factors). Recently, a study of interns on call showed that improving rest conditions (maximum 16 consecutive hours of work and 60 hours per week) greatly reduced many types of medical mistakes, of which several were serious [93]. Taken together, the connection between sleepiness and accidents is far less strong in industry compared with transport work. Still, several studies have tried to evaluate the costs to society of alertness-related accidents and loss of performance (which does not necessarily reflect only the costs of shift work). One estimate exceeds $40 billion per year in the United States [94].

Sleep

The picture of sleepiness in shift workers is not complete without considering sleep. The dominating health problem reported by shift workers is disturbed sleep and wakefulness. At least three fourths of the shift working population is affected [15]. When comparing individuals with a very negative attitude to shift work with those with a very positive one, the strongest discriminator seems to be the ability to obtain sufficient quality of sleep during daytime [20]. EEG studies of rotating shift workers and similar groups have shown that day sleep is 1 to 4 hours shorter than night sleep [23,25,30–33]. The shortening is caused by the fact that sleep is terminated after only 4 to 6 hours without the individual being able to return to sleep. The sleep loss is primarily taken out of stage 2 sleep (basic sleep) and stage rapid eye movement sleep (dream sleep). Stages 3 and 4 (deep sleep) do not seem to be affected. Furthermore, the time taken to fall asleep (sleep latency) is usually shorter. Also, night sleep before a morning shift is reduced, but the termination is through artificial means and the awakening usually difficult and unpleasant [60,95–97].

Interestingly, day sleep does not seem to improve much across series of night shifts [98,99]. It appears, however, that night workers sleep slightly better (longer) than rotating workers on the night shift [100–102]. The long-term effects of shift work on sleep are rather poorly understood. Dumont and coworkers [103] found that the amount of sleep-wake and related disturbances in present day workers was positively related to their previous experience of night work. Guilleminault and coworkers [104] found an overrepresentation of former shift workers with different clinical sleep-wake disturbances appearing at a sleep clinic. Recently, the present author's group has shown that in pairs of twins discordant on night work exposure, the exposed twin reports somewhat deteriorated sleep quality and health after retirement [105].

Sleepiness is mainly determined by circadian phase, time awake, and amount of sleep. No study has attempted to dissect the relative contributions of these factors in shift work. Shift work sleep duration is around 5.5 to 6 hours after the night shift and several laboratory studies have found that this amount of sleep curtailment may affect sleepiness marginally [106–109]. The effect of the circadian trough and extended wakefulness (often up to 20 hours) seem more powerful contributors [12,110].

Jet lag

Another type of circadian rhythm sleep disorder is jet lag [16,17], reviewed in Reid and Zee [18]. One of the first reports was that of Post and Gatty [111] describing the out-of-phase problems during a flight across the globe. It involves disturbed sleep and wakefulness for some days after rapid transportation across several time zones [112]. Sleepiness seem to be the major component of jet lag, but also sleep, bowel movements, the need to urinate, and other symptoms form part of the syndrome [113–115]. The correlation between the global perceptions of jet lag is highest for sleepiness.

The reason for jet lag is that the biologic clock adjusts slowly to a shift of the light-dark pattern [112]. For some days sleep is placed at a circadian phase that interferes with sleep, and wakefulness (and work) is placed at a circadian phase (the trough) when alertness is impaired. The effects differ depending on the direction of flight [116–118]. Westward flights across 4 to 10 time zones result in pronounced evening sleepiness and extremely early awakenings. Eastward flights result in difficulties falling asleep and noon sleepiness. The effects of the westward flight are milder than those of eastward flights, but the adjustment takes longer time. The reason for the latter is probably that the traveler is exposed to light during the daytime at the destination. The circadian trough, which occurs around noon to early afternoon after a 6- to 8-hour time zone crossing, coincides with maximum light exposure as does both the phase-delaying pretrough time and the phase-advancing posttrough time. Neither a phase delay nor phase advance occurs, and adjustment becomes slow.

To illustrate the effects of time zone crossings on sleepiness, Fig. 3 shows the results from a study of 25 cabin crew with sleep diaries and actigraphs during the days before, during, and after a westward flight across nine time zones (Copenhagen–Los Angeles) [113]. The two days at home exhibit the normal pattern with values below or around 4 during the day and values around 6 toward bedtime. On the outbound day, the sleepiness level fell to almost 2 because of the high activation level immediately before and during the early stages of the flight. The end of the flight shows values close to 8 and the evening values in Los Angeles almost reach 9. This level exceeds what is normally seen in night shift work. The latter is caused by the extended time awake in combination with being awake close to the circadian trough. Most air crew go to bed around 2100 hours' local time, corre-

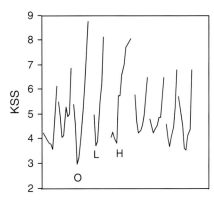

Fig. 3. Mean sleepiness in air crew before, during, and after a westward flight across nine time zones (Copenhagen to Los Angeles). Ratings are made from awakening to bedtime. H, homebound flight day; L, layover day in Los Angeles; O, outbound flight day.

sponding to 0600 hours' Scandinavian (biologic) time. The second day in Los Angeles, sleepiness is moderate, although high levels (level 8) are reached toward the end of the day. On the day of the return flight sleepiness is moderate during the day but reaches very high levels toward the end of the flight and before getting to bed in Copenhagen. During the first recovery day a normal, but slightly increased day level is seen. Complete recovery in terms of low daytime alertness appears on Day 3.

Whereas long duration effects of rapid time zone travel seldom have been reported, the effect of being out of phase and sleep loss may affect performance and well-being. A number of countermeasures have been developed. Probably the most common countermeasure is a hypnotic taken at bedtime at the destination after transmeridian flights [119]. After the eastward flight sleep may be difficult to initiate, particularly on the second day after arrival. After a westward flight the problem is early awakenings, which makes a longer half-life hypnotic more suitable than a short half-life one. Also rather widespread in the United States is the use of melatonin, taken before bedtime on the new destination, but mainly in connection with eastward flights [120]. Westward flights cause pronounced sleepiness in the evening on the destination and melatonin is normally not needed. Formal bright light treatment is less common but seems efficient [121]. It may be most useful before an eastward flight when early morning light treatment one or several days before the flight makes a phase advance easier. It needs to be followed-up with afternoon exposure to light at the destination, together with morning darkness (to avoid a phase delay). The latter may be difficult to adhere to, however, for social reasons. Light treatment before westward flights should be applied in the late evening and evening exposure to light (natural or through bright light devices) at the destination speeds up adjustment.

It should be emphasized that air crew and business travelers who spend 1 to 3 days at the destination may want to avoid jet lag after returning home. This requires remaining on home base time during the layover [122], particularly after westward flights to which adjustment is rapid. Essentially, this means that one should avoid afternoon light at the destination and go to bed at normal home base time, approximately 5:00 PM, and rise at 1:00 AM. At this time artificial light exposure may help to prevent adjustment.

Delayed sleep phase syndrome

Delayed sleep phase syndrome (DSPS) is the most common of the intrinsic circadian rhythm disorders, even if the prevalence figures are unknown. It mainly affects adolescents or young adults, however, and may involve around 7% [123]. It is characterized by difficulties falling asleep at "normal" bedtimes, but a normal sleep onset and sleep duration if bedtime is delayed by several hours [16,17], reviewed in [18]. Wyatt has recently reviewed the area [124]. The problem remains for several months and is not caused by shift work, jet lag, or other temporary delays of the sleep-wake schedule. It was first described by Weitzman and co-workers [125].

With regard to sleepiness, patients complain of high alertness in the evening and complain of difficulties awakening in the morning, and feeling sleepy for a long period after awakening. Studies of life quality [126] have shown rather low levels because of the difficulties functioning in the morning, and during parts of the rest of the day. The weekend usually leads to a remission, when the preferred sleep-wake timing can be adhered to. The extreme evening orientation is also reflected in high "owl" scores on "owl-lark" (morningness-eveningness) questionnaires [127].

Rather few polysomnographic studies have been performed, but they suggest that sleep is essentially normal when the patient sleeps at preferred bedtimes [125,128]. Recently, however, Watanabe and coworkers [129] found reduced sleep efficiency and slow wave sleep compared with age-matched controls (sleeping at their habitual time). Also, the percentage of stage 1 was increased as was sleep latency. Interestingly, the time of the temperature nadir occurred earlier in DSPS and the earlier the nadir the lower the amount of slow wave sleep. This suggests more

than a delayed circadian phase (ie, a disturbance in the relation between circadian phase and sleep).

It may not only be a circadian phase delay behind the DSPS, but there also seems to exist a different phase angle between the melatonin phase and awakening. Patients wake up later than controls in relation to their respective melatonin phases [130]. Sleep onset did not have a different phase angle, however, and it was suggested that the delayed awakening may be blocking exposure to light during the phase advance portion of the phase-response curve [131].

With respect to sleepiness there seems to be a virtual absence of polysomnography (Multiple Sleep Latency Test) results, but also few studies of self-rated sleepiness. Thorpy and coworkers [128], however, showed maximum sleepiness in the morning and a reduction of sleepiness across the day. It was suggested that the morning sleepiness contributed to the educational difficulties associated with the diagnosis. Dahlitz and coworkers [132] found low levels of alertness around noon (not on awakening) and a peak around 6:00 to 7:00 PM.

The mechanism has not been clearly identified. One possibility is an abnormally long circadian period that makes it difficult to make the daily adjustments required to remain synchronized with the day-night cycle [123]. Another explanation may be a deviating entrainment response (eg, a short circadian advance portion of the phase response curve or an abnormally long delay portion) [133]. In addition, social preferences for timing of activity may also reduce the exposure to morning daylight, preventing a phase-advance response. Interestingly, individuals with a long free-running period have a reduced response to morning light. Possibly, this might reduce any phase-advance response in individuals with delayed sleep phase because this group suffers from severely curtailed sleep during normal work weeks. Delayed sleep phase patients also seem to respond less to sleep loss during the subjective day [134], which presumably makes it difficult to use the sleep loss during the working week to result in a sleep pressure that overcomes the circadian interference at normal bedtimes.

Some of the precipitating factors may be irregular work-rest patterns with considerable use of the night for activity [135]. In many cases, stress and other major changes also may be seen before the diagnosis.

Circadian pathology may then be related to mutations or drastic changes in genes, like natural polymorphisms, such as was found for the *Clock* gene [136] and was related to diurnal preference. Ebisawa and coworkers [137] also found a polymorphism in the human Per3 gene in DSPS. Archer and coworkers [138] found a length polymorphism in the same gene such that the longer allele was associated with morningess and the shorter with eveningess. The shorter allele was strongly associated with the DSPS patients, who in most cases were homozygous.

Treatments for DSPS include "chronotherapy," delaying the bedtime by 3 hours per day until a suitable bedtime has been reached and maintained [139]. The method seems to work but presents practical problems socially and may lead to the development of the non–24-hour sleep-wake syndrome. Timed bright (>2000 lux) light therapy is another relatively successful treatment that reduces morning sleepiness and phase advances sleep onset [140]. It involves exposure to bright light for 1 or 2 hours in the morning and leads to a phase advance of sleep and reduction of sleepiness in the morning [61]. Evening administration of the hormone melatonin also causes a phase advance that has been used in the treatment of DSPS [141,142].

Advanced sleep phase syndrome

The advanced sleep phase syndrome is essentially the reverse of the DSPS in the sense that it involves a phase advance of sleep and wakefulness of several hours [16,17], reviewed in [18]. Sleepiness appears early in the evening and if sleep is started then it has a normal onset, duration, and architecture [143]. Even if there is some impairment in functioning, this mainly concerns social activities and not work; the syndrome may have less severe consequences than DSPS. The prevalence is small but has been estimated at 1% of middle-aged groups [144]. It is virtually unknown outside this age range; however, some familial cases have been identified [145]. About 25% of the United States population complains of problems with early awakening (www.sleepfoundation.org).

In one of the few studies of sleepiness Lack and Lushington [146] studied a group (mean age 47 years) of early morning awakening insomniacs (waking up at 4.49 AM) and normal controls under constant conditions. The results showed that sleepiness started to rise already around noon and was much higher than that of the control group during the afternoon-evening. The sleep propensity rhythm, rectal temperature, and urinary melatonin showed similar phase advances.

The mechanism is unknown, but may involve similar paths as those of DSPS. Advanced sleep phase syndrome patients score the opposite of DSPS patients on "owl-lark" questionnaires [127]. Clearly, there is a genetic component involved. One study in three extended families who reported advanced bedtimes and times of rising showed a strong autosomal-dominant trait with high penetrance [145]. The melatonin and temperature rhythms were phase advanced and the period was shortened in one of the patients who were subjected to an isolation study. Advanced sleep phase is related to a mutation in the hPer2 gene [147].

Treatment may involve bright light exposure in the evening [148], which seems to have good results on sleep and sleepiness. Chronotherapy through advancing sleep gradually day by day has been tried [143].

Non–24-hour sleep-wake syndrome

This syndrome is also called "free-running" or hypernychthemeral syndrome, and involves a drift of the sleep period of 1 to 2 hours per day [16,17], reviewed in [18]. Attempts to retain entrainment to the day-night alternation results in reports of insomnia, early morning awakening, and excessive sleepiness during the daytime. These symptoms occur only when the sleep is out of phase with normal sleep hours. When the sleep hours are plotted against days there is a gradual daily delay of 1 to 2 hours, making sleep cover the 24 hours 3 to 4 weeks [149–151]. Very little polysomnographic data are available and all information on sleepiness seems to derive from anamnestic interviews. If sleep latency may be used to reflect sleepiness, maximum sleepiness occurs around the acrophase as is expected [152]. There is a need for systematic data on the sleepiness pattern across days.

The syndrome mainly occurs in blind people without photic entrainment [149,152]. Most totally blind individuals have free-running circadian rhythms and complain of sleep disturbances [153]. The absence of photic entrainment is probably the main reason for the syndrome, but some blind maintain a normal sleep wake pattern, either because they get sufficient entrainment from activity or because they have remnants of light perception even if this is not detected by the visual system [154]. The few sighted individuals who exhibit the syndrome may have a long endogenous circadian period [155] or have a decreased sensitivity to light. Among treatment approaches melatonin before bedtime has had some success [156,157].

Irregular sleep-wake syndrome

Irregular sleep-wake syndrome involves several sleep episodes per day, an apparent lack of circadian regulation of sleep, and wakefulness [16,17], reviewed in [18]. Sleepiness occurs out of phase with the light-dark cycle but no systematic description of sleepiness is available. The prevalence is unknown but is probably low, although it may be seen rather frequently in institutionalized elderly [158].

The mechanism is probably a dysfunctional circadian system or lack of normal light and dark stimuli or physical activity [114]. The latter study found increased sleep-wake instability when the daylight period grew shorter in the fall. Bright light, sleep hygiene, and physical activity have been tried as treatment [159].

References

[1] Hastings MH, Reddy AB, Maywood ES. A clockwork web: circadian timing in brain and periphery, in health and disease. Nat Rev Neurosci 2003;4:649–61.

[2] Reppert SM, Weaver DR. Comparing clockworks: mouse versus fly. J Biol Rhythms 2000; 15:357–64.

[3] Field MD, Maywood ES, O'Brien JA, et al. Analysis of clock proteins in mouse SCN demonstrates phylogenetic divergence of the circadian clockwork and resetting mechanisms. Neuron 2000;25:437–47.

[4] Vitaterna MH, King DP, Chang AM, et al. Mutagenesis and mapping of a mouse gene. Clock, essential for circadian behavior. Science 1994;264:719–25.

[5] Czeisler CA. The effect of light on the human circadian pacemaker. In: Chadwick D, Ackrill K, editors. Circadian clocks and their adjustment. Chichester: Ciba Foundation; 1995. p. 254–302.

[6] Aschoff J, Wever R. Spontanperiodik des menschen bei ausschlus aller zeitgeber. Naturwissenschaften 1962;49:337–42.

[7] Aschoff J, Gerecke U, Wever R. Desynchronization of human circadian rhythms. Jpn J Physiol 1967;17:450–7.

[8] Czeisler CA, Duffy JF, Shanahan TL, et al. Stability, precision, and near-24-hour period of the human circadian pacemaker. science 1999;284: 2177–81.

[9] Czeisler CA, Weitzman ED, Moore-Ede MC, et al. Human sleep: its duration and organization depend on its circadian phase. Science 1980;210:1264–7.

[10] Åkerstedt T, Gillberg M. Experimentally displaced sleep: effects on sleepiness. Electroencephalogr Clin Neurophysiol 1982;54:220–6.

[11] Dijk DJ, Duffy JF, Czeisler CA. Circadian and sleep-wake dependent aspects of subjective alertness and cognitive performance. J Sleep Res 1992;1:112–7.

[12] Dijk D-J, Czeisler CA. Contribution of the circadian pacemaker and the sleep homeostat to sleep propensity, sleep structure, electroencephalographic slow waves, and sleep spindle activity in humans. J Neurosci 1995;15:3526–38.

[13] Czeisler C, Dijk D-J, Duffy J. Entrained phase of the circadian pacemaker serves to stabilize alertness and performance throughout the habitual waking day. In: Ogilvie R, Harsh J, editors. Sleep onset normal and abnormal processes. Washington: American Psychological Association; 1995. p. 89–110.

[14] Åkerstedt T. Shift work and disturbed sleep/wakefulness. Occup Med 2003;53:89–94.

[15] Åkerstedt T. Sleepiness as a consequence of shift work. Sleep 1988;11:17–34.

[16] APA. Diagnostic and statistical manual of mental disorders. 4th edition. Washington: American Psychiatric Association; 2000.

[17] AASM. International classification of sleep disorders—diagnostic and coding manual. Chicago: American Academy of Sleep Medicine; 2001.

[18] Reid KJ, Zee PC. Circadian rhythm disorders. Semin Neurol 2004;24:315–25.

[19] Drake CL, Roehrs T, Richardson G, et al. Shift work sleep disorder: prevalence and consequences beyond that of symptomatic day workers. Sleep 2004;27:1453–62.

[20] Axelsson J, Åkerstedt T, Kecklund G, et al. Tolerance to shift work: how does it relate to sleep and wakefullness? Int Arch Occup Environ Health 2004;77:121–9.

[21] Torsvall L, Åkerstedt T. Sleepiness on the job: continuously measured EEG changes in train drivers. Electroencephalogr Clin Neurophysiol 1987;66:502–11.

[22] Kecklund G, Åkerstedt T. Sleepiness in long distance truck driving: an ambulatory EEG study of night driving. Ergonomics 1993;36: 1007–17.

[23] Mitler MM, Miller JC, Lipsitz JJ, et al. The sleep of long-haul truck drivers. N Engl J Med 1997; 337:755–61.

[24] Rosekind MR, Graeber RC, Dinges DF, et al. Crew factors in flight operations. IX: Effects of planned cockpit rest on crew performance and alertness in long haul operations. Moffett Field (CA): NASA Technical Memorandum; 1995.

[25] Torsvall L, Åkerstedt T, Gillander K, et al. Sleep on the night shift: 24-hour EEG monitoring of spontaneous sleep/wake behavior. Psychophysiology 1989;26:352–8.

[26] Landrigan CP, Rothschild JM, Cronin JW, et al. Effect of reducing interns' work hours on serious medical errors in intensive care units. N Engl J Med 2004;351:1838–48.

[27] Gillberg M, Kecklund G, Åkerstedt T. Sleepiness and performance of professional drivers in a truck simulator: comparisons between day and night driving. J Sleep Res 1996;5:12–5.

[28] Gillberg M, Kecklund G, Göransson B, et al. Operator performance and signs of sleepiness during day and night work in a simulated

thermal power plant. Int J Ind Ergon 2003;31: 101–9.

[29] Åkerstedt T, Peters T, Anund A, et al. Impaired alertness and performance while driving home from the night shift: a driving simulator study. J Sleep Res 2005;14:17–20.

[30] Foret J, Lantin G. The sleep of train drivers: an example of the effects of irregular work schedules on sleep. In: Colquhoun WP, editor. Aspects of human efficiency: diurnal rhythm and loss of sleep. London: The English Universities Press; 1972. p. 273–81.

[31] Foret J, Benoit O. Structure du sommeil chez des travailleurs à horaires alternants. Electroencephalogr Clin Neurophysiol 1974;37:337–44.

[32] Matsumoto K. Sleep patterns in hospital nurses due to shift work: an EEG study. Waking Sleeping 1978;2:169–73.

[33] Tilley AJ, Wilkinson RT, Drud M. Night and day shifts compared in terms of the quality and quantity of sleep recorded in the home and performance measured at work: a pilot study. In: Reinberg A, Vieux N, Andlauer P, editors. Night and shift work: biological and social aspects, vol. 30. Oxford: Pergamon Press; 1981. p. 187–96.

[34] Roehrs T, Roth T. Multiple Sleep Latency Test: technical aspects and normal values. J Clin Neurophysiol 1992;9:63–7.

[35] Åkerstedt T, Gillberg M. Subjective and objective sleepiness in the active individual. Int J Neurosci 1990;52:29–37.

[36] Cajochen C, Khalsa SBS, Wyatt JK, et al. EEG and ocular correlates of circadian melatonin phase and human performance decrements during sleep loss. Am J Physiol 1999;277: R640–9.

[37] Horne JA, Baulk SD. Awareness of sleepiness when driving. Psychophysiology 2004;41: 161–5.

[38] Drapeau C, Carrier J. Fluctuation of waking electroencephalogram and subjective alertness during a 25-hour sleep-deprivation episode in young and middle-aged subjects. Sleep 2004;27: 55–60.

[39] Bjerner B. Alpha depression and lowered pulse rate during delayed actions in a serial reaction test. Acta Physiol Scand 1949;19(Suppl 65): 1–93.

[40] Daniel RS. Electroencephalographic pattern quantification and the arousal continuum. Psychophysiology 1966;2:146–60.

[41] Torsvall L, Åkerstedt T. Extreme sleepiness: quantification of EOG and spectral EEG parameters. Int J Neurosci 1988;38:435–41.

[42] O'Hanlon JF, Beatty J. Concurrence of electroencephalographic and performance changes during a simulated radar watch and some implications for the arousal theory of vigilance. In: Mackie RR, editor. Vigilance. New York: Plenum Press; 1977. p. 189–202.

[43] Reyner LA, Horne JA. Falling asleep whilst driving: are drivers aware of prior sleepiness? Int J Legal Med 1998;111:120–3.

[44] Dinges DF, Mallis MM. Managing fatigue by drowsiness detection: can technological promises be realized. In: Hartley L, editor. Managing fatigue in transportation. Oxford: Elsevier Science; 1998. p. 209–30.

[45] Liberson WT, Liberson CW. EEG records, reaction times, eye movements, respiration, and mental content during drowsiness. In: Wortis J, editor. Recent advances in biological psychiatry. Soc of Biol Psych, Annual Convention 20. New York: Society of Biological Psychology; 1965. p. 295–302.

[46] Fruhstorfer H, Langanke P, Meinzer K, et al. Neurophysiological vigilance indicators and operational analysis of a train vigilance monitoring device: a laboratory and field study. In: Mackie RR, editor. Vigilance. New York: Plenum Press; 1977. p. 147–62.

[47] Lobb ML, Stern JA. Pattern of eyelid motion predictive of decision errors during drowsiness: oculomotor indices of altered states. Int J Neurosci 1986;30:17–22.

[48] Santamaria J, Chiappa KH. The EEG of drowsiness in normal adults. J Clin Neurophysiol 1987; 4:327–82.

[49] Wierwille WW, Ellsworth LA. Evaluation of driver drowsiness by trained raters. Accid Anal Prev 1994;26:571–81.

[50] Torsvall L, Åkerstedt T. Eye closure, sleepiness and EEG spectra. In: Koella WP, Rüther E, Schulz H, editors. Sleep 1984. Stuttgart: Gustav Fischer Verlag; 1985. p. 300–1.

[51] Thiis-Evensen E. Shift work and health. Ind Med Surg 1958;27:493–7.

[52] Andersen JE. Three-shift work. Copenhagen: Socialforskningsinstitutet; 1970.

[53] Verhaegen P, Maasen A, Meers A. Health problems in shift workers. In: Johnson LC, Tepas DJ, Colquhoun WP, et al, editors. Biological rhythms and shift work. New York: Spectrum; 1981. p. 271–82.

[54] Paley MJ, Tepas DI. Fatigue and the shiftworker: firefighters working on a rotating shift schedule. Hum Factors 1994;36:269–84.

[55] Prokop O, Prokop L. Ermüdung und einschlafen am steuer. Zbl Verkehrsmed 1955;1:19–30.

[56] Coleman RM, Dement WC. Falling asleep at work: a problem for continuous operations. Sleep Res 1986;15:265.

[57] Johns MW. A new method for measuring daytime sleepiness: the Epworth sleepiness scale. Sleep 1991;14:540–5.

[58] Lowden A, Kecklund G, Axelsson J, et al. Change from an 8-hour shift to a 12-hour shift, attitudes, sleep, sleepiness and performance. Scand J Work Environ Health 1998;24(Suppl 3):69–75.

[59] Härmä M, Sallinen M, Ranta R, et al. The effect of an irregular shift system on sleepiness at work in train drivers and railway traffic controllers. J Sleep Res 2002;11:141–51.

[60] Tilley AJ, Wilkinson RT, Warren PSG, et al. The sleep and performance of shift workers. Hum Factors 1982;24:624–41.

[61] Kecklund G, Åkerstedt T, Lowden A. Morning work: effects of early rising on sleep and alertness. Sleep 1997;20:215–23.

[62] Eastman CI, Stewart KT, Mahoney MP, et al. Shift work: dark goggles and bright light improve circadian rhythm adaption to night-shift work. Sleep 1994;17:535–43.

[63] Bjorvatn B, Kecklund G, Åkerstedt T. Rapid adaptation to night work at an oil platform, but slow readaptation following return home. J Occup Environ Med 1998;40:601–8.

[64] Gillberg M, Kecklund G, Åkerstedt T. Relations between performance and subjective ratings of sleepiness during a night awake. Sleep 1994;17: 236–41.

[65] Dorrian J, Lamond N, Dawson D. The ability to self-monitor performance when fatigued. J Sleep Res 2000;9:137–44.

[66] Rogers NL, Dinges DF. Subjective surrogates of performance during night work. Sleep 2003;26: 790–1.

[67] Dinges DF. The nature of sleepiness: causes, contexts, and consequences. In: Stunkard A, Baum A, editors. Perspectives in behavioral medicine: eating, sleeping, and sex. Hillsdale: Lawrence Erlbaum; 1989. p. 147–79.

[68] Yang C-M, Lin F-W, Spielman AJ. A standard procedure enhances the correlation between subjective and objective measures of sleepiness. Sleep 2004;27:329–32.

[69] Folkard S, Åkerstedt T. Trends in the risk of accidents and injuries and their implications for models of fatigue and performance. Aviat Space Environ Med 2004;75:A161–7.

[70] Harris W. Fatigue, circadian rhythm and truck accidents. In: Mackie RR, editor. Vigilance. New York: Plenum Press; 1977. p. 133–46.

[71] Hamelin P. Lorry driver's time habits in work and their involvement in traffic accidents. Ergonomics 1987;30:1323–33.

[72] Langlois PH, Smolensky MH, Hsi BP, et al. Temporal patterns of reported single-vehicle car and truck accidents in Texas, USA during 1980–1983. Chronobiol Int 1985;2:131–46.

[73] Horne JA, Reyner LA. Sleep related vehicle accidents. BMJ 1995;310:565–7.

[74] NTSB. Factors that affect fatigue in heavy truck accidents. National Transportation Safety Board Safety Study. NTSB/SS-95/01. Washington (DC): National Transportation Safety Board; 1995.

[75] NTSB. Grounding of the US tankship Exxon Valdez on Bligh Reef, Prince William Sound near Valdez, Alaska, March 24, 1989. National Transportation Safety Board. Maritime Accident Report. NTSB/MAR-90/04. Washington (DC): National Transportation Safety Board; 1990.

[76] NTSB. Evaluation of US Department of Transportation: efforts in the 1990s to address operation fatigue. Washington: National Transportation Safety Board; 1999.

[77] Bjerner B, Holm Å, Swensson Å. Diurnal variation of mental performance: a study of three-shift workers. Br J Ind Med 1955;12:103–10.

[78] Brown RC. The day and night performance of teleprinter switchboard operators. Occupational Psychology 1949;23:121–6.

[79] Wojtczak-Jaroszowa J, Pawlowska-Skyga K. Night and shift work I: Circadian variations in work. Med Pr 1967;18:1–10.

[80] Wojtczak-Jaroszowa J, Jarosz D. Time-related distribution of occupational accidents. J Safety Res 1987;18:33–41.

[81] Ong CN, Phoon WO, Iskandar N, et al. Shiftwork and work injuries in an iron and steel mill. Appl Ergon 1987;18:51–6.

[82] Andlauer P. The effect of shift working on the workers' health. European Productivity Agency, TU Information Bulletin 1960:90:29.

[83] Quaas M, Tunsch R. Problems of disablement and accident frequency in shift and night work. Stockholm (Sweden): Studia Laboris et Salutis; 1972.

[84] Smith P. A study of weekly and rapidly rotating shift workers. Int Arch Occup Environ Health 1979;43:211–20.

[85] Totterdell P, Spelten E, Smith L, et al. On-shift and daily variations in self-reported and performance measures in rotating shift and permanent night nurses. Work Stress 1995;9:187–97.

[86] Folkard S. Effects on performance efficiency. In: Colquhoun P, Costa G, Folkard S, et al, editors. Shiftwork: problems and solutions. Frankfurt am Main: Peter Lang; 1996. p. 65–87.

[87] Colquhoun WP, Blake MJF, Edwards RS. Experimental studies of shift work. I: A comparison of rotating and stabilized 4-hour systems. Ergonomics 1968;11:437–53.

[88] Folkard S. Circadian rhythms and human memory. In: Brown FM, Graeber RC, editors. Rhythmic aspects of behaviour. Hillsdale: Lawrence Erlbaum Associates; 1982. p. 241–72.

[89] Dawson D, Reid K. Fatigue, alcohol and performance impairment. Nature 1997;388:235.

[90] Mitler MM, Carskadon MA, Czeisler CA, et al. Catastrophes, sleep and public policy: consensus report. Sleep 1988;11:100–9.

[91] Smith L, Folkard S, Poole CJM. Increased injuries on night shift. Lancet 1994;344:1137–9.

[92] Åkerstedt T, Fredlund P, Gillberg M, et al. A prospective study of fatal occupational accidents: relationship to sleeping difficulties and occupational factors. J Sleep Res 2002;11:69–71.

[93] Lockley SW, Cronin JW, Evans EE, et al. Effect of reducing interns' weekly work hours on sleep and attentional failures. N Engl J Med 2004; 351:1829–37.

[94] Leger D. The cost of sleep-related accidents: a report for the National Commission on Sleep Disorders Research. Sleep 1994;17:84–93.

[95] Dahlgren K. Adjustment of circadian rhythms

and EEG sleep functions to day and night sleep among permanent night workers and rotating shift workers. Psychophysiology 1981;18:381–91.

[96] Åkerstedt T, Kecklund G, Knutsson A. Spectral analysis of sleep electroencephalography in rotating three-shift work. Scand J Work Environ Health 1991;17:330–6.

[97] Kecklund G. Sleep and alertness: effects of shift work, early rising, and the sleep environment (PhD-thesis). Stress Research Report 1996;252: 1–94.

[98] Foret J, Benoit O. Shiftwork: the level of adjustment to schedule reversal assessed by a sleep study. Waking Sleeping 1978;2:107–12.

[99] Dahlgren K. Long-term adjustment of circadian rhythms to a rotating shiftwork schedule. Scand J Work Environ Health 1981;7:141–51.

[100] Kripke DF, Cook B, Lewis OF. Sleep of night workers: EEG recordings. Psychophysiology 1971;7:377–84.

[101] Bryden G, Holdstock TL. Effects of night duty on sleep patterns of nurses. Psychophysiology 1973;10:36–42.

[102] Tepas DI, Walsh JK, Moss PD, et al. Polysomnographic correlates of shift worker performance in the laboratory. In: Reinberg A, Vieux N, Andlauer P, editors. Night and shift work: biological and social aspects. Oxford: Pergamon Press; 1981. p. 179–86.

[103] Dumont M, Montplaisir J, Infante-Rivard C. Insomnia symptoms in nurses with former permanent nightwork experience. In: Koella WP, Obal F, Schulz H, et al, editors. Sleep '86. Stuttgart: Gustav Fischer Verlag; 1988. p. 405–6.

[104] Guilleminault C, Czeisler S, Coleman R, et al. Circadian rhythm disturbances and sleep disorders in shift workers (EEG Suppl No. 36). In: Buser PA, Cobb WA, Okuma T, editors. Kyoto symposia. Amsterdam: Elsevier; 1982. p. 709–14.

[105] Ingre M, Åkerstedt T. Effect of accumulated night work during the working lifetime, on subjective health and sleep in monozygotic twins. J Sleep Res 2004;13:45–8.

[106] Wilkinson RT, Edwards RS, Haines E. Performance following a night of reduced sleep. Psychon Sci 1966;5:471–2.

[107] Härmä M, Suvanto S, Popkin S, et al. A dose-response study of total sleep time and the ability to maintain wakefulness. J Sleep Res 1998;7: 167–74.

[108] Jewett ME, Dijk D-J, Kronauer RE, et al. Dose-response relationship between sleep duration and human psychomotor vigilance and subjective alertness. Sleep 1999;22:171–9.

[109] Van Dongen HP, Maislin G, Mullington JM, et al. The cumulative cost of additional wakefulness: dose-response effects on neurobehavioral functions and sleep physiology from chronic sleep restriction and total sleep deprivation. Sleep 2003;26:117–26.

[110] Folkard S, Åkerstedt T. A three process model of the regulation of alertness and sleepiness. In: Ogilvie R, Broughton R, editors. Sleep, arousal and performance: problems and promises. Boston: Birkhäuser; 1991. p. 11–26.

[111] Post W, Gatty H. Around the world in eight days. London: John Hamilton; 1931.

[112] Haimov I, Arendt J. The prevention and treatment of jet lag. Sleep Med Rev 1999;3:229–40.

[113] Lowden A, Åkerstedt T. Sleep and wake patterns in aircrew on a 2-day layover on westward long distance flights. Aviat Space Environ Med 1998; 69:596–602.

[114] Spitzer RL, Terman M, Williams JB, et al. Jet lag: clinical features, validation of a new syndrome-specific scale, and lack of response to melatonin in a randomized, double-blind trial. Am J Psychiatry 1999;156:1392–6.

[115] Waterhouse J, Nevill A, Edwards B, et al. The relationship between assessments of jet lag and some of its symptoms. Chronobiol Int 2003; 20:1061–73.

[116] Nicholson AN, Pascoe PA, Spencer MB, et al. Nocturnal sleep and daytime alertness of aircrew after transmeridian flights. Aviat Space Environ Med 1986;57:B42–52.

[117] Sasaki M, Kurosaki Y, Mori A, et al. Patterns of sleep-wakefulness before and after transmeridian flight in commercial airline pilots. Aviat Space Environ Med 1986;57:B29–42.

[118] Wegmann HM, Gundel A, Naumann M, et al. Sleep, sleepiness and circadian rhythmicity in aircrews operating on transatlantic routes. Aviat Space Environ Med 1986;57:53–64.

[119] Stone BM, Turner C. Promoting sleep in shift-workers and intercontinental travelers. Chronobiol Int 1997;14:133–43.

[120] Arendt J, Skene DJ. Melatonin as a chronobiotic. Sleep Med Rev 2005;9:25–39.

[121] Samel A, Wegmann H-M. Bright light: a countermeasure for jet lag? Chronobiol Int 1997;14: 173–83.

[122] Lowden A, Åkerstedt T. Retaining home base sleep hours to prevent jet lag in connection with a westward flight across 9 time zones. Chronobiol Int 1998;15:365–76.

[123] Regestein QR, Monk TH. Delayed sleep phase syndrome: a review of its clinical aspects. Am J Psychiatry 1995;152:602–8.

[124] Wyatt JK. Delayed sleep phase syndrome: pathophysiology and treatment options. Sleep 2004;27:1195–203.

[125] Weitzman ED, Czeisler CA, Coleman RM, et al. Delayed sleep phase syndrome: a chronobiologic disorder with sleep onset insomnia. Arch Gen Psychiatry 1981;38:737–46.

[126] Nagtegaal JE, Laurant MW, Kerkhof GA, et al. Effects of melatonin on the quality of life in patients with delayed sleep phase syndrome. J Psychosom Res 2000;48:45–50.

[127] Horne JA, Östberg O. A self-assessment questionnaire to determine morningness-eveningness in human circadian rhythms. Int J Chronobiol 1976;4:77–110.

[128] Thorpy MJ, Korman E, Spielman AJ, et al. Delayed sleep phase syndrome in adolescents. J Adolesc Health Care 1988;9:22–7.

[129] Watanabe T, Kajimura N, Kato M, et al. Sleep and circadian rhythm disturbances in patients with delayed sleep phase syndrome. Sleep 2003;26:657–61.

[130] Shibui K, Uchiyama M, Okawa M. Melatonin rhythms in delayed sleep phase syndrome. J Biol Rhythms 1999;14:72–6.

[131] Minors DS, Waterhouse JM, Wirtz-Justice A. A human phase-response curve to light. Neurosci Lett 1991;133:36–40.

[132] Dahlitz M, Alvarez B, Vignau J, et al. Delayed sleep phase syndrome response to melatonin. Lancet 1991;337:1121–4.

[133] Czeisler CA, Richardson GS, Zimmerman MC, et al. Entrainment of human circadian rhythms by light-dark cycles. Photochem Photobiol 1981;34:239–47.

[134] Uchiyama M, Okawa M, Shibui K, et al. Poor recovery sleep after sleep deprivation in delayed sleep phase syndrome. Psychiatry Clin Neurosci 1999;53:195–7.

[135] Yamadera H, Takahashi K, Okawa M. A multicenter study of sleep-wake rhythm disorders: clinical features of sleep-wake rhythm disorders. Psychiatry Clin Neurosci 1996;50:195–201.

[136] Katzenberg D, Young T, Finn L, et al. A CLOCK polymorphism associated with human diurnal preference. Sleep 1998;21:569–76.

[137] Ebisawa T, Uchiyama M, Kajimura N, et al. Association of structural polymorphisms in the human period 3 gene with delayed sleep phase syndrome. EMBO Rep 2001;2:342–6.

[138] Archer SN, Robilliard EL, Skene DJ, et al. A length polymorphism in the circadian clock gene Per3 is linked to delayed sleep phase syndrome and extreme diurnal preference. Sleep 2003;26:413–5.

[139] Czeisler CA, Richardson GS, Coleman RM, et al. Chronotherapy: resetting the circadian clocks of patients with delayed sleep phase insomnia. Sleep 1981;4:1–21.

[140] Rosenthal NE, Joseph-Vanderpool JR, Levendosky AA, et al. Phase-shifting effects of bright morning light as treatment for delayed sleep phase syndrome. Sleep 1990;13:354–61.

[141] Dagan Y, Yovel I, Hallis D, et al. Evaluating the role of melatonin in the long-term treatment of delayed sleep phase syndrome (DSPS). Chronobiol Int 1998;15:181–90.

[142] Yang CM, Spielman AJ, D'Ambrosio P, et al. A single dose of melatonin prevents the phase delay associated with a delayed weekend sleep pattern. Sleep 2001;24:272–81.

[143] Moldofsky H, Musisi S, Phillipson EA. Treatment of a case of advanced sleep phase syndrome by phase advance chronotherapy. Sleep 1986;9:61–5.

[144] Schrader H, Bovim G, Sand T. The prevalence of delayed and advanced sleep phase syndromes. J Sleep Res 1993;2:51–5.

[145] Jones CR, Campbell SS, Zone SE, et al. Familial advanced sleep-phase syndrome: a short-period circadian rhythm variant in humans. Nat Med 1999;5:1062–5.

[146] Lack LC, Lushington K. The rhythms of human sleep propensity and core body temperature. J Sleep Res 1996;5:1–11.

[147] Toh KL, Jones CR, He Y, et al. An hPer2 phosphorylation site mutation in familial advanced sleep phase syndrome. Science 2001;291:1040–3.

[148] Lack L, Wright H, Kemp K, et al. The treatment of early-morning awakening insomnia with 2 evenings of bright light. Sleep 2005;28:616–23.

[149] Elliott AL, Mills JN, Waterhouse JM. A man with too long a day. J Physiol 1971;212:30–1.

[150] Weber AL, Cary MS, Connor N, et al. Human non-24-hour sleep-wake cycles in an everyday environment. Sleep 1980;2:347–54.

[151] Kamgar-Parsi B, Wehr TA, Gillin JC. Successful treatment of human non-24-hour sleep-wake syndrome. Sleep 1983;6:257–64.

[152] Klein T, Martens H, Dijk D-J, et al. Chronic non-24-hour circadian rhythm sleep disorder in a blind man with a regular 24-hour sleep-wake schedule. Sleep 1993;16:333–43.

[153] Miles LEM, Raynal DM, Wilson MA. Blind man living in normal society has circadian rhythms of 24.9 hours. Science 1977;198:421–3.

[154] Czeisler CA, Shanahan TL, Klerman EB, et al. Suppression of melatonin secretion in some blind patients by exposure to bright light. N Engl J Med 1995;332:6–11.

[155] Uchiyama M, Okawa M, Shibui K, et al. Altered phase relation between sleep timing and core body temperature rhythm in delayed sleep phase syndrome and non-24-hour sleep-wake syndrome in humans. Neurosci Lett 2000;294:101–4.

[156] Folkard S, Arendt J, Aldhous M, et al. Melatonin stabilizes sleep onset time in a blind man without entrainment of cortisol or temperature rhythms. Neurosci Lett 1990;113:193–8.

[157] Lockley SW, Skene DJ, James K, et al. Melatonin administration can entrain the free-running circadian system of blind subjects. J Endocrinol 2000;164(1):R1–6.

[158] Regestein QR, Morris J. Daily sleep patterns observed among institutionalized elderly residents. J Am Geriatr Soc 1987;35:767–72.

[159] Naylor E, Penev PD, Orbeta L, et al. Daily social and physical activity increases slow-wave sleep and daytime neuropsychological performance in the elderly. Sleep 2000;23:87–95.

ELSEVIER
SAUNDERS

SLEEP
MEDICINE
CLINICS

Sleep Med Clin 1 (2006) 31–45

Sleep Deprivation and Sleepiness Caused by Sleep Loss

Scott M. Leibowitz, MD[a], Maria-Cecilia Lopes, MD[a,b],
Monica L. Andersen, PhD[b], Clete A. Kushida, MD, PhD[a,*]

- Sleep deprivation research
  Animal studies
  Human studies
- Evaluating and quantifying sleepiness
  Multiple Sleep Latency Test
  Maintenance of Wakefulness Test
  Psychomotor Vigilance Test
  Questionnaires
- Interactions between clinical sleep disorders and sleep loss
  Sleep disorders that result in sleep loss
- Summary
- References

Sleep deprivation (SD) and sleep loss have become increasingly prevalent in western society as societal demands on productivity increase. This increase in productivity, however, does not come without a cost. Although sleep is considered a luxury by some, it has become progressively more apparent that sleep is an essential part of health and wellness. The National Highway Traffic Safety Administration estimates that drowsiness is the primary causal factor in 100,000 police-reported crashes each year, resulting in 76,000 injuries and 1500 deaths, representing 1% to 3% of all police-reported crashes and 4% of fatalities, whereas other studies quote even higher percentages [1].

Because sleep is an integral aspect of the function of diurnal organisms, SD has a dramatic impact on multiple physiologic processes. These processes are often dependent on sleep for normal restoration. Over a thousand studies on SD have been published over the last century. These studies have

been performed to understand better the consequences of SD and to use SD as a tool to derive a better understanding of the elusive function of sleep. This article summarizes the animal and human models of SD and clinical disorders that cause either sleep curtailment or fragmented sleep that results in a functional SD that, in turn, yields excessive daytime sleepiness (EDS).

Sleep deprivation research

Animal studies

Numerous studies have been performed in animals involving SD and its resultant consequences [2,3]. Most of these consequences are believed to be under the control of central nervous system neurotransmitter systems. Central nervous system neurotransmitters, such as catecholamines, acetylcholine, serotonin, and γ-aminobutyric acid, either alone or

[a] Stanford Sleep Disorders Clinic, Stanford University Center of Excellence for Sleep Disorders, 401 Quarry Road, Suite 3301, Stanford, CA 94305–5730, USA
[b] Department of Psychobiology, Universidade Federal de Sao Paulo, EPM-UNIFESP, Rua Napoleao de Barros, 925, 20 Andar, CEP-04042-002 Sao Paulo, Brazil
* Corresponding author.
E-mail address: clete@stanford.edu (C.A. Kushida).

1556-407X/06/$ – see front matter © 2006 Elsevier Inc. All rights reserved.
sleep.theclinics.com

doi:10.1016/j.jsmc.2005.11.010

in transsynaptic relationships, have been implicated in several behavioral alterations in the sleep-deprived animal [4]. It could well be predicted that the behavioral alterations observed to occur after SD are the result of changes in functionality of brain neurotransmitters.

Experiments with selective paradoxical SD (PSD) (or rapid eye movement [REM]) using the water tank technique have shown that this procedure is able to alter some behaviors (ie, behavioral sensitization, locomotor and stereotypic activity) in the same way certain drugs can by acting on a number of different neurotransmitter systems [5,6]. Most of the instrumental methods used to induce PSD are modifications of the single method developed by Jouvet and coworkers [7] for cats, and later adapted for rats by Cohen and Dement [8] by placing a rat onto a narrow platform surrounded by water. To eliminate the restriction of movement and allow the animal to ambulate, the multiple platform method was developed, in which one rat is placed inside a large water tank containing several platforms [9]. This method was further modified by Nunes and Tufik [10] to eliminate the social isolation experienced by the animal. In this paradigm, 10 animals on 14 narrow platforms were used, avoiding both social isolation and movement restriction.

The neurochemical basis for the constellation of behavioral changes following PSD is not completely clear, but many observations suggest a major role for central dopamine in these processes because supersensitivity in brain dopamine receptors was observed after 96-hour sleep-deprived rats [11,12]. Notwithstanding, because sleep is regulated by circadian and homeostatic processes, the circadian pacemaker, located in the suprachiasmatic nuclei of the hypothalamus, has been proposed to regulate the timing and consolidation of the sleep-wake cycle, whereas a homeostatic mechanism governs the accumulation of sleep debt and sleep recovery [13]. In a study performed by Easton and coworkers [13] following SD, suprachiasmatic nuclei–lesioned mice exhibited an attenuated increase in non-REM (NREM) sleep time, whereas an increase in NREM electroencephalographic delta power was seen, similar to that of the sham controls. These changes seem to indicate that the suprachiasmatic nuclei consolidates the sleep-wake cycle by generating a signal of arousal during the dark period (ie, the active period), thereby having the capacity to alter the amount of baseline sleep. In addition, compared with controls cats, an important increase in Fos expression, one of the so-called "clock genes," was observed in neurons in the preoptic area of sleep-deprived cats by both gentle and stressful methods, the preoptic area being a primary region of the brain involved in sleep. These data indicate that *c-fos* expression can be used as a marker of a type of putative homeostatic mechanism regulating sleep [14].

The identification of the molecular correlates of sleep and wakefulness is essential in understanding the restorative processes occurring during sleep, the cellular mechanisms underlying sleep regulation, and the functional consequences of sleep loss [15]. Indeed, little is known about this complex area of science. Recently, Naidoo and coworkers [16] demonstrated the induction of key regulatory proteins in a cellular protective pathway, the unfolded protein response, following 6 hours of induced wakefulness in mice. Prolonging wakefulness beyond certain duration induces the unfolded protein response indicating a physiologic limit to wakefulness.

Sleep loss has been associated with an alteration in the regulation of the hypothalamic-pituitary-adrenal axis, stress hormone release [17], and rapid autonomic activation [18]. Using the rat as model species, Meerlo and coworkers [19] investigated hypothalamic-pituitary-adrenal axis activity during and after SD and the effect of sleep loss on the subsequent hypothalamic-pituitary-adrenal response to a novel stressor. The results showed that sleep loss not only is a mild activator of the hypothalamic-pituitary-adrenal axis, but also affects the ability of the hypothalamic-pituitary-adrenal axis to respond at pre-SD levels in response to subsequent stress. Alterations in hypothalamic-pituitary-adrenal axis regulation may appear gradually in both conditions of long periods of total SD and after repeated sleep curtailment.

In this fashion, SD in animals causes several behavioral changes that may produce a conditional state that eventually becomes lethal [2], but lacks specific localization and is reversible with sleep; all of which implies mediation by a biochemical abnormality [20]. Metabolic and immunologic consequences of SD point to a high potential for an antioxidant imbalance that results from SD [21]. It has been hypothesized that SD represents an oxidative challenge for the brain and that sleep may have a protective role against oxidative damage [22]. A recent study in long-term SD animals, however, found no evidence of oxidative damage at the lipid level, the protein level, in the cerebral cortex, or in peripheral tissues. Furthermore, no consistent change in antioxidant enzymatic activities was found after prolonged SD, nor was any evidence of increased oxidant production in the brain or in peripheral tissues in these animals. According to this study, findings do not support the assumption that prolonged wakefulness may cause oxidative damage, or that it may represent an oxidative stress for the brain or peripheral tissues, such as the liver and skeletal muscle [23].

Paradoxically, there is some evidence that at times SD may result in a positive consequence. One example of these positive consequences is the antidepressant effect caused by SD in clinically depressed patients. Indeed, total SD (TSD) has been found to be an effective treatment for mood disorders [23]. This mechanism is thought to occur through an enhancement in several neurotransmitter pathways, including dopaminergic transmission [24]. SD, in particular PSD, has also shown a facilitatory effect on the occurrence of genital reflexes in male rats [25,26].

Despite abundant data regarding the various neural activities that characterize the two states of sleep, the constellation of intricate behavioral and neuropharmacologic consequences of SD remain to be elucidated. If sleep serves important biologic and vital functions, it is not surprising that deprivation of sleep leads to relevant consequences. In fact, SD is a potentially useful strategy for studying the function of sleep. Still, little is known about how SD affects the physiologic functions of the brain and the body.

Human studies

A considerable debate over the need for sleep in modern humans has been the center of attention in many studies. Although sleep occupies approximately one third of each person's lifetime, there is an ever more frequent and marked increase in the time spent awake. The prevalence of sleep disorders is increasing in modern societies where constant exposure to artificial light and interactive activities, such as television or the Internet, are combined with socioeconomic pressure that drives us to into a 24-hour society.

Deprivation of sleep in humans is widely believed to impair health, whereas sleep is thought to have powerful restorative properties. Much literature documents the negative effects of SD on a wide range of psychomotor tasks and cognitive performance [27,28]. In addition, total sleep restriction in humans is associated with increased daytime sleepiness, decreased performance, and hormonal and metabolic disturbances [29].

Emerging research has shown that sleepiness, defined as the tendency to fall asleep, is not only determined by sleep pressure and time of day, but also by physiologic and cognitive arousal [30]. In this sense, although the function of sleep remains largely unknown, some of the most exciting and contentious hypotheses are that sleep contributes importantly to memory. A large number of studies offer a substantive body of evidence supporting the role of sleep in "sleep-dependent memory processing" [31]. In experimental models, paradoxical sleep (PS) has been shown to be necessary for cortical synaptic plasticity and for the acquisition of spatial and nonspatial memory [32], whereas PSD produced impairment of the acquisition of inhibitory avoidance [33,34]. Both human and animal studies support the idea that memory consolidation of waking experiences occurs during sleep.

Common symptoms associated with sleep fragmentation and SD include increased objective sleepiness (as measured by the Multiple Sleep Latency Test [MSLT] and the Maintenance of Wakefulness Test [MWT]); decreased psychomotor performance on a number of tasks including tasks involving short-term memory, reaction time, or vigilance; and degraded mood. Differences in degrees of sleepiness seem to be related more to the degree of sleep loss or fragmentation rather than to the type of sleep disturbance [35]. Both sleep fragmentation and SD can exacerbate sleep pathology by increasing the severity of sleep apnea in terms of frequency of apneic events and duration of apneic events after sleep loss [36].

The neurocognitive changes caused by restricted sleep, including EDS and altered mood, may result in work-related injuries and motor vehicle accidents [37]. Evidence links sleep loss to hormonal changes that could result in obesity [38] and total SD leads to marked hyperphagia [39]. Over the past 40 years, self-reported sleep duration in the United States has decreased by almost 2 hours. With the epidemic of obesity in this country, this finding correlates remarkably with the fact that short sleep duration in young, healthy men is associated with decreased leptin levels, increased ghrelin levels, and increased hunger and appetite [40].

Sleep is hypothesized to be a restorative process that is integral for the optimal functioning of the immune system. Severity of disordered sleep in depressed and alcoholic subjects correlates with a decline in natural and cellular immunity and is associated with alterations in the complex cytokine network [41]. Sleep loss has a role in mediating these immune changes as experimentally induced partial night SD has shown. These experiments have replicated sleep loss similar in nature to sleep loss found in clinical samples. Through this experimental sleep loss, a pattern of immune alteration was induced in these subjects, similar to that found in depressed and alcoholic patients [41]. Recently, a high-sensitivity C-reactive protein, a stable marker of inflammatory marker of cardiovascular risk, has been reported to be elevated after acute total and short-term partial SD [42]. This finding suggests that sleep loss may be one of the ways that inflammatory processes are activated and contribute to the association of sleep complaints and short sleep duration, and cardiovascular morbidity observed in epidemiologic surveys.

Both NREM and REM SD lead to specific compensatory rebound, suggesting that these states fulfill certain physiologic needs. In view of impaired performance that is seen after SD, a recovery function of sleep seems likely. The timing of this recovery is restricted to a narrow time interval within the 24-hour day (ie, the night). Generally, nocturnal sleep in humans is considered to be a consequence of the impact of the hypothalamic circadian pacemaker on sleep propensity. The interaction between the homeostatic recovery process and the circadian pacemaker has been described in the two-process model of sleep regulation [43].

SD seems to disrupt vital biologic processes necessary for optimal cognitive functioning and physical health, yet the ways in which the myriad of functions of the brain and body are compromised from SD are not fully understood. There is pressure in modern society to carry out an increasing variety of responsibilities during waking hours, and the expectations that these responsibilities can be achieved tends to push sleep into the background. This trend toward SD and irregular sleep-wake patterns leads to impairment in concentration and memory. This decrement in function likely reduces the quality of life of the sleep-deprived individual, and diminishes the ability to fulfill the expectations of enjoying and completing anticipated activities of work and leisure. The balance may have to swing back toward awareness that adequate and regular hours of sleep are required to promote a state of well-being during wakefulness.

Evaluating and quantifying sleepiness

It has been well established that the cumulative effect of SD or sleep fragmentation results in EDS [44–47]. To quantify degrees of sleepiness across individuals, many subjective and objective measures of EDS have been developed. These measures do not necessarily take into account the cause of the EDS. Regardless of the cause, these measures need to be reliable and reproducible to be an accurate representation of EDS in both a clinical and research environment.

Multiple Sleep Latency Test

To evaluate objectively the degree of sleepiness of an individual, the MSLT has become the most commonly used test. Because the MSLT is based on a simple intuitive approach toward sleepiness, it has achieved widespread acceptance in the evaluation of EDS. The MSLT consists of four or five 20-minute naps with routine polysomnographic monitoring; the patient is asked not to resist sleep. The primary assessments made by the MSLT are the rapidity of sleep onset, which correlates to degree of sleepiness [48–50], and to establish the presence of sleep-onset REM periods, which may be indicative of narcolepsy [51,52]. Typical sleep latencies in the normal adult are between 10 and 20 minutes, whereas pathologic sleepiness is manifested by a latency of less than 5 minutes [45]. This shortened sleep latency is associated with impaired performance in patients with significant EDS and in sleep-deprived normal subjects [53]. Latencies between 5 and 10 minutes indicate moderate sleepiness, and may or may not be associated with pathologic conditions [54].

As a diagnostic test for narcolepsy, the MSLT should be performed immediately following a nocturnal polysomnogram to exclude other causes of EDS from either sleep fragmentation or insufficient sleep. If the polysomnogram is remarkable for other causes of EDS, these conditions should be adequately treated before an evaluation of EDS with an MSLT is pursued.

Maintenance of Wakefulness Test

As an alternative to the physiologically based evaluation of sleepiness of the MSLT, Mitler and colleagues developed the MWT [55]. This test was designed for use with patients whose sleepiness during the day might adversely affect performance or safety. The reasoning behind the MWT was that a person who has little difficulty with falling asleep inappropriately should be able to stay awake in a quiet, sedentary situation, such as during the MWT trial. The MWT involves instruction to remain awake while sitting in a comfortable position in a partially reclining chair or propped-up in bed for either 20 or 40 minutes. This laboratory situation parallels circumstances in which sleep onset occurs inadvertently while a person is passive and sedentary in a nonstimulating environment. In the MWT there is no task other than to remain awake. During the MWT, an individual is monitored for electroencephalographic sleep onset during four to six sessions, scheduled at 2-hour intervals commencing 2 hours after awakening from the previous night's sleep. The MSLT measures a propensity to sleep, a physiologic sleepiness, whereas the MWT measures the ability to stay awake, a manifest sleepiness [56]. Although these two tests do measure degrees of sleepiness, studies have had mixed results when correlating these tests to each other as an objective assessment tool for sleepiness [57–59]. These differences may relate to the fact that the two tests measure fundamentally different end points.

Psychomotor Vigilance Test

Although the MSLT and the MWT adequately assess the clinical degree of sleepiness, neither test evaluates the degree of psychomotor or neurocognitive impairment that results from sleepiness and SD. The psychomotor vigilance test (PVT) is a test that was developed to evaluate objectively the ability of an individual to sustain attention and to respond in a timely fashion to salient signals or cues, usually in research settings. The PVT is administered by requiring an individual to respond to a small, bright red light stimulus (LED-digital counter) by pressing a response button when the stimulus appears. This action stops the stimulus counter and displays the reaction time in milliseconds for a 1-second period. The subject is instructed to respond as quickly as possible, but not to press the button too soon (which causes a false start warning to be displayed). The PVT was designed in such a way that is has only very minor learning effects [60,61], a necessary prerequisite for any test of psychomotor function. The PVT has demonstrated a learning effect on the order of a one- to three-trial learning curve [62], whereas other simple learning tasks, such as the digit symbol substitution task, may have on the order of a 30- to 60-trial learning curve [63]. When the PVT is administered, the interval between stimuli varies randomly from 2 to 10 seconds, and the task duration is typically 10 minutes. This duration allows approximately 90 reaction times per trial to be evaluated. The sensitivity of the PVT can be increased by increasing the task durations (eg, 20 minutes). This manipulation can be useful when studying the assessment of interventions purporting to reduce sleepiness (eg, various pharmacologic agents, naps, work-rest schedules) or when evaluating more subtle degrees of sleepiness [64].

There have been extensive studies validating the PVT as an assay for neurocognitive effects of sleep loss. It has been tested under a variety of conditions, including TSD, chronic partial SD, and sleep fragmentation. Irrespective of the mode of sleep loss, the PVT has been shown to represent accurately the cumulative effects of sleep loss on sustained attention and psychomotor decrement, in both the acute and chronic form. Additionally, the PVT has been shown to represent accurately the effectiveness of countermeasures to sleep loss (eg, naps, stimulants). The PVT has also been used to quantify daytime functioning levels in patients suffering from obstructive sleep apnea syndrome (OSAS), in relation to drowsy driving and in alcohol intoxication protocols. Although not routinely used in clinical practice, there is clearly a role for the PVT is assessing baseline functioning of certain at-risk individuals.

Questionnaires

The most commonly used tool in clinical practice for screening and evaluating patients for sleepiness of any cause comes in the form of patient questionnaires. Questionnaires are, by definition, subjective evaluation of an individual's symptoms. In effect, it is merely an extension of the routine medical history, and unfortunately most subjective questionnaires have not proved to be a reliable surrogate for the MSLT when evaluated methodologically. In fact, several investigators have reported weak or no association between sleep latency on the MSLT and subjective scales [30–32,65–68]. Questionnaires can, at minimum, be a useful screening tool and a starting point to qualify and quantify the complaint of EDS.

One of the first questionnaires to be designed and validated specifically to measure sleepiness is the Stanford Sleepiness Scale [69]. The Stanford Sleepiness Scale was constructed as a seven-point rating scale of equal-appearing intervals from wide awake to devastatingly sleepy, and subsequently validated against SD [Box 1]. Studies have shown the Stanford Sleepiness Scale to be a reliable means of rating sleepiness in healthy, sleep-deprived individuals. Patients with chronic sleepiness seem to lose the ability to assess their internal level of sleepiness accurately [70].

The most commonly used questionnaire among sleep specialists to evaluate EDS is the Epworth Sleepiness Scale [Table 1] developed by Johns

---

> ***Box 1:* The Stanford Sleepiness Scale**
>
> The subject is to choose the statement that best describes his or her state.
>
> 1. Feeling active and vital, alert, wide awake
> 2. Functioning at high level, but not at peak, able to concentrate
> 3. Relaxed, awake, not at full alertness, responsive
> 4. A little foggy, not at peak, let down
> 5. Fogginess, beginning to lose interest in remaining awake, slowed down
> 6. Sleepiness, prefer to be lying down, fighting sleep, woozy
> 7. Almost in reverie, sleep onset soon, lost struggle to remain awake
>
> *From* Hoddes E, Zarcone V, Smythe H, et al. Quantification of sleepiness: a new approach. Psychophysiology 1973;10(4):431–6; with permission.

Table 1: The Epworth Sleepiness Scale

Each question is answered with a number from 0 (not at all likely to fall asleep) to 3 (very likely to fall asleep). This yields a total of 0 (minimum) to 24 (maximum), and scores above 10 are thought to warrant investigation.

How likely are you to doze off or fall asleep in the following situations, in contrast to feeling just tired? This refers to your usual way of life in recent times. Even if you have not done some of these things recently, try to work out how they would have affected you. Use the following scale to choose the most appropriate number for each situation:

0: would *never* doze
1: *slight* chance of dozing
2: *moderate* chance of dozing
3: *high* chance of dozing

Activity	Chance of Dozing
Sitting and reading	_____
Watching television	_____
Sitting inactive in a public place (meeting, theater, and so forth)	_____
As a passenger in a car for 1 hour without a break	_____
Lying down in the afternoon when circumstances permit	_____
Sitting and talking to someone	_____
Sitting quietly after lunch without alcohol	_____
In a car, while stopped for a few minutes in traffic	_____
TOTAL	_____

From Johns MW. A new method for measuring daytime sleepiness: the Epworth sleepiness scale. Sleep 1991;14(6): 540–5; with permission.

[71]. The Epworth Sleepiness Scale has eight specific real-life situations listed and the patient is asked to rate the likelihood of falling asleep during any of these activities, evaluating a behavior rather than an internal state. A score of 10 or more usually warrants further investigation. Of any questionnaire to evaluate EDS, the Epworth Sleepiness Scale has undergone the most studies to assess its ability to predict sleep latency in the MSLT. The results of these studies are mixed, and at best, a small statistical significance was found between the Epworth Sleepiness Scale to the sleep latency on the MSLT [72,73].

Finally, the Sleep-Wake Activity Inventory was rigorously developed using a stepwise regression analysis with the mean sleep latency. Because of its comprehensive and complex approach to the evaluation of EDS, it is extensive, with 59 items in the questionnaire. This scale seems to be sensitive to different levels of sleepiness, and also seems reliably to reflect improvements associated with treatment [74]. Its usefulness is probably best reserved for clinical research protocols evaluating various aspects of EDS.

Interactions between clinical sleep disorders and sleep loss

Sleep disorders are hugely prevalent in the United States. In the 2005 National Sleep Foundation "Sleep in America" poll, over 75% of respondents reported having had at least one symptom of a sleep problem a few nights a week or more within the past year [75]. Although not all of these complaints may constitute a sleep disorder, this statistic underscores the prevalence of this problem in the United States.

There is a large spectrum of sleep disorders that may result in curtailed total sleep time or sleep fragmentation. Often, these disorders share the same final pathway of resultant EDS. A subset of patients with significant objective measures of sleep disruption and poor sleep quality, however, may not complain of frank sleepiness. Studies have shown that the severity of EDS may not correlate directly with severity of sleep disruption [69,76]. Many theories have been postulated as to why these discrepancies are seen, but none have been verified and further studies are needed. This section describes a variety of clinical sleep disorders that may result in SD, and sleep disorders associated with sleep fragmentation, both of which may result in EDS.

Sleep disorders that result in sleep loss

Insomnia

Insomnia is a markedly common complaint in society. The cause of insomnia is multifactorial and often several coexisting factors exist in the individual suffering from insomnia. The Spielman model describes three important conditions that exist, which facilitate the evolution of the insomnia process: (1) predisposing, (2) precipitating, and (3) perpetuating factors [77]. These conditions are usually present in some form in an individual suffering from acute or chronic insomnia.

There are several subtypes of insomnia of differing causes. These include psychophysiologic insomnia, adjustment insomnia, idiopathic insomnia, paradoxical insomnia, insomnia caused by drug or substance, or insomnia caused by a medical condition. More than one subtype of insomnia can exist simultaneously and the distinction between subtypes can at times be difficult to make. Subsequently, the clinical history is an essential component in the evaluation of the patient who presents with this complaint.

According to the newly revised International Classification of Sleep Disorders-2 [78], there is a minimum criterion required to make the diagnosis of psychophysiologic insomnia. These include

- The patient's symptoms meet the basic clinical criteria of insomnia plus a decrease in function while awake.
- The symptoms are present for at least 1 month.
- Maladaptive sleep associations (conditioned alerting behavior in the bedroom at sleep times or "trying too hard to sleep") are reported.
- The patient reports evidenced somatic tension, excessive focus on sleep, or heightened anxiety about sleep.
- Difficulty falling asleep at bedtime or during planned naps is reported. This difficulty may be absent during other monotonous activities, however, when not intending to sleep.
- The patient may report that it is easier to sleep away from home than at home.
- Intrusive thoughts at bedtime (mental arousal) are typical.
- Absence of other medical-sleep disorder responsible for the complaint.
- Polysomnography with prolonged sleep latency and awakenings with subsequent reduced sleep efficiency.

Sleep laboratory testing has limited value in distinguishing insomniacs from normal sleepers [79]. There are, however, several studies that have demonstrated that sleep fragmentation and SD can exacerbate sleep pathology by increasing the pathophysiology of sleep apnea [80]. Moreover, chronic insomnia, in particular the inability to maintain sleep as opposed to difficulties initiating sleep, may be a consequence of coexisting sleep disorders, such as sleep-disordered breathing [81–83]. Additionally, polysomnography may play a role in distinguishing sleep state misperception from true psychophysiologic insomnia. Sleep state misperception is a condition where individuals perceive themselves as not sleeping but are clearly sleeping by electroencephalogram criteria for sleep.

Other monitoring methods, such as actigraphy or sleep logs, have been proved useful; however, there is great variability in the consistency of these tools in accurately representing sleep in insomnia patients. This variability is caused by the fact that actigraphy cannot identify periods of wakefulness in bed without movement, and subjective sleep scales and sleep logs may inaccurately represent the severity of sleeplessness. Nonetheless, these tools may provide information that is practical and useful to the practicing physician.

Because sleep is regulated by a circadian pacemaker, insomnia may develop in the setting of disturbances between the coupling of sleep and this pacemaker [84]. More commonly, however, insomnia is triggered by a psychologic disturbance and often persists despite the elimination or improvement of the initial perceived stress, anxiety, or depressive symptomatology [85,86].

Although it has been established that insomnia is a risk factor for the development of psychiatric disorders, the possibility that chronic insomnia can be associated with significant medical morbidity has not been well-explored. The effect of chronic insomnia on the cardiovascular system, including hypertension, coronary artery disease, and stroke, is still unclear.

Therapeutic goals in treating insomnia are generally to improve the quality or quantity of nighttime sleep. Adjunctive interventions, such as melatonin or bright light, have been recommended with mixed results in some forms of chronic insomnia [87]. The focus of psychotherapeutic and behavioral treatments is to reduce emotional and physiologic arousal that prevents sleep initiation and maintenance, and the underlying factors of hyperarousal present throughout the 24-hour sleep-wake period, in accordance with the two-model process proposed by Borbely [88]. A task force appointed by the American Academy of Sleep Medicine showed that 70% to 80% of patients treated with nonpharmacologic interventions derive benefit from this modality of treatment [89]. Using behavioral techniques, such as sleep restriction and stimulus control, either before or during bedtime, has been shown significantly to improve insomnia complaints [90]. After 8 weeks of sleep restriction treatment, insomnia patients have reported an increase in total sleep time and improvement in sleep latency, total wake time, sleep efficiency, and subjective assessment of their insomnia [88]. Use of adjunctive pharmacologic intervention may be useful on a short-term basis, but its long-term use remains controversial [91,92].

Interestingly, despite consistent SD in this patient population, insomnia patients tend to complain less of sleepiness than of being "tired." This is demonstrated by the report that insomnia patients have a difficult time napping despite SD [93]. Although not well understood, this finding has been explained by the hyperarousal theory. This theory states that the basis of chronic insomnia stems from a generalized hyperarousal that these patients experience throughout the day and night. In support of this theory, neuroimaging studies of insomnia patients have shown an increase in brain metabolism as compared with controls representing increased cortical activation, leading to increased arousal states [94]. Furthermore, it has been found that MSLT sleep latencies are increased in insomniacs as compared with normal sleepers [93]. This fact tends to support the theory that insomnia is correlated with central nervous system hyperarousal that exists throughout the 24-hour day.

Insufficient sleep and voluntary sleep restriction

The evolution of human society has resulted in many significant changes in human behavior. One significant change in the culture is that nighttime activity has become a prominent part of society. Bedtimes occurring later in the night are normal for many people, and as a result these individuals may obtain an inadequate amount of sleep. Insufficient sleep syndrome can be defined by the lack of sufficient sleep to support normal alert wakefulness. This condition is the most common cause of EDS in the general population [95]. It may result from societal constraints, voluntary sleep restriction, shift work, or circadian rhythm disturbances. In addition to sleepiness, insufficient sleep may be associated with such symptoms as irritability, problems with concentration, or fatigue.

Studies have shown that despite subjectively adequate daytime sleep, shift workers lose an average of 5 to 7 hours of sleep per week as compared with their diurnal worker counterparts [96]. Additionally, studies have consistently shown that individuals who engage in consistent night shift work experience more disrupted sleep and sleepiness during waking hours as compared with day workers in the absence of shift work sleep disorder [97,98].

Circadian rhythm disorders

Circadian rhythm disorders are chronic conditions that occur when biologically governed sleep patterns are not aligned with environmental cues for sleep and wakefulness. As a result of these desynchronized phases, sleep time is often curtailed and resultant EDS occurs. These disorders are manifest when a patient cannot sleep at a suitable time or desires to sleep at an unsuitable time. There are a variety of different circadian rhythm disturbances, although the most common are the advanced sleep phase syndrome, which is characterized by propensity to fall asleep in the early evening with subsequent early awakening; the delayed sleep phase syndrome, characterized by inability to fall asleep at early times with subsequent inability to awake at an early time; jet lag, where an individual's internal

circadian rhythm is desynchronized with the external environment because of travel over several time zones; and shift work sleep disorder, where work demands the constant adjustment and readjustment of sleep and circadian patterns resulting in EDS during work hours and curtailed, fragmented sleep in off-hours.

Patients with circadian rhythm disturbances may effectively shift their biologic clock by the appropriate timing of bright light therapy (phototherapy). To shift the circadian phase, bright light may be applied either in the evening for advanced sleep phase syndrome, or in the morning, for delayed sleep phase syndrome, and the concomitant avoidance of bright light in the morning and the evening, respectively [99]. The use of properly timed melatonin administration also seems to have an impact on phase-shifting [100]. Both light and exogenous melatonin have been found to affect the desynchronized circadian phase seen in jet lag and shift work. Melatonin treatment, when timed appropriately, has been shown to improve sleep, and in some cases hasten adaptation to the new phase [101]. Regardless of this intervention, however, the individual adjusts to the destination time zone, on average within 1 hour per day with eastward travel and 30 minutes per day with westward travel [102].

Regular, fixed wake times with fixed daytime and nighttime routines helps to reinforce the phase shift. The severity of difficulty in initiating or maintaining sleep is variable between subjects, as are other symptoms, such as excessive sleepiness, decrements in subjective daytime alertness, and performance. Circadian disorders can be associated with some somatic symptoms, and there seems to be an individual susceptibility component regarding clinical severity of the symptomatology of these disorders.

Sleep fragmentation caused by sleep disorders

There are several disorders that may lead to fragmented, interrupted sleep. Fragmented sleep, usually in the form of microfragmentation, is described as an electroencephalogram recording that demonstrates cortical microarousals. These microarousals may originate from a breathing disturbance (OSAS, central sleep apnea, mixed sleep apnea, upper airway resistance syndrome [or snoring]), or from abnormal movements during sleep, most commonly in the form of periodic limb movements of sleep (PLMS). Frequently, the patient is unaware of these problems, but at times may lead to frank awakenings. Microarousal activity has been demonstrated to produce sleepiness or daytime performance deficits when induced by various sensory stimuli in normal subjects and has been postulated to disrupt the normal restorative processes of sleep. Subsequently, it can be concluded that clinically, sleep fragmentation is a correlate of SD [103,104].

Sleep fragmentation does not always lead to frank EDS; this is most evident in children. Although children with sleep-related breathing disorder (SRBD) are generally sleepier than children without fragmented sleep [105,106], and the degree of sleepiness in these children tends to increase with severity of SRBD [107], children with SRBD more often tend to display externalizing hyperactive-type behaviors as opposed to EDS [108,109]. In addition, recent evidence strongly suggests that children with primary snoring, in the absence of clinically defined obstructive sleep apnea, have demonstrated neurobehavioral deficits as compared with children who do not snore, seemingly because of increased susceptibility to sleep fragmentation [110]. Behavioral problems, such as attention-deficit hyperactivity disorder associated with sleep fragmentation, have also been described in children with PLMS. A significant portion of children diagnosed with attention-deficit hyperactivity disorder have been found to have PLMS, and conversely a substantial number of children with PLMS were also found to have attention-deficit hyperactivity disorder [111,112].

The prevalence of sleep-disordered breathing in North America is extremely high, with an estimated 20% of adults with mild to asymptomatic disease and at least 5% of adults with significant disease [113]. In children, primary snoring has been found to have prevalence between 10% and 25% between the ages of 3 and 12 years [114,115], whereas the OSAS has been found to have prevalence between 1% and 3% in the general pediatric population [116].

The OSAS is a condition where repetitive obstructive respiratory events occur during sleep because of upper airway obstruction, with subsequent microarousals occurring at the termination of a respiratory event [117,118]. OSAS has been found to disrupt the normal pattern and distribution of sleep stage activity, known as "sleep architecture." These alterations have been described as reductions in slow wave sleep (stages 3 and 4) and REM sleep percentages, with corresponding increases in lighter sleep (stages 1 and 2). Interestingly, sleep-related electroencephalogram alterations do not consistently correlate with measures of sleepiness severity [119]. Additionally, it has been demonstrated that patient's with OSAS complain more often of fatigue and "lack of energy" than of frank sleepiness [120].

In addition to OSAS, two other types of SRBD subtypes have been described: central sleep apnea

and mixed sleep apnea [121]. Central sleep apnea occurs when the drive to breathe during sleep is intermittently absent, whereas mixed sleep apnea begins as a central event but transitions to an obstructive event as respiratory effort begins in the midst of airflow cessation. Although central apnea seems to be a unique physiologic event, mixed apnea seems to be essentially obstructive events where respiratory effort is undetected at the beginning of the apnea. Although both types of apnea are associated with EDS because of frequent arousals and fragmented sleep, patients with pure central sleep apnea less commonly complain of this problem as compared with OSAS [122,123]. Central sleep apnea may be seen in infants with immature central respiratory control system, whereas in adults it may occur with cerebrovascular or neuromuscular disease, hypoventilation syndromes, or in association with the Cheyne-Stokes breathing. It is notably present in patients with low cardiac output heart failure [124].

Upper airway resistance syndrome is a condition that exists within the SRBD spectrum of diseases, where there is increased effort in breathing during periods of increased upper airway resistance, without the presence of frank hypopnea or apnea [125]. Like OSAS, these patients have frequent microarousals associated with increased respiratory effort and may have resultant EDS. Snoring is the first symptom often reported by patients later diagnosed with OSAS or upper airway resistance syndrome. Snoring does imply an increased resistance of the upper airway during sleep, although data are mixed regarding the true consequences of snoring with regard to EDS.

PLMS are described as repetitive flexions of the toes, feet, legs, thighs, or the arms during sleep, lasting 0.5 to 5 seconds in duration, with four or more movements in sequence, separated by an interval of more than 5 seconds than and less than 90 seconds [126]. Cortical microarousals may be associated with these events. Cross-sectional studies have shown a prevalence of PLMS 3.9% to 5% in the adult population [127] and about 1.2% in children [128], in the absence of other sleep disorders. The data are not entirely clear about the impact of PLMS on sleep disturbance and subsequent daytime functioning in adults. When PLMS occur at rates of five or more per hour of sleep, there seems to be a correlation with EDS and periodic limb movement disorder may be diagnosed [129]. Several studies have shown conflicting evidence about this correlation. These studies have shown no consistent correlation between the number of PLMS-arousal complexes per hour of sleep and EDS, as measured by MSLT [130,131]. Clearly, the significance of PLMS and associated arousals remains poorly understood and thoughtful clinical correlation is required to understand the significance of each individual case.

Neurologic and medical disorders resulting in sleep loss

EDS is a common complaint in patients with disorders of the central or peripheral nervous systems. These complaints may be the result of a variety of influences; however, often it is caused by fragmented sleep. In some chronic neurologic diseases, EDS may be the predominate complaint rather than the primary neurologic dysfunction in question. In many toxic or metabolic encephalopathic processes, it may be the primary clinical feature. Structural brain lesions, including strokes, tumors, cysts, abscesses, hematomas, vascular malformations, hydrocephalus, and multiple sclerosis plaques, are known to produce EDS. The cause of the EDS in these patients is not always clear, but it seems that in many of these patients somnolence may result either from direct involvement of discrete brain regions or because of effects on sleep continuity (eg, nocturnal seizure activity or secondary SRBD).

Various neurodegenerative disorders and dementias, such as Parkinson's disease, Alzheimer's disease, and multiple system atrophy, have all been shown commonly to have sleep disruption and EDS [132–134]. Patients with neuromuscular disorders or peripheral neuropathies have an increased incidence of SRBD (OSAS or central sleep apnea); pain; and PLMS. Because of these coexisting disorders, these patients may develop EDS from disrupted sleep [135]. It has also been observed that patients with myotonic dystrophy often suffer from EDS, even in the absence of sleep-disordered breathing [136].

Chronic medical conditions are another source of significant sleep disturbance and may manifest clinically as either EDS or fatigue. Patients with fibromyalgia frequently characterize their sleep as being restless, light, and nonrefreshing [137]. These patients have a characteristic electroencephalogram finding during sleep described as alpha intrusion or "alpha-delta" sleep [138]. This unique electroencephalogram pattern is described as alpha-frequency waveforms, a characteristic rhythm of quiet wakefulness, which in this setting is seen to occur during slow wave or delta sleep. In addition to fibromyalgia, this electroencephalogram finding is frequently seen in rheumatoid arthritis and chronic fatigue syndrome [138–140]. Although studies have shown a positive correlation between the frequency of alpha-delta sleep and severity of overnight pain in fibromyalgia patients, studies have also demonstrated an inverse correlation between frequency of alpha-delta sleep and subjective sleep depth and refreshing sleep [141,142].

Heart failure is another chronic medical condition where patients have difficulty with sleep continuity. A recent study has shown that at least 21% of patients with congestive heart failure complained of EDS and 48% of patients complained of being awake more than 30 minutes during the course of the night [143]. Patients with severe congestive heart failure often have highly fragmented sleep, with frequent arousals and sleep changes [144]. Additionally, more than half of patients with heart failure suffer from SRBDs [145].

Endocrine disorders are another prominent chronic disease group where patients may complain of EDS. It has been long established that sleepiness is a distinct complaint in patients with hypothyroidism. Additionally, there are considerable data to show that hypothyroidism is a risk factor for the development of OSAS [146]. It has not been established whether the sleepiness that hypothyroid patients experience is caused by primary central effect of the hypothyroid state on sleep or if it is caused by coexisting SRBD. Patients with acromegaly have also been shown to have an increased prevalence of sleep apnea, with rates between to 39% and 58.8% in various studies [147,148]. Patients with growth hormone deficiency consistently report a reduced level of energy, fatigue, and impaired sleep quality [149].

Summary

SD has dramatic impact on daily function and quality of life. There are both animal and human studies of SD that have been conducted to understand better the physiologic impact of SD and the vital role of sleep. SD has been shown to have significant impact on neurocognitive functioning and psychomotor skills. There is a clear homeostatic, biologic drive for sleep as evidenced by compensatory sleep and sleep distribution observed with recovery sleep. SD and sleep disorders that cause either sleep curtailment or fragmented sleep may have a significant impact on society because of the resultant EDS. Much is known about the physiologic changes and consequences of SD, although it is clear that there is still much to learn about this interesting area of human behavior.

References

[1] Lyznicki JM, Doege TC, Davis RM, et al. Sleepiness, driving, and motor vehicle crashes. JAMA 1998;279:1908–13.
[2] Kushida C. Sleep deprivation: basic science, physi-

ology, and behavior. Lung Biology in Health and Disease 2005;192:1–46.

[3] Kushida C. Sleep deprivation: clinical issues, pharmacology, and sleep loss effects. Lung Biology in Health and Disease 2005;193:195–385.

[4] Farooqui SM, Brock JW, Zhou J. Changes in monoamines and their metabolite concentrations in REM sleep-deprived rat forebrain nuclei. Pharmacol Biochem Behav 1996;54:385–91.

[5] Frussa-Filho R, Gonçalves MTM, Andersen ML, et al. Paradoxical sleep deprivation potentiates amphetamine-induced behavioural sensitization by increasing its conditioned component. Brain Res 2004;1003:188–93.

[6] Andersen ML, Perry JC, Tufik S. Acute cocaine effects in paradoxical sleep deprived male rats. Prog Neuropsychopharmacol Biol Psychiatry 2005;29:245–51.

[7] Jouvet D, Vilmont P, Delorme F, et al. Etude de la privation sélective de la phase paradoxale de sommeil chez le chat. Compt Rend Soc Biol 1964;158:756–9.

[8] Cohen HB, Dement WC. Sleep: changes in threshold to electroconvulsive shock in rats after deprivation of paradoxical phase. Science 1965;150:1318–9.

[9] Van Hulzen ZJM, Coenen AML. Paradoxical sleep deprivation and locomotor activity in rats. Physiol Behav 1981;27:741–4.

[10] Nunes GP, Tufik S. Validation of the modified multiple platform method (MMP) of paradoxical sleep deprivation in rats. Sleep Res 1994; 22:419.

[11] Tufik S, Lindsey CJ, Carlini EA. Does REM sleep deprivation induce a supersensitivity of dopaminergic receptors in the rat brain? Pharmacology 1978;16:95–108.

[12] Nunes GP, Tufik S, Nobrega JN. Autoradiographic analysis of D1 and D2 dopaminergic receptors in rat brain after paradoxical sleep deprivation. Brain Res Bull 1994;34:435–56.

[13] Easton A, Meerlo P, Bergmann B, et al. The suprachiasmatic nucleus regulates sleep timing and amount in mice. Sleep 2004;27:1307–18.

[14] Ledoux L, Sastre JP, Buda C, et al. Alterations in c-fos expression after different experimental procedures of sleep deprivation in the cat. Brain Res 1996;735:108–18.

[15] Cirelli C. How sleep deprivation affects gene expression in the brain: a review of recent findings. J Appl Physiol 2002;92:394–400.

[16] Naidoo N, Giang W, Galante RJ, et al. Sleep deprivation induces the unfolded protein response in mouse cerebral cortex. J Neurochem 2005;92:1150–7.

[17] Andersen ML, Martins PJF, D'Almeida V, et al. Endocrinological alterations during sleep deprivation and recovery in male rats. J Sleep Res 2005;14:83–90.

[18] Cauter EV. Sleep loss, jet lag, and shift work. In: Fink G, editor. Encyclopedia of stress, vol. 1. San Diego: Academic Press; 2000. p. 447–8.

[19] Meerlo P, Koehl M, van der Borght K, et al. Sleep restriction alters the hypothalamic-pituitary-adrenal response to stress. J Neuroendocrinol 2002;14:397–402.

[20] Rechtschaffen A, Bergmann BM, Everson CA. Sleep deprivation in the rat: III. Total sleep deprivation. Sleep 1989;12:1–4.

[21] Everson CA, Laatsch CD, Hogg N. Antioxidant defense responses to sleep loss and sleep recovery. Am J Physiol Regul Integr Comp Physiol 2005;288:R374–83.

[22] Inoue S, Honda K, Komoda Y. Sleep as neuronal detoxification and restitution. Behav Brain Res 1995;69:91–6.

[23] Benedetti F, Serretti A, Colombo C, et al. Dopamine receptor D2 and D3 gene variants are not associated with the antidepressant effect of total sleep deprivation in bipolar depression. Psychol Res 2003;118:241–7.

[24] Ebert D, Albert R, Hammon G, et al. Eye blink rate and depression. Is the antidepressant effect of sleep deprivation mediated by the dopamine system? Neuropsychopharmacol 1996;15: 332–9.

[25] Andersen ML, Bignotto M, Tufik S. Influence of paradoxical sleep deprivation and cocaine on development of spontaneous penile reflexes in rats of different ages. Brain Res 2003;968:130–8.

[26] Andersen ML, Bignotto M, Tufik S. Hormone treatment facilitates penile erection in castrated rats after sleep deprivation and cocaine. J Neuroendocrinol 2004;16:154–9.

[27] Harrison Y, Horne JA. Sleep loss impairs short and novel language tasks having a prefrontal focus. J Sleep Res 1998;7:95–100.

[28] Mu G, Nahas Z, Johnson KA, et al. Decreased cortical response to verbal working memory following sleep deprivation. Sleep 2005;28:55–67.

[29] Vgontzas AN, Zoumakis E, Bixler EO, et al. Adverse effects of modest sleep restriction on sleepiness, performance, and inflammatory cytokines. J Clin Endocrinol Metab 2004;89: 2119–26.

[30] De Valck E, Cluydts R, Pirrera S. Effect of cognitive arousal on sleep latency, somatic and cortical arousal following partial sleep deprivation. J Sleep Res 2004;13:295–304.

[31] Walker MP, Stickgold R. Sleep-dependent learning and memory consolidation. Neuron 2004; 44:121–33.

[32] Romcy-Pereira R, Pavlides C. Distinct modulatory effects of sleep on the maintenance of hippocampal and medial prefrontal cortex LTP. Eur J Neurosci 2004;20:3453–62.

[33] Bueno OFA, Lobo LL, Oliveira MGM, et al. Dissociated paradoxical sleep deprivation effects on inhibitory avoidance and conditioned fear. Physiol Behav 1994;56:775–9.

[34] Silva RH, Abílio VC, Takatsu AL, et al. Role of hippocampal oxidative stress in memory deficits induced by sleep deprivation in mice. Neuropharmacology 2004;46:895–903.

[35] Bonnet MH, Arand DL. Clinical effects of sleep

fragmentation versus sleep deprivation. Sleep Med Rev 2003;7:293–5.

[36] Persson HE, Svanborg E. Sleep deprivation worsens obstructive sleep apnea: comparison between diurnal and nocturnal polysomnography. Chest 1996;109:645–50.

[37] Santos HER, De Mello MT, Pradella-Hallinan M, et al. Sep and sleepiness among Brazilian shift-work bus drivers. Chronobiol Int 2004;21:881–8.

[38] Vorona RD, Winn MP, Babineau TW, et al. Overweight and obese patients in a primary care population report less sleep than patients with a normal body mass index. Arch Intern Med 2005;165:15–6.

[39] Everson CA, Bergmann BM, Rechtschaffen A. Sleep deprivation in the rat: II. Total sleep deprivation. Sleep 1989;12:13–21.

[40] Spiegel K, Tasali E, Penev P, et al. Brief communication: sep curtailment in health young men is associated with decreased leptin levels, elevated ghrelin levels, and increased hunger and appetite. Ann Intern Med 2004;7:141–52.

[41] Irwin M. Effects of sleep and sleep loss on immunity and cytokines. Behav Brain Immun 2002;16:503–12.

[42] Meier-Ewert HK, Ridker PM, Rifai N, et al. Effect of sleep loss on C-reactive protein, an inflammatory marker of cardiovascular risk. J Am Coll Cardiol 2004;44:1529–30.

[43] Beersma DG. Models of human sleep regulation. Sleep Med Rev 1998;2:31–43.

[44] Rosenthal L, Roehrs TA, Rosen A, et al. Level of sleepiness and total sleep time following various time in bed conditions. Sleep 1993;16:226–32.

[45] Carskadon MA, Dement WC. Cumulative effects of sleep restriction on daytime sleepiness. Psychophysiology 1981;18:107–13.

[46] Chugh DK, Weaver TE, Dinges DF. Neurobehavioral consequences of arousals. Sleep 1996;19:S198–201.

[47] Philip P, Stoohs R, Guilleminault C. Sleep fragmentation in normals. Sleep 1994;17:242–7.

[48] Carskadon MA, Dement WC. Effects of total sleep loss on sleep tendency. Percept Mot Skills 1979;48:495–506.

[49] Chervin RD, Kraemer HC, Guilleminault C. Correlates of sleep latency on the multiple sleep latency test in a clinical population. Electroencephalogr Clin Neurophysiol 1995;95:147–53.

[50] Richardson GS, Carskadon MA, Flagg W, et al. Excessive daytime sleepiness in man: multiple sleep latency measurement in narcoleptic and control subjects. Electroencephalogr Clin Neurophysiol 1978;45:621–7.

[51] Amira SA, Johnson TS, Logowitz NB. Diagnosis of narcolepsy using the multiple sleep latency test: analysis of current laboratory criteria. Sleep 1985;8:325–31.

[52] Aldrich MS, Chervin RD, Malow BA. Value of the multiple sleep latency test (MSLT) for the diagnosis of narcolepsy. Sleep 1997;20:620–9.

[53] Carskadon MA, Dement WC. Sleep loss in elderly volunteers. Sleep 1985;83:207–21.

[54] Van den Hoed J, Kraemer H, Guilleminault C, et al. Disorders of excessive daytime somnolence: polygraphic and clinical data for 100 patients. Sleep 1981;4:23–7.

[55] Mitler MM, Gujavarty KS, Browman CP. Maintenance of wakefulness test: a polysomnographic technique for evaluation treatment efficacy in patients with excessive somnolence. Electroencephalogr Clin Neurophysiol 1982;53:658–61.

[56] Mitler MM. Maintenance of Wakefulness Test (MWT). In: Kushida CA, editor. Sleep deprivation: Clinical issues, pharmacology and sleep loss effects. Lung Biology in Health and Disease 2005;193:325–8.

[57] US Modafinil in Narcolepsy Multicenter Study Group. Randomized trial of modafinil for the treatment of pathological somnolence in narcolepsy. Ann Neurol 1998;43:88–97.

[58] Sangal RB, Thomas L, Mitler MM. Disorders of excessive sleepiness: treatment improves ability to stay awake but does not reduce sleepiness. Chest 1992;102:699–703.

[59] Sangal RB, Thomas L, Mitler MM. Maintenance of wakefulness test and multiple sleep latency test: measurement of different abilities in patients with sleep disorders [see comments]. Chest 1992;101:898–902.

[60] Dinges DF, Pack F, Williams K, et al. Cumulative sleepiness, mood disturbance, and psychomotor vigilance performance decrements during a week of sleep restricted to 4–5 hours per night. Sleep 1997;20:267–77.

[61] Jewett ME, Dijk DJ, Kronauer RE, et al. Dose-response relationship between sleep duration and human psychomotor vigilance and subjective alertness. Sleep 1999;22:171–9.

[62] Kribbs NB, Dinges DF. Vigilance decrement and sleepiness. In: Harsh JR, Ogilvie RD, editors. Sleep onset mechanisms. Washington: American Psychological Association; 1994. p. 113–25.

[63] Van Dongen HPA, Dinges DF. Circadian rhythms in fatigue, alertness and performance. In: Kryger MH, Roth T, Dement WC, editors. Principles and practice of sleep medicine. Philadelphia: WB Saunders; 2000. p. 391–9.

[64] Dinges DF, Weaver T. Effects of modafinil on sustained attention performance and quality of life in OSA patients with residual sleepiness while being treated with nCPAP. Sleep Med 2003;4:393–402.

[65] Seidel WF, Balls S, Cohen S, et al. Daytime alertness in relation to mood, performance and nocturnal sleep in chronic insomniacs and non-complaining sleepers. Sleep 1984;7:230–8.

[66] Pressman MR, Fry JM. Relationship of autonomic nervous system activity to daytime sleepiness and prior sleep. Sleep 1989;12:239–45.

[67] Hoch CC, Reynolds CF, Jennings R, et al. Daytime sleepiness and performance among

healthy 80 and 20 year olds. Neurobiol Aging 1991;13:353–6.

[68] Harnish MJ, Chard SR, Orr WC. Relationship between measures of objective and subjective sleepiness. Sleep Res 1996;25:492.

[69] Hoddes E, Dement WC, Zarcone V. The development and use of the Stanford Sleepiness Scale (SSS). Psychophysiology 1972;1:150–7.

[70] Herscovitch J, Broughton R. Sensitivity of the Stanford Sleepiness Scale to the effects of cumulative sleep deprivation and recovery oversleeping. Sleep 1981;4:83–92.

[71] Johns MW. A new method of sleepiness: the Epworth sleepiness scale. Sleep 1991;14:540–5.

[72] Sangal RB, Sangal JM, Belisle C. MWT and ESS measure different abilities in 41 patients with snoring and daytime sleepiness. Sleep Res 1997; 26:493.

[73] Chervin R, Aldrich MS, Pickett R, et al. Comparison of the results of Epworth Sleepiness Scale and multiple sleep latency test. J Psychosom Res 1997;42:145–55.

[74] Rosenthal L, Roehr TA, Roth T. The sleep-wake activity inventory: a self-report measure of daytime sleepiness. Biol Psychiatry 1993;34:810–20.

[75] Sleep in America poll. National Sleep Foundation; 2005. Available at: http://www.sleepfoundition.org/_content/hottopics/2005_summary_of_findings.pdf. Accessed January 12, 2006.

[76] Engleman HM, Kingshott RN, Martin SE, et al. Cognitive function in the sleep apnea/hypopnea syndrome (SAHS). Sleep 2000; 23(Suppl 4):S102–8.

[77] Spielman A, Caruso L, Glovinsk P. A behavioral perspective on insomnia treatment. Psychiatry Clin North Am 1987;10:541–53.

[78] American Academy of Sleep Medicine. The international classification of sleep disorders. 2nd edition. Diagnostic and coding manual. Westchester (IL): American Academy of Sleep Medicine; 2005.

[79] Vgontzas AN, Bixler EO, Kales A, et al. Validity and clinical utility of sleep laboratory criteria for insomnia. Int J Neurosci 1994;77:11–21.

[80] Bonnet MH, Arand DL. Clinical effects of sleep fragmentation versus sleep deprivation. Sleep Med Rev 2003;7:297–310.

[81] Guilleminault C, Stoohs R, Clerk A, et al. A cause of excessive daytime sleepiness: the upper airway resistance syndrome. Chest 1993;104: 781–7.

[82] Guilleminault C, Black JE, Palombini L, et al. A clinical investigation of obstructive sleep apnea syndrome (OSAS) and upper airway resistance syndrome (UARS) patients. Sleep Med 2000;1: 51–6.

[83] Halasz P, Terzano M, Parrino L, et al. The nature of arousal in sleep. J Sleep Res 2004;13:1–23.

[84] Czeisler CA, Richardson GS. Detection and assessment of insomnia. Clin Ther 1991;13:663–79.

[85] Kales A, Kales JD. Evaluation and treatment of insomnia. New York: Oxford University Press; 1984.

[86] Ford DE, Kamerow DB. Epidemiologic study of sleep disturbances and psychiatric disorders. JAMA 1989;262:1479–84.

[87] Postolache TT, Oren DA. Circadian phase shifting, alerting, and antidepressant effects of bright light treatment. Clin Sports Med 2005; 24:381–413.

[88] Borbely AA. A two process model of sleep regulation. Hum Neurobiol 1982;1:195–204.

[89] Morin CM, Hauri PJ, Espie CA, et al. Non-pharmacologic treatment of chronic insomnia. Sleep 1999;22:1134–56.

[90] Spielman AJ, Yang CM, Glovinsky PB. Assessment techniques for insomnia. In: Kriger MK, Ruth T, Dement WC, editors. Principles and practice of sleep medicine. 3rd edition. Philadelphia: WB Saunders; 2000. p. 1239–50.

[91] National Institutes of Health. Drugs and insomnia: the use of medication to promote sleep. JAMA 1984;18:2410–4.

[92] National Institutes of Health. Consensus development conference statement: the treatment of sleep disorders of older people. Sleep 1991;14: 169–77.

[93] Bonnet MH, Arand DL. The consequences of a week of insomnia. Sleep 1996;19:453–61.

[94] Nofzinger EA, Buysse DJ, Germain A, et al. Functional neuroimaging evidence for hyperarousal in insomnia. Am J Psychiatry 2004;161: 2126–8.

[95] Spiegel K, Tasali E, Penev P, et al. Brief communication: sleep curtailment in healthy young men is associated with decreased leptin levels, elevated ghrelin levels, and increased hunger and appetite. Ann Intern Med 2004; 141:846–50.

[96] Monk TH. Shift work. In: Kryger MH, Roth T, Dement WC, editors. Principles and practices of sleep medicine. 3rd edition. Philadelphia: WB Saunders; 2000. p. 602–3.

[97] Akerstedt T. Sleepiness as a consequence of shift work. Sleep 1988;11:17–34.

[98] Budnick LD, Lerman SE, Baker TL, et al. Sleep and alertness in a 12-hour rotating shift work environment. J Occup Med 1994;36: 1295–300.

[99] Chesson Jr AL, Littner M, Davila D, et al. Practice parameters for the use of light therapy in the treatment of sleep disorders. Standards of Practice Committee, American Academy of Sleep Medicine. Sleep 1999;22:641–60.

[100] Skene DJ. Optimization of light and melatonin to phase-shift human circadian rhythms. J Neuroendocrinol 2003;15:438–41.

[101] Arendt J, Skene DJ, Middleton B, et al. Efficacy of melatonin treatment in jet lag, shift work, and blindness. J Biol Rhythms 1997;12: 604–17.

[102] Waterhouse J, Reilly T, Edwards B. The stress of travel. J Sports Sci 2004;22:946–65.

[103] Philip P, Stoohs R, Guilleminault C. Sleep fragmentation in normals. Sleep 1994;17:242–7.

[104] Chugh DK, Weaver TE, Dinges DF. Neurobehavioral consequences of arousals. Sleep 1996;19:S198–201.

[105] Melendres CS, Lutz JM, Rubin ED, et al. Daytime sleepiness and hyperactivity in children with suspected sleep-disordered breathing. Pediatrics 2004;114:768–75.

[106] Golan N, Shahar E, Ravid S, et al. Sleep disorders and daytime sleepiness in children with attention-deficit/hyperactive disorder. Sleep 2004;27:261–6.

[107] Gozal D, Wang M, Pope DW. Objective sleepiness measure in pediatric obstructive sleep apnea. Pediatrics 2001;108:693–7.

[108] Rosen CL, Storfer-Isser A, Taylor HG, et al. Increased behavioral morbidity in school-aged children with sleep-disordered breathing. Pediatrics 2004;114:1640–8.

[109] Chervin RD, Archbold KH, Dillon JE, et al. Inattention, hyperactivity, and symptoms of sleep-disordered breathing. Pediatrics 2002;109:449–56.

[110] O'Brien LM, Mervis CB, Holbrook CR, et al. Neurobehavioral implications of habitual snoring in children. Pediatrics 2004;114:44–9.

[111] Picchietti DL, England SJ, Walters AS, et al. Periodic limb movements disorder and restless legs syndrome in children with attention-deficit hyperactivity disorder. J Child Neurol 1998;13:588–94.

[112] Picchietti DL, Walters AS. Moderate to severe periodic limb movements disorder in childhood and adolescence. Sleep 1999;22:297–300.

[113] Young T, Peppard PE, Gottlieb DJ. Epidemiology of obstructive sleep apnea: a population health perspective. Am J Respir Crit Care Med 2002;165:1217–39.

[114] Ali NJ, Pitson DJ, Stradling JR. Snoring, sleep disturbance, and behaviour in 4–5 year olds. Arch Dis Child 1993;68:360–6.

[115] Castronovo V, Zucconi M, Nosetti L, et al. Prevalence of habitual snoring and sleep-disordered breathing in preschool-aged children in an Italian community. J Pediatr 2003;142:377–82.

[116] Redline S, Tishler PV, Schluchter M, et al. Risk factors for sleep-disordered breathing in children: associations with obesity, race, and respiratory problems. Am J Respir Crit Care Med 1999;159:1527–32.

[117] Guilleminault C, Tilkian A, Dement WC. The sleep apnea syndromes. Annu Rev Med 1976;27:465–84.

[118] Bassiri AG, Guilleminault C. Clinical features of evaluation of obstructive sleep apnea-hypopnea syndrome. In: Kryger MH, Roth T, Dement WC, editors. Principles and practices of sleep medicine. 3rd edition. Philadelphia: WB Saunders; 2000. p. 868–78.

[119] Guilleminault C, Do Kim Y, Chowdhuri S, et al. Sleep and daytime sleepiness in upper airway resistance syndrome compared to obstructive sleep apnoea syndrome. Eur Respir J 2001;17:838–47.

[120] Chervin RD. Sleepiness, fatigue, tiredness, and lack of energy in obstructive sleep apnea. Chest 2000;118:372–9.

[121] Gastaut H, Tassinari CA, Duron B. Polygraphic study of the episodic diurnal and nocturnal (hypnic and respiratory) manifestations of the Pickwick syndrome. Brain Res 1966;1:167–86.

[122] Guilleminault C, van den Hoed J, Mitler M. Clinical overview of the sleep apnea syndromes. In: Guillemininault C, Dement W, editors. Sleep apnea syndromes. New York: Alan R Liss; 1978. p. 1–11.

[123] Bradley TD, McNicholas WT, Rutherford R, et al. Clinical physiological heterogeneity of the central sleep apnea syndrome. Am Rev Respir Crit Care Med 1986;134:217–21.

[124] Findley LJ, Zwillich CW, Ancoli-Israel S, et al. Cheyne-Stokes breathing during sleep in patients with left ventricular heart failure. South Med J 1985;78:11–5.

[125] Chesson AL, Wise M, Davila D, et al. Practice parameters for the treatment of restless legs syndrome and periodic limb movement disorder. Sleep 1999;22:961–8.

[126] American Academy of Sleep Medicine. Sleep related movement disorders. In: The international classification of sleep disorders. Diagnostic and coding manual. 2nd edition. Westchester (IL): American Academy of Sleep Medicine; 2005.

[127] Ohayon MM, Roth T. Prevalence of restless legs syndrome and periodic limb movement disorder in the general population. J Psychosom Res 2002;53:547–54.

[128] Kirk VG, Bohn S. Periodic limb movements in children: prevalence in a referred population. Sleep 2004;27:313–5.

[129] American Sleep Disorders Association. International classification of sleep disorders, revised: diagnostic and coding manual. Rochester (MN): American Sleep Disorders Association; 1997.

[130] Mendelson WB. Are periodic leg movements associated with clinical sleep disturbance? Sleep 1996;19:219–23.

[131] Chervin RD. Periodic limb movements and sleepiness in patients evaluated for sleep-disordered breathing. Am J Respir Crit Care Med 2001;164:1454–8.

[132] Askenasy JJM. Sleep in Parkinson's disease. Acta Neurol Scand 1993;87:167–70.

[133] Chokroverty S. Sleep and degenerative neurologic disorders. Neurol Clin 1996;14:807–26.

[134] Trenkwalder C. Sleep dysfunction in Parkinson's disease. Clin Neurosci 1998;5:107–14.

[135] George CFP. Neuromuscular disorders. In: Kryger MH, Roth T, Dement WC, editors. Principles and practice of sleep medicine. 3rd edition. Philadelphia: WB Saunders; 2000. p. 1087–92.

[136] Gibbs JW, Ciafaloni E, Radtke RA. Excessive daytime somnolence and increased rapid eye

movement pressure in myotonic dystrophy. Sleep 2002;25:662–5.

[137] Campbell SM, Clark S, Tindall EA, et al. Clinical characteristics of fibrositis. I: A blinded controlled study of symptoms and tender points. Arthritis Rheum 1983;26:817–25.

[138] Hyyppa MT, Kronhom E. Nocturnal motor activity in fibromyalgia patients with poor sleep quality. J Psychosom Res 1995;39:85–91.

[139] Modolfsky H, Saskin P, Lue FA. Sleep and symptoms in fiborsitis syndrome after a febrile illness. J Rheumatol 1988;15:1701–4.

[140] Moldolfsky H, Lue FA, Smythe H. Alpha EEG sleep and morning symptoms of rheumatoid arthritis. J Rheumatol 1983;10:373–9.

[141] Perlis ML, Giles DE, Bootzin RR, et al. Alpha sleep and information processing, perception of sleep, pain, and arousability in fibromyalgia. Int J Neurosci 1997;89:265–80.

[142] Moldolfsky H, Lue FA. The relationship of alpha delta EEG frequencies to pain and mood in "fibrositis" patients with chlorpromazine and L-tryptophan. Electroencephalogr Clin Neurophysiol 1980;50:71–80.

[143] Brostrom A, Stromber A, Dahlsrom U, et al. Sleep difficulties, daytime sleepiness, and health-related quality of life in patients with chronic heart failure. J Cardiovasc Nurs 2004; 19:232–42.

[144] Yamashiro Y, Kryger MH. Sleep in heart failure. Sleep 1993;16:513–23.

[145] Javaheri S, Parker TJ, Liming JD, et al. Sleep apnea in 81 ambulatory male patients with stable heart failure: types and their prevalences, consequences, and presentations. Circulation 1998;97:2154–9.

[146] Resta O, Panacciulli N, Di Gioia G, et al. High prevalence of previously unknown subclinical hypothyroidism in obese patients referred to a sleep clinic for sleep disordered breathing. Nutr Metab Cardiovasc Dis 2004;14:248–53.

[147] Blanco Perez JJ, Blanco-Ramos MA, Zamarron Sanz C, et al. Acromegaly and sleep apnea. Arch Bronconeumol 2004;40:355–9.

[148] Rosenow F, Reuter S, Deuss U, et al. Sleep apnoea in treated acromegaly: relative frequency and predisposing factors. Clin Endocrinol 1996;45:563–9.

[149] Bjork S, Jonsson B, Westphal O, et al. Quality of life of adults with growth hormone deficiency: a controlled study. Acta Paediatr Scand Suppl 1998;356:55–9.

ELSEVIER
SAUNDERS

SLEEP
MEDICINE
CLINICS

Sleep Med Clin 1 (2006) 47–61

Narcolepsy

Seiji Nishino, MD, PhD

- Symptoms of narcolepsy
  Sleepiness or excessive daytime sleepiness
  Cataplexy
  Hypnagogic or hypnopompic
   hallucinations
  Sleep paralysis
- Narcolepsy evaluation
  Polysomnography, nocturnal and daytime
   sleep studies
  Cerebrospinal fluid hypocretin-1
   assessment
  HLA testing
- Idiopathic hypersomnia and other primary
  excessive daytime sleepiness
- Pathophysiology of narcolepsy

Pathophysiologic consideration of the
 symptoms of narcolepsy
HLA, immune system, and narcolepsy
Deficiency in hypocretin (orexin)
 transmission in canine and human
 narcolepsy
Symptomatic case of narcolepsy and
 excessive daytime sleepiness and the
 hypocretin system
Hypocretin-orexin system and sleep
 regulation
- Treatments of narcolepsy
- Future directions
- References

Narcolepsy is characterized by excessive daytime sleepiness (EDS), cataplexy, and other dissociated manifestations of rapid eye movement (REM) sleep (hypnagogic hallucinations and sleep paralysis). Narcolepsy is currently treated with amphetamine-like central nervous system stimulants (for EDS) and antidepressants (for cataplexy). Some other classes of compounds, such as modafinil (a nonamphetamine wake-promoting compound for EDS) and γ-hydroxybutyrate (a short-acting sedative for EDS and fragmented nighttime sleep and cataplexy), given at night are also used. The major pathophysiology of human narcolepsy has recently been revealed by the extended discoveries of narcolepsy genes in animal models: about 90% of human narcolepsy-cataplexy has been found to be hypocretin-orexin ligand deficient. This directly led to the development of new diagnostic tests (ie, cerebrospinal fluid [CSF] hypocretin measures). Hypocretin replacement is also likely to be a new therapeutic option for hypocretin-deficient narcolepsy, but this is still not available in humans. In this article the clinical, pharmacologic, and pathophysiologic aspects of narcolepsy and related disorders are discussed.

Symptoms of narcolepsy

Narcolepsy is a syndrome of unknown etiology (prevalence = 1 in 2000 [1,2]) characterized by EDS that is often profound. About 95% of narcoleptic cases are sporadic, but it also occurs in familial forms. Narcolepsy usually occurs in association with cataplexy and other symptoms, which commonly include hypnagogic or hypnopompic hallucinations, sleep paralysis, automatic behavior, and disrupted nocturnal sleep [Table 1] [3]. Symptoms most often begin between adolescence and young adulthood. Narcolepsy may also occur earlier in childhood, however, or not until the third or fourth decade of life. Quality-of-life studies suggest that

Sleep and Circadian Neurobiology Laboratory, Center for Narcolepsy, Stanford University School of Medicine, 1201 Welch Road, RM213, Palo Alto, CA 94304, USA
E-mail address: nishino@stanford.edu

1556-407X/06/$ – see front matter © 2006 Elsevier Inc. All rights reserved.   doi:10.1016/j.jsmc.2005.11.008
sleep.theclinics.com

Table 1: Clinical characteristics of narcolepsy-cataplexy, narcolepsy without cataplexy, and idiopathic hypersomnia

| | Daytime sleepiness | | Other symptoms | MSLT | | HLA DQB1*0602 positivity | Low CSF hypocretin levels (<110 pg/mL) |
	Duration awaken	Refreshed		Sleep latency	SOREMPS		
Narcolepsy-cataplexy	Short (<30 min)	(+)	Cataplexy REM sleep-related symptoms	<8 min[a]	≥2	>90%	85%–90% (>90% in HLA positive)
Narcolepsy without cataplexy	Short (<30 min)	(+)	Cataplexy (–) REM sleep-related symptoms	<8 min[a]	≥2	40%–50%	10%–20% (almost all HLA positive)
Idiopathic hypersomnia with long sleep time	Long (>30 min)	(–)	Cataplexy (–) Prolonged nighttime sleep (>10 h) Autonomic nervous dysfunction	<8 min[a]	≤1	No consistent results	Normal
Idiopathic hypersomnia without long sleep time	Varied	(–)	Cataplexy (–) No prolonged nighttime sleep (<10 h) Autonomic nervous dysfunction	<8 min[a]	≤1	No consistent results	Normal

Abbreviations: CSF, cerebrospinal fluid; MSLT, Multiple Sleep Latency Test; REM, rapid eye movement; SOREMPS, sleep-onset REM sleep periods.
[a] Less than 8 minutes (instead of 10 minutes) is considered for the 2nd revision of ICSD.

the impact of narcolepsy is equivalent to that of Parkinson's disease [4]. Although EDS is not specific for narcolepsy, and is seen in other primary and secondary EDS disorders (eg, sleep apnea syndrome), cataplexy is generally regarded as pathognomonic. Occurrence of cataplexy is tightly associated with loss of hypocretin neurotransmission [5], and it rarely occurs as an isolated symptom. Cataplexy occasionally occurs in conjunction with other neurologic conditions, such as Niemann-Pick type C disease, but the pathophysologic links in these neurologic conditions with the hypocretin abnormalities are not yet well established [6].

Sleepiness or excessive daytime sleepiness

Similar to other sleep disorders, the EDS of narcolepsy presents itself with an increased propensity to fall asleep, nod, or easily doze in relaxed or sedentary situations, or a need to exert extra effort to avoid sleeping in these situations [7]. Additionally, irresistible or overwhelming urges to sleep commonly occur from time to time during wakeful periods in the untreated patient with narcolepsy. These so-called "sleep attacks" are not instantaneous lapses into sleep, as is often thought by the general public, but represent the episodes of profound sleepiness experienced by those with marked sleep deprivation or other severe sleep disorders. In addition to frank sleepiness, the EDS of narcolepsy (as in other sleep disorders) can cause related symptoms, including poor memory, reduced concentration, and irritability. Narcoleptic subjects feel refreshed after a short nap, but this does not last long and they become sleepy again within a few hours [see Table 1]. Narcolepsy may consist of an inability to maintain wakefulness combined with the intrusion of REM sleep–associated phenomena (hallucinations, sleep paralysis, and possibly cataplexy) into wakefulness.

Cataplexy

Cataplexy is the partial or complete loss of bilateral muscle tone in response to a strong emotion [7]. Reduced muscle tone may be minimal, occur in a few muscle groups, and cause minimal symptoms (eg, bilateral ptosis, head drooping, slurred speech, or dropping things from the hand), or it may be so severe that total body paralysis occurs, resulting in complete collapse. Cataplectic events usually last from a few seconds to 2 or 3 minutes, but occasionally continue longer [8]. The patient is usually alert and oriented during the event despite the inability to respond. Positive emotions, such as laughter, more commonly trigger cataplexy than negative emotions. Any strong emotion, however, is a potential trigger [9]. Startling stimuli, stress,

physical fatigue, or sleepiness may also be important triggers or factors that exacerbate cataplexy.

In a broader classification, diagnosing narcolepsy does not require cataplexy if REM sleep abnormalities (ie, sleep-onset REM sleep periods during Multiple Sleep Latency Test [MSLT]) are objectively documented [see Table 1]. According to epidemiologic studies, cataplexy is found in 60% to 100% of patients with narcolepsy. This large range is caused by the fact that the definition of narcolepsy may vary among each study (and by use of different diagnostic criteria). The onset of cataplexy is most frequently simultaneous with or within a few months of the onset of EDS, but in some cases cataplexy may not develop until many years after the initial onset of EDS [8].

Hypnagogic or hypnopompic hallucinations

These phenomena may be visual, tactile, auditory, or multisensory events, usually brief but occasionally continuing for a few minutes, that occur at the transition from wakefulness to sleep (hypnagogic) or from sleep to wakefulness (hypnopompic) [7]. Hallucinations may contain elements of dream sleep and consciousness combined, and is often bizarre or disturbing to patients.

Sleep paralysis

Sleep paralysis is the inability to move, lasting from a few seconds to a few minutes, during the transition from sleep to wakefulness or from wakefulness to sleep [7]. Episodes of sleep paralysis may alarm patients, particularly those who experience the sensation of being unable to breathe. Although accessory respiratory muscles may not be active during these episodes, diaphragmatic activity continues and air exchange remains adequate.

Other commonly reported symptoms include automatic behavior; absent-minded behavior or speech that is often nonsensical, which the patient does not remember; and fragmented nocturnal sleep with frequent awakenings during the night. Hypnagogic hallucinations, sleep paralysis, and automatic behavior are not specific to narcolepsy and occur in other sleep disorders (and in healthy individuals); however, these symptoms are far more common and occur with much greater frequency in narcolepsy [7].

Narcolepsy evaluation

Polysomnography, nocturnal and daytime sleep studies

Nocturnal polysomnography is not essential in the diagnostic work-up when straightforward cataplexy accompanies EDS. It remains an important part of the evaluation process, however, primarily to exclude other conditions that occur in narcolepsy at a higher than normal rate (obstructive sleep apnea, periodic limb movement syndrome, and REM sleep behavior disorder) and could add to the sleepiness or nocturnal sleep disruption the patient may be experiencing [10]. Additionally, sleep-onset REM sleep periods during nocturnal polysomnography may be witnessed and is also supportive for the diagnosis.

Daytime nap studies (in the form of the MSLT) usually demonstrate substantially reduced sleep latency and sleep-onset REM sleep periods in patients with narcolepsy. Average MSLT sleep latencies for narcolepsy with cataplexy is approximately 2 to 3 minutes [11]; however, substantial variability across and within patients can be seen, and the mean sleep latency of less than 8 minutes during MSLT is used for 2nd revision of the International Classification of Sleep Disorders (ICSD) [see Table 1] [3]. Sleep-onset REM sleep periods are also not specific for narcolepsy, but the occurrence of two or more of these events during the MSLT, in the setting of objectively marked sleepiness and without any other explanation for their occurrence (eg, sleep deprivation, REM-suppressant medication rebound, altered sleep schedule, obstructive sleep apnea, or delayed sleep-phase syndrome) is suggestive of narcolepsy.

Cerebrospinal fluid hypocretin-1 assessment

Many (about 90% of narcolepsy-cataplexy subjects) patients with narcolepsy have very low or undetectable levels of hypocretin-1–orexin A in the CSF [5,12]. Such low levels of CSF hypocretin-1 are relatively specific for narcolepsy-cataplexy, but are also seen in a few other neurologic conditions, such as a subset of patients with Guillain-Barré syndrome and Ma2-positive paraneoplastic syndrome [13,14]. Because these conditions are clinically distinct from narcolepsy, low CSF hypocretin levels in these conditions do not confound their diagnostic values. When used to assess patients for narcolepsy, low CSF hypocretin-1 seems to be a more specific test than the MSLT [see Table 1]. Low CSF hypocretin-1 levels (less than 110 pg/mL) were also included for the 2nd revision of ICSD. Previously, no specific and sensitive diagnostic test for narcolepsy based on the pathophysiology of the disease was available, and the final diagnosis was often delayed for several years after the disease onset, which is typically during adolescence [15]. Many patients with narcolepsy and related EDS disorders are likely to obtain immediate benefit from this new specific diagnostic test.

HLA testing

A very strong but incomplete correlation exists between narcolepsy (with cataplexy) and the HLA subtype DQB1* 0602, yet this subtype is very common in the general population (approximately 20% in the combined United States population) and is neither specific nor sensitive for narcolepsy [2]. HLA testing is not useful in confirming or excluding the diagnosis of narcolepsy, and may lead a clinician to inappropriate diagnostic conclusions (see the pathophysiology of narcolepsy section later).

Idiopathic hypersomnia and other primary excessive daytime sleepiness

Less common forms of hypersomnia include the idiopathic and recurrent hypersomnia [16]. Idiopathic hypersomnia is marked by excessive nocturnal sleep of good quality and by EDS that is not as severe as in the narcoleptic patients (but not refreshing after naps) and that is not REM sleep–related [see Table 1]. The best characterized recurrent hypersomnia is the Kleine-Levin syndrome, a pervasive functional disorder of the hypothalamus characterized by hypersexuality, binge eating, and irritability associated with periods of EDS and sleep periods as long as 18 to 20 hours [17,18]. For details of clinical symptoms and treatments of these primary EDS, refer to the article by Black and coworkers [16].

Pathophysiology of narcolepsy

Pathophysiologic consideration of the symptoms of narcolepsy

The similarity between cataplexy and REM sleep atonia (the presence of frequent episodes of hypnagogic hallucinations and of sleep paralysis, and the propensity for narcoleptics to go directly from wakefulness into REM sleep [ie, sleep-onset REM sleep periods]) suggests that narcolepsy is primarily a "disease of REM sleep" [19]. This hypothesis may, however, be too simplistic and does not explain the presence of sleepiness during the day and the short latency to both non-REM and REM sleep during nocturnal and nap recordings. Another complementary hypothesis is that narcolepsy results from the disruption of the control mechanisms of both sleep and wakefulness, of the vigilance-state boundary problems [20]. According to this hypothesis, a cataplectic attack represents an intrusion of REM sleep atonia during wakefulness, whereas the hypnagogic hallucinations appear as dream-like imagery taking place in the waking state, especially at sleep onset in patients who frequently have sleep-onset REM sleep periods.

Cataplexy is associated with an inhibition of the monosynaptic H-reflex and the polysynaptic deep tendon reflexes [21]. In control subjects, it is only during REM sleep that the H-reflex is totally suppressed. This finding highlights the relationship between the inhibition of motor processes during REM sleep and the sudden atonia and areflexia seen during cataplexy. Studies in canine narcolepsy, however, suggest that the mechanisms for the induction of cataplexy are different from those for REM sleep [22]. Furthermore, an extended human study confirmed that cataplexy correlates much more highly to hypocretin-deficient narcolepsy (see later), in contrast to other REM sleep–related phenomena [5]. Cataplexy may be viewed as somewhat distinct from other REM-related symptoms and as a hypocretin-deficiency pathologic phenomenon. The fact that patients with other sleep disorders, such as sleep apnea, and even healthy controls can manifest sleep-onset REM sleep periods, hypnagogic hallucinations, and sleep paralysis when their sleep-wake patterns are sufficiently disturbed, yet these subjects never develop cataplexy, provides further support to the proposal that cataplexy may be unrelated to other REM-associated symptoms [23–26]. Although cataplexy and REM sleep atonia have great similarity and possibly share a common executive system, it is not necessary for the regulatory mechanism of both states to be identical. The mechanism of emotional triggering of cataplexy remains undetermined.

HLA, immune system, and narcolepsy

An abundant amount of research into the HLA association in narcolepsy has already been conducted, which has yielded important discoveries. The research, however, has yet to provide clinically meaningful information. This work is only very briefly addressed in this article. A remarkably high HLA association with narcolepsy was discovered in the early 1980s [27]. Since the time of this initial finding, a variety of research across multiple ethnic groups has corroborated the existence of this strong HLA association. The most specific marker of narcolepsy in a number of different ethnic groups studied to date is DQB1*0602 [2]. This association is seen in an average of approximately 90% of those with unequivocal cataplexy [28]. Importantly, this association is substantially lower (only approximately 40%) in individuals who have received the diagnosis of narcolepsy, but do have cataplexy [see Table 1].

The strong association between HLA type and narcolepsy with cataplexy raises the possibility that narcolepsy is an autoimmune disease [29].

Some earlier studies testing a variety of serologic tests in narcoleptics yielded higher levels of antistreptolysine 0 and anti-DNase antibodies in narcoleptics than in controls [30,31]. There is, however, no strong evidence of the inflammatory processes or immune abnormalities associated with narcolepsy [29], and studies have found no classical autoantibodies and no increase in oligoclonal CSF bands in narcoleptics [32]. Typical autoimmune pathologies (erythrocyte sedimentation rates, serum immunoglobulin levels, C-reactive protein levels, complement levels, and lymphocyte subset ratios) are apparently normal in narcoleptic patients [33]. Recent studies by Black and coworkers [34] examined the presence of many neuron-specific and organ-specific autoantibodies but no antibody was associated with narcolepsy patients (HLA DQB1*0602 positive and negative). Furthermore, the same authors tested for IgG reactive to preprohypocretin and its major cleavage products (including hypocretin-1 and -2) in serum or CSF in DQB1*0602-positive narcoleptic subjects with cataplexy, but found no evidence for IgG reactive to preprohypocretin or its cleavage products in narcoleptic subjects [35].

Deficiency in hypocretin (orexin) transmission in canine and human narcolepsy

Narcolepsy has been described in several animal species including dogs, and most recently in genetically engineered mice and rat models. Canine narcolepsy is a naturally occurring model, with both sporadic (17 breeds) and familial forms (Doberman, Labrador, and Dachshund). In Doberman pinschers and Labrador retrievers, the disease is transmitted as a recessive-autosomal trait with complete penetrance [36].

In 1999, using positional cloning and gene-targeting strategies, two groups independently revealed the pathogenesis of narcolepsy in animals. The lack of the hypothalamic neuropeptide hypocretin-orexin ligand (preprohypocretin-orexin gene knockout mice) [37] or mutations in one of the two hypocretin-orexin receptor genes (hypocretin receptor 2 [*hcrtr 2*] gene in autosomal-recessive canine narcolepsy) [38] was observed to result in narcolepsy. After extensive screening (especially in familial and early onset human narcolepsy), it was demonstrated that mutations in hypocretin-related genes are rare: only a single case with early onset (6 months of age) was found to be associated with a single point mutation in the preprohypocretin gene [39]. This result was, however, not surprising considering the fact that most human narcolepsy cases are sporadic. Even in rare familial cases of narcolepsy, it is unlikely that a high pene-

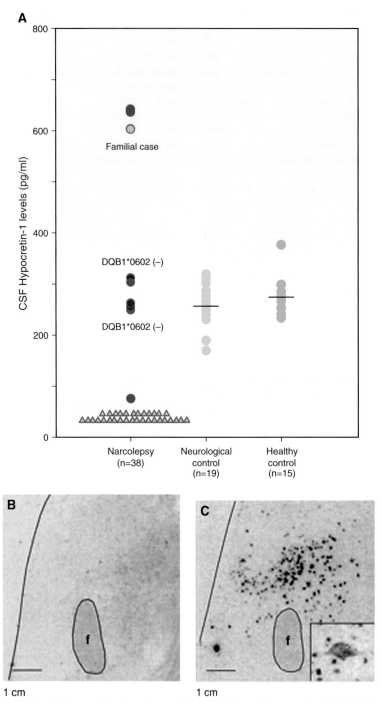

Fig. 1. CSF hypocretin-1 levels in narcoleptic and control subjects. Preprohypocretin mRNA in situ hybridization in the hypothalamus of control and narcoleptic subjects. (*A*) CSF hypocretin-1 levels are undetectably low in most narcoleptic subjects (84.2%). Note that two HLA DqB1*0602 negative and one familial cases have normal or high CSF hypocretin levels. Preprohypocretin transcripts are detected in the hypothalamus of control (*C*) but not narcoleptic subjects (*B*). Melanin concentrating hormone transcripts are detected in the same region in control and narcoleptic sections (data not shown). F, fornix.

trant single gene (like hypocretin-related genes) is involved.

Despite the lack of genetic abnormalities in the hypocretin system, it was found that most (85%–90%) patients with narcolepsy-cataplexy have low or undetectable hypocretin-1 ligand in their CSF [Fig. 1] [12,40]. This hypocretin deficiency is tightly associated with the occurrence of cataplexy and HLA DQ1*0602 positivity [5,41,42]. Post-mortem human studies (using a few brains) have confirmed hypocretin ligand deficiency (both hypocretin-1 and -2) in the narcoleptic brain [see Fig. 1] [39,43]. Hypocretin deficiency has also been observed in sporadic cases of canine narcolepsy (seven out of seven currently studied; the results of four cases are reported), suggesting that the pathophysiology in these animals mirrors that of most human cases [44].

It should also be noted that even when a very strict criteria for cataplexy is applied, about 10% of narcolepsy-cataplexy patients have normal CSF hypocretin-1 [5,40,41]. Whether or not hypocretin neurotransmission is abnormal in these rarer cases is unknown. Considering the fact that hypocretin production and hypocretin neurons seemed to be normal in hypocretin receptor 2–mutated narcoleptic Dobermans [44], it is possible that deficiencies in hypocretin receptors and a downstream pathway may exist in some of these patients. This cannot, however, be tested currently.

Although the cause of hypocretin deficiency in humans still needs to be determined, the fact that most human narcolepsy-cataplexy subjects are hypocretin ligand deficient suggests that hypocretin agonists may be promising in the treatment of narcolepsy (see pharmacology section later).

Symptomatic case of narcolepsy and excessive daytime sleepiness and the hypocretin system

The symptoms of narcolepsy can also occur during the course of other neurologic conditions (ie, symptomatic narcolepsy). A recent meta-analysis counted 116 symptomatic cases of narcolepsy reported in the literature (cases meet with the ICSD criteria for narcolepsy and are also associated with a significant underlying neurologic disorder that accounts for EDS and temporal associations) [6]. As several authors previously reported, inherited disorders (N = 38), tumors (N = 33), and head trauma (N = 19) are the three most frequent causes for symptomatic narcolepsy. Of the 116 cases, 10 are associated with multiple sclerosis, one case of acute disseminated encephalomyelitis, and relatively rare cases were reported with vascular disorders (N = 6), encephalitis (N = 4), and degeneration (N = 1), and heredodegenerative disorder (three cases in a family). EDS without cataplexy or any REM sleep ab-

normalities is also often associated with these neurologic conditions, and defined as symptomatic cases of EDS.

Although it is difficult to rule out the comorbidity of idiopathic narcolepsy in some cases, review of the literature reveals numerous unquestionable cases of symptomatic narcolepsy [6]. These include cases with HLA-negative or late onset, and cases in which the occurrences of the narcoleptic symptoms are parallel with the rise and fall of the causative disease. Interestingly, a review of these cases (especially those with brain tumors) illustrates a clear picture that the hypothalamus is most often involved [6].

CSF hypocretin-1 measurement was also performed in a limited number of symptomatic cases of narcolepsy and EDS [6]. Reduced CSF hypocretin-1 levels were seen in most symptomatic narcolepsy cases of EDS with various etiologies and EDS in these cases is sometimes reversible with an improvement of the causative neurologic disorder and an improvement of the hypocretin status. It is also noted that some symptomatic EDS cases (with Parkinson's disease and the thalamic infarction) appeared, but they are not linked with hypocretin ligand deficiency. In contrast to idiopathic narcolepsy cases, an occurrence of cataplexy is not tightly associated with hypocretin ligand deficiency in symptomatic cases.

Because CSF hypocretin measures are still experimental, cases with sleep abnormalities and cataplexy are habitually selected for CSF hypocretin measures. The fact that all or most cases with low CSF hypocretin-1 levels with central nervous system interventions exhibit EDS and cataplexy warrants further study.

Hypocretin-orexin system and sleep regulation

Hypocretins and orexins were only recently discovered (in 1998, 1 year before the cloning of the canine narcolepsy gene) by two independent research groups. One group called the peptides "hypocretin" because of their primary hypothalamic localization and similarities with the hormone secretin [45]. The other group called the molecules "orexin" after observing that central administration of these peptides increased appetite in rats [46]. Hypocretins-1 and -2 are produced exclusively by a well-defined group of neurons localized in the lateral hypothalamus. The neurons project to the olfactory bulb, cerebral cortex, thalamus, hypothalamus, and brainstem, particularly the locus coeruleus, raphe nucleus, and to the cholinergic nuclei (the laterodorsal tegmental and pedunculopontine tegmental nuclei) and cholinoceptive sites

A

human*/bovine/rat/mouse*
hypocretin-1 (Orexin A)

rat/mouse* hypocretin-2 (Orexin B)

human* hypocretin-2 (Orexin B)

<EPLPDCCRQKTCSCRLYELLHGAGNHAAGILTL–NH₂
RPGPPGLQGRLQRLLQANGNHAAGILTM–NH₂
RSGPPGLQGRLQRLLQASGNHAAGILTM–NH₂

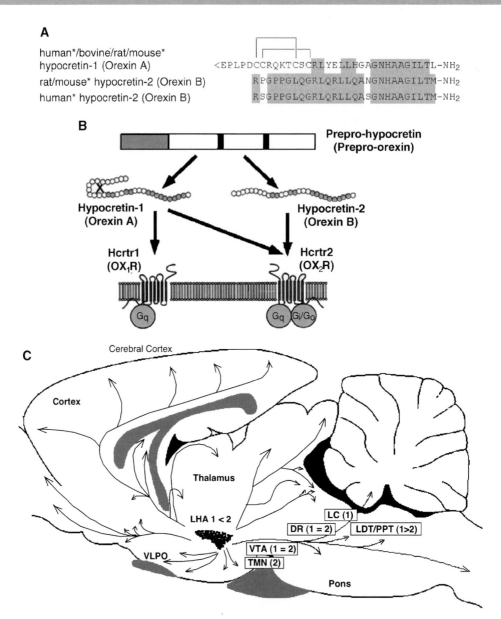

Fig. 2. (A) Structures of mature hypocretin-1 (orexin-A) and hypocretin-2 (orexin-B) peptides. (B) Schematic representation of the hypocretin (orexin) system. (C) Projections of hypocretin neurons in the rat brain and relative abundances of hypocretin receptor 1 and 2. (A) The topology of the two intrachain disulfide bonds in orexin-A is indicated in this sequence. Amino acid identities are indicated by shaded areas. Asterisks indicate that human and mouse sequences were deduced from the respective cDNA sequences and not from purified peptides. Hypocretin-1 (orexin-A) and hypocretin-2 (orexin-B) are derived from a common precursor peptide, prepro-hypocretin (prepro-orexin). (B) The actions of hypocretins are mediated by two G protein–coupled receptors named hypocretin receptor 1 (hcrtr-1) and hypocretin receptor 2 (hcrtr-2), also known as orexin-1 (OX₁R) and orexin-2 (OX₂R) receptors, respectively. Hcrtr 1 is selective for hypocretin-1, whereas hcrtr 2 is nonselective for both hypocretin-1 and hypocretin-2. Hcrtr 1 is coupled exclusively to the G_q subclass of heterotrimeric G proteins, whereas in vitro experiments suggest that hcrtr 2 couples with $G_{i/o}$, or G_q. (*Adapted from* Sakurai T. Roles of orexins in the regulation of feeding and arousal. Sleep Medicine 2002;3:S3–S9; with permission.) (C) Hypocretin-containing neurons project to these previously identified monoaminergic and cholinergic and cholinoceptive regions where the hypocretin receptors are enriched. Impairments of hypocretin input may result in cholinergic and monoaminergic imbalance and generation of narcoleptic symptoms. BF, basal forebrain; DR, dorsal raphe; LC, locus coeruleus; LDT, laterodorsal tegmental nucleus; LHA, lateral hypothalamic area; PPT, pedunculopontine tegmental nucleus; PRF, pontine reticular formation; SN, substantia nigra; TMN, tuberomamillary nucleus; VLPO, ventrolateral preoptic nucleus; VTA, ventral tegmental area.

(eg, pontine reticular formation), thought to be important for sleep regulation [Fig. 2] [47].

A series of recent studies have now shown that the hypocretin system is a major excitatory system that affects the activity of monoaminergic (dopamine, norepinephrine, serotonin [5-HT], and histamine) and cholinergic systems with major effects on vigilance states [see Fig. 2] [48,49]. It is likely that a deficiency in hypocretin neurotransmission induces an imbalance between these classical neurotransmitter systems, with primary effects on sleep-state organization and vigilance [see Fig. 2]. Indeed, dopamine or norepinephrine contents have been reported to be high in several brain structures in narcoleptic Dobermans, and in human narcolepsy brains, postmortem [7,50]. These changes are possibly caused by compensatory mechanisms, because the drugs that enhance dopaminergic neurotransmission (eg, amphetamine-like stimulants and modafinil [for EDS]) and norepinephrine neurotransmission (eg, noradrenaline uptake blockers [for cataplexy]), are needed to subside the symptoms of narcolepsy [7]. Histamine is another monoamine implicated in the control of vigilance, and the histaminergic system is also likely indirectly to mediate the wake-promoting effects of hypocretin [51–53]. Interestingly, brain histamine contents both in hcrtr-2 gene mutated and ligand-deficient narcoleptic dogs are dramatically reduced [54]. It is interesting further to evaluate the involvement of the histaminergic system in the pathophysiology of narcolepsy and therapeutic applications of histaminergic compounds [55].

Many measurable activities (brain and body) and compounds manifest rhythmic fluctuations over the 24-hour period. Whether hypocretin tone changes with zeitgeber time was assessed by measuring extracellular hypocretin-1 levels in the rat brain CSF across 24-hour periods, using in vivo dialysis [56–58]. The results demonstrate the involvement of a slow diurnal pattern of hypocretin neurotransmission regulation (as in the homeostatic or circadian regulation of sleep). Hypocretin levels increase during the active periods and are highest at the end of the active period, and the levels decline with the onset of sleep. Furthermore, sleep deprivation increases hypocretin levels [56–58].

Recent electrophysiologic studies have shown that hypocretin neurons are active during wakefulness, and reduce the activity during slow wave and REM sleep, but an increase in neuronal activity is associated with body movements or phasic REM activity [59,60]. In addition to this short-term change, the results of microdialysis experiments also suggest that basic hypocretin neurotransmission fluctuates across the 24-hour period, and slowly builds up during the active period. Adrener-gic locus coeruleus neurons are typical wake-active neurons involved in vigilance control, and it has been recently demonstrated that basic firing activity of wake-active locus coeruleus neurons also significantly fluctuates across various circadian times [61].

Several acute manipulations, such as exercise, low glucose use in the brain, and forced wakefulness, increase hypocretin levels [48,57,62]. It is hypothesized that a build-up and acute increase of hypocretin levels may counteract homeostatic sleep propensity that typically increases during the daytime and during forced wakefulness [57]. Because of the lack of increase in hypocretin tone, narcoleptic subjects may not be able to stay awake for a prolonged period and do not respond to various alerting stimuli. Conversely, reduction of the hypocretin tone at sleep onset may contribute to the profound deep sleep that normally inhibits REM sleep at sleep onset, and the lack of this system in narcolepsy may allow the occurrence of REM sleep at sleep onset.

Treatments of narcolepsy

Nonpharmacologic treatments (ie, by behavioral modification) are often reported to be useful additions to the clinical management of narcoleptic patients [63–66]. Regular napping usually relieves sleepiness for 1 to 2 hours [63] and is the treatment of choice for some patients, but this often has negative social and professional consequences. Exercising to avoid obesity, keeping a regular sleep-wake schedule, and having a supportive social environment (eg, patient group organizations and support groups) are also helpful. In almost all cases, however, pharmacologic treatment is needed, and 94% of patients reported using medications in a recent survey by a patient group organization [67].

For EDS, amphetamine-like central nervous system stimulants or modafinil (nonamphetamine stimulant, mechanisms of action is debated) are most often used. These compounds possess wake-promoting effects in narcoleptic subjects and in control populations, but very high doses are required to normalize abnormal sleep tendency during daytime for narcolepsy [68]. For consolidating nighttime sleep, benzodiazepine hypnotics or γ-hydroxybutyrate are occasionally used, and nighttime administration of γ-hydroxybutyrate reduces EDS and cataplexy during daytime [69,70]. γ-Hydroxybutyrate was once classified as a schedule I control substance in 2000, but has been recently approved for the treatment of narcolepsy. Because amphetamine-like stimulants and modafinil have little effect on cataplexy, tricyclic antidepressants, such as imipramine or clomipramine,

Table 2: Current pharmacologic treatment for human narcolepsy and its related disorders

Compound	Mode of action	Usual daily doses	Half-life (h)	Side effects and notes
Wake-promoting compounds for EDS				
Sympathomimetic stimulants				
D-amphetamine sulfate	Dopamine enhancer (dopamine release/ Dopamine uptake inhibition)	5–60 mg	16–30	Irritability, mood changes, headaches, palpitations, tremors, excessive sweating, insomnia
Methylphenidate HCl	Dopamine enhancer	10–60 mg	~3	Same as amphetamines, less reduction of appetite or increase in blood pressure
Pemoline[a]	Dopamine enhancer	20–115 mg	11–13	Less sympathomimetic effect, milder stimulant, slower onset of action, occasionally produces liver toxicity
Nonamphetamine wake-promoting compounds				
Modafinil	Unknown, inhibits dopamine uptake inhibition	100–400 mg	11–14	No peripheral sympathomimetic action, headaches, nausea
Short acting hypnotics				
γ-hydroxybutyric acid	Unknown, may act γ-aminobutyric acid–B or specific γ-hydroxybutyric acid receptors, reduces dopamine release	6–9 g (divided nightly)	~2	Sedation, nausea

[a] Potentially hepatotoxic; frequent liver function monitoring required.

are used in addition to control cataplexy [7,71,72]. These compounds can cause a number of side effects, however, such as dry mouth, constipation, or impotence. γ-Hydroxybutyrate is also used for the treatment of cataplexy, but the mechanisms of actions of γ-hydroxybutyrate remain unknown. The antidepressants and γ-hydroxybutyrate used are also effective for the other REM sleep phenomena.

Most of these therapeutic compounds for narcolepsy are known to act on the monoaminergic systems [Tables 2 and 3]. The compounds effective for EDS mostly target the presynaptic enhancement of dopaminergic neurotransmission (dopamine release and dopamine uptake inhibition) [73,74], whereas anticataplectics are mostly mediated by enhancement of noradrenergic neurotransmission [73]. Animal data suggest that these compounds are effective for EDS and cataplexy,

regardless of hypocretin receptor dysfunction and ligand deficiency [7,75,76], and are likely to act on downstream pathways of hypocretin neurotransmission. A series of anatomic and functional findings suggested that these monoaminergic systems are likely to mediate effects of hypocretin on vigilance and muscle tonus control [47,49,52,77–80]. In addition, the loss of hypocretin input possibly induces monoaminergic dysfunction [49,50].

Current pharmacologic treatments are rather symptomatic treatments and are not satisfactory for many patients because they bring undesirable side effects and drug tolerance. Furthermore, most patients need to take two different classes of compounds to manage both EDS and cataplexy, creating a variety of complications [7,71,72]. For these reasons, people have awaited an ideal treatment that is more directly pathophysiologically

Table 3: Antidepressants currently used as anticataplectic agents

Antidepressants compound	Usual daily doses	Half-life (hours)	Notes and side-effects
Tricyclics			
Imipramine	10–100 mg	5–30	(NE>5-HT>DA) Dry mouth, anorexia, sweating, constipation, drowsiness
Desipramine	25–200 mg	10–30	(NE » 5-HT>DA) A desmethyl metabolite of imipramine, effects and side effects similar to those of imipramine
Protryptiline	5–60 mg	55–200	(NE>5-HT>DA) Reported to improve vigilance measures, anticholinergic effects
Clomipramine	10–150 mg	15–60	(5-HT>NE»DA) Digestive problem, dry mouth, sweating, tiredness, impotence; anticholinergic effects; desmethyl-chlomipramine (NE»5-HT>DA) is an active metabolite
SSRIs			
Fluoxetine	20–60 mg	24–72	No anticholinergic or antihistaminergic effects, good anticataplectic effect but less potent than clomipramine; active metabolite norfluoxetine has more adrenergic effects
Fluvoxamine	50–300 mg	15	No active metabolite, pharmacologic profile similar to fluoxetine, less active than clomipramine, gastrointestinal side effects
NSRIs			
Venlafaxine	150–375 mg	4	New serotonergic and adrenergic uptake blocker; no anticholinergic effects, effective on cataplexy and sleepiness, nausea
Milnaciplan	30–50 mg	8	New serotonergic and adrenergic uptake blocker; no anticholinergic or antihistaminergic effects, effective on cataplexy
NRI[a]			
Atomotetin	40–60 mg[b]	5.2	Normally indicated for attention-deficit hyperactivity disorder

Abbreviations: NRI, norepinephrine reuptake inhibitor; NSRI, norepinephrine-serotonin reuptake inhibitor; SSRI, selective serotonin reuptake inhibitor.
[a] Reboxetine is another NRI, but is not available in the United States.
[b] Doses for treatments for ADHD and suggested to start with smaller doses for anticataplectic treatment. γ-Hydroxybutyric acid (sodium oxybate) is also reported to be effective on cataplexy and may act by γ-aminobutyric acid–B or by specific γ-hydroxybutyric acid receptors. Reduces dopamine release.

oriented. Hypocretin-orexin peptides or its mimetic are the most promising agent for this ligand-deficient condition. Unfortunately, however, large molecular peptides do not penetrate to the brain efficiently [81] and oral administration is not applicable for neuropeptides. Nonpeptide agonists need to be developed. Because most hypocretin receptors are G-protein coupled, 7-transmembraine receptors [see Fig. 2], as most neuropeptide receptors are, this deployment may be possible in the near future.

Future directions

The observation of low CSF hypocretin-1 levels is very specific for narcolepsy when compared with other sleep or neurologic disorders. Measuring CSF hypocretin-1 is rapidly becoming a new diagnostic tool for the condition. The availability of this test is also challenging the view of the nosology of narcolepsy. As emphasized by Honda [8], narcolepsy with cataplexy may be a more homogeneous etiologic entity, as reflected by low CSF hypocretin, to be differentiated from narcolepsy without cataplexy or the related syndrome of idiopathic hypersomnia, with generally normal hypocretin levels. In the 2nd revised ICSD, narcolepsy with cataplexy and narcolepsy without cataplexy are coded separately. Low CSF hypocretin-1 is also considered as a positive diagnostic result for narcolepsy-cataplexy.

Because most narcolepsy-cataplexy subjects (about 90% of idiopathic cases) are hypocretin ligand deficient, hypocretin agonists may be promising in the treatment of narcolepsy. In this respect, the development of small-molecular and centrally penetrant (ie, nonpeptide) hypocretin agonists is likely to be necessary [81]. A consideration is the possible absence of functional hypocretin receptors many years after the disease onset. If hypocretin-deficient patients are able to respond to hypocretin agonists and symptoms are subsided, cell transplantation, using embryonic hypothalamic cells or neural stem cells, and gene therapy (preprohypocretin-orexin gene transfer using various vectors) might also be used to cure the disease in the future.

Although cataplexy is now known to be tightly associated with hypocretin-deficiency in narcolepsy, the pathophysiologic mechanisms underlying the occurrence of cataplexy are largely unknown. The observation that prepubertal narcolepsy-cataplexy cases are almost always hypocretin deficient suggests that hypocretin deficiency occurs before cataplexy onset [82]. Considering the fact that acute ablation of hypocretin ligands by focal hypothalamic lesions associated with immune-related inflammatory encephalopathies, such as in multiple sclerosis and acute disseminated encephalomyelitis, rarely induce cataplexy [83], chronic and selective loss of hypocretin ligand may be required to exhibit cataplexy. The mechanisms of emotional induction of cataplexy remain to be studied.

The causes and mechanisms of the ligand deficiency in human narcolepsy remain unknown, but it is believed to be a result of acquired cell death of hypocretin neurons [43]. This is likely because (1) the onset of most sporadic cases of human narcolepsy is around puberty, later than those for the genetic animal models, (2) the only know human hypocretin gene mutation had a very early onset at 6 months of age; and (3) postnatal ablation of hypocretin neurons in mice [84] induces a phenotype that most resembles human narcolepsy. The mechanisms of the hypocretin cell death, especially in relation to HLA positivity, should be determined to prevent or rescue the disease. The current hypothesis, that narcolepsy is an autoimmune disease, is still unsubstantiated.

Hypocretins are involved in various other hypothalamic functions, such as feeding, energy homeostasis, and neuroendocrine regulation [48,49]. Narcolepsy now seems to be a more complex condition than simply a sleep disorder [85]. The disease is likely to be associated with various hypothalamic dysfunctions caused by hypocretin deficiency. Narcolepsy is an important model to study the fundamental hypothalamic mechanisms linking sleep regulation, energy homeostasis, or feeding [85].

References

[1] Hublin C, Kaprio J, Partinene M, et al. The prevalence of narcolepsy: an epidemiological study of the Finnish twin cohort. Ann Neurol 1994;35: 709–16.

[2] Mignot E. Genetic and familial aspects of narcolepsy. Neurology 1998;50:S16–22.

[3] American Academy of Sleep Medicine. ICSD-2-International classification of sleep disorders. Diagnostic and coding manual. 2nd edition. Westchester (IL): American Academy of Sleep Medicine; 2005.

[4] Beusterien KM, Rogers AE, Walsleben JA, et al. Health-related quality of life effects of modafinil for treatment of narcolepsy. Sleep 1999;22: 757–65.

[5] Mignot E, Lammers GJ, Ripley B, et al. The role of cerebrospinal fluid hypocretin measurement in the diagnosis of narcolepsy and other hypersomnias. Arch Neurol 2002;59:1553–62.

[6] Nishino S, Kanbayashi T. Symptomatic narcolepsy, cataplexy and hypersomnia, and their implications in the hypothalamic hypocretin/ orexin system. Sleep Med Rev 2005;9:269–310.

[7] Nishino S, Mignot E. Pharmacological aspects of

human and canine narcolepsy. Prog Neurobiol 1997;52:27–78.

[8] Honda Y. Clinical features of narcolepsy: Japanese experience. In: Honda Y, Juji T, editors. HLA in narcolepsy. New York: Springer-Verlag; 1988. p. 24–57.

[9] Gelb M, Guilleminault C, Kraemer H, et al. Stability of cataplexy over several months-information for the design of therapeutic trials. Sleep 1994;17:265–73.

[10] Overeem S, Mignot E, van Dijk JG, et al. Narcolepsy: clinical features, new pathophysiologic insights, and future perspectives. J Clin Neurophysiol 2001;18:78–105.

[11] Group USXMS. A randomized, double blind, placebo-controlled multicenter trial comparing the effects of three doses of orally administered sodium oxybate with placebo for the treatment of narcolepsy. Sleep 2002;25:42–9.

[12] Nishino S, Ripley B, Overeem S, et al. Hypocretin (orexin) deficiency in human narcolepsy. Lancet 2000;355:39–40.

[13] Nishino S, Kanbayashi T, Fujiki N, et al. CSF hypocretin levels in Guillain-Barre syndrome and other inflammatory neuropathies. Neurology 2003;61:823–5.

[14] Overeem S, Dalmau J, Bataller L, et al. Hypocretin-1 CSF levels in anti-Ma2 associated encephalitis. Neurology 2004;62:138–40.

[15] Alaila SL. Life effects of narcolepsy: measures of negative impact, social support and psychological well-being. In: Goswanmi M, Pollak CP, Cohen FL, et al, editors. Loss, grief and care: psychosocial aspects of narcolepsy, vol. 5. New York: Haworth Press; 1992. p. 1–22.

[16] Black JE, Brooks SN, Nishino S. Narcolepsy and syndromes of primary excessive daytime somnolence. Semin Neurol 2004;24:271–82.

[17] Smolik P, Roth B. Kleine-Levin syndrome ethiopathogenesis and treatment. Acta Univ Carol Med Monogr 1988;128:5–94.

[18] Billiard M. Kleine Levin syndrome. In: Krieger MH, Roth T, Dement WC, editors. Principles and practice of sleep medicine. Philadelphia: WB Saunders; 1989. p. 377–8.

[19] Dement W, Rechtschaffen A, Gulevich G. The nature of the narcoleptic sleep attack. Neurology 1966;16:18–33.

[20] Broughton R, Valley V, Aguirre M, et al. Excessive daytime sleepiness and pathophysiology of narcolepsy-cataplexy: a laboratory perspective. Sleep 1986;9:205–15.

[21] Guilleminault C, Wilson RA, Dement WC. A study on cataplexy. Arch Neurol 1974;31:255–61.

[22] Nishino S, Riehl J, Hong J, et al. Is narcolepsy REM sleep disorder? Analysis of sleep abnormalities in narcoleptic Dobermans. Neurosci Res 2000;38:437–46.

[23] Bishop C, Rosenthal L, Helmus T, et al. The frequency of multiple sleep onset REM periods among subjects with no excessive daytime sleepiness. Sleep 1996;19:727–30.

[24] Aldrich MS, Chervin RD, Malow BA. Value of the multiple sleep latency test (MSLT) for the diagnosis of narcolepsy. Sleep 1997;20:620–9.

[25] Fukuda K, Miyasita A, Inugami M, et al. High prevalence of isolated sleep paralysis: Kanashibari phenomenon in Japan. Sleep 1987;10:279–86.

[26] Ohayon MM, Priest RG, Caulet M, et al. Hypnagogic and hypnopompic hallucinations: pathological phenomena? Br J Psychiatry 1996;169:459–67.

[27] Juji T, Satake M, Honda Y, et al. HLA antigens in Japanese patients with narcolepsy: all the patients were DR2 positive. Tissue Antigens 1984;24:316–9.

[28] Mignot E, Hayduk R, Black J, et al. HLA class II studies in 509 narcoleptic patients. Sleep Res 1997;26:433.

[29] Mignot E, Guilleminault C, Grumet FC, et al. Is narcolepsy an autoimmune disease? In: Smirne S, Francesci M, Ferini-Strambi L, et al, editors. Proceedings of the Third Milano International Symposium, September 18–19 Sleep, Hormones, and the Immune System. Milan: Masson; 1992. p. 29–38.

[30] Billiard M, Laaberki MF, Reygrobellet C, et al. Elevated antibodies to streptococcal antigens in narcoleptic subjects. Sleep Res 1989;18:201.

[31] Montplaisir J, Poirier G, Lapierre O, et al. Streptococcal antibodies in narcolepsy and idiopathic hypersomnia. Sleep Res 1989;18:271.

[32] Frederickson S, Carlander B, Billiard M, et al. CSF immune variable in patients with narcolepsy. Acta Neurol Scand 1990;81:253–4.

[33] Matsuki K, Juji T, Honda Y. Immunological features of narcolepsy in Japan. In: Honda Y, Juji T, editors. HLA in narcolepsy. New York: Springer-Verlag; 1988. p. 150–7.

[34] Black III JL, Krahn LE, Pankratz VS, et al. Search for neuron-specific and nonneuron-specific antibodies in narcoleptic patients with and without HLA DQB1*0602. Sleep 2002;25:719–23.

[35] Black III JL, Silber MH, Krahn LE, et al. Studies of humoral immunity to preprohypocretin in human leukocyte antigen DQB1*0602-positive narcoleptic subjects with cataplexy. Biol Psychiatry 2005;58:504–9.

[36] Mignot E, Wang C, Rattazzi C, et al. Genetic linkage of autosomal recessive canine narcolepsy with a mu immunoglobulin heavy-chain switch-like segment. Proc Natl Acad Sci U S A 1991;88:3475–8.

[37] Chemelli RM, Willie JT, Sinton CM, et al. Narcolepsy in orexin knockout mice: molecular genetics of sleep regulation. Cell 1999;98:437–51.

[38] Lin L, Faraco J, Li R, et al. The sleep disorder canine narcolepsy is caused by a mutation in the hypocretin (orexin) receptor 2 gene. Cell 1999;98:365–76.

[39] Peyron C, Faraco J, Rogers W, et al. A mutation in a case of early onset narcolepsy and a generalized absence of hypocretin peptides in human narcoleptic brains. Nat Med 2000;6:991–7.

[40] Nishino S, Ripley B, Overeem S, et al. Low CSF

hypocretin (orexin) and altered energy homeo-stasis in human narcolepsy. Ann Neurol 2001; 50:381–8.

[41] Krahn LE, Pankratz VS, Oliver L, et al. Hypocretin (orexin) levels in cerebrospinal fluid of patients with narcolepsy: relationship to cataplexy and HLA DQB1*0602 status. Sleep 2002;25:733–6.

[42] Kanbayashi T, Inoue Y, Chiba S, et al. CSF hypocretin-1 (orexin-A) concentrations in narco-lepsy with and without cataplexy and idiopathic hypersomnia. J Sleep Res 2002;11:91–3.

[43] Thannickal TC, Moore RY, Nienhuis R, et al. Reduced number of hypocretin neurons in hu-man narcolepsy. Neuron 2000;27:469–74.

[44] Ripley B, Fujiki N, Okura M, et al. Hypocretin levels in sporadic and familial cases of canine narcolepsy. Neurobiol Dis 2001;8:525–34.

[45] De Lecea L, Kilduff TS, Peyron C, et al. The hypocretins: hypothalamus-specific peptides with neuroexcitatory activity. Proc Natl Acad Sci U S A 1998;95:322–7.

[46] Sakurai T, Amemiya A, Ishii M, et al. Orexins and orexin receptors: a family of hypothalamic neuropeptides and G protein-coupled receptors that regulate feeding behavior. Cell 1998;92: 573–85.

[47] Peyron C, Tighe DK, van den Pol AN, et al. Neu-rons containing hypocretin (orexin) project to multiple neuronal systems. J Neurosci 1998;18: 9996–10015.

[48] Willie JT, Chemelli RM, Sinton CM, et al. To eat or to sleep? Orexin in the regulation of feeding and wakefulness. Annu Rev Neurosci 2001;24: 429–58.

[49] Taheri S, Zeitzer JM, Mignot E. The role of hypo-cretins (orexins) in sleep regulation and narco-lepsy. Annu Rev Neurosci 2002;25:283–313.

[50] Nishino S, Fujiki N, Ripley B, et al. Decreased brain histamine contents in hypocretin/orexin receptor-2 mutated narcoleptic dogs. Neurosci Lett 2001;313:125–8.

[51] Huang ZL, Qu WM, Li WD, et al. Arousal effect of orexin A depends on activation of the hista-minergic system. Proc Natl Acad Sci U S A 2001; 98:9965–70.

[52] Yamanaka A, Tsujino N, Funahashi H, et al. Orexins activate histaminergic neurons via the orexin 2 receptor. Biochem Biophys Res Com-mun 2002;290:1237–45.

[53] Eriksson KS, Sergeeva O, Brown RE, et al. Orexin/ hypocretin excites the histaminergic neurons of the tuberomammillary nucleus. J Neurosci 2001; 21:9273–9.

[54] Nishino S, Sakurai E, Nevisimalova S, et al. CSF histamine content is decreased in hypocretin-deficient human narcolepsy. Sleep 2002;25:A476.

[55] Shiba T, Fujiki N, Wisor J, et al. Wake promoting effects of thioperamide, a histamine H3 antago-nist in orexin/ataxin-3 narcoleptic mice. Sleep 2004;27(suppl):A241.

[56] Fujiki N, Yoshida Y, Ripley B, et al. Changes in CSF hypocretin-1 (orexin A) levels in rats across

24 hours and in response to food deprivation. Neuroreport 2001;12:993–7.

[57] Yoshida Y, Fujiki N, Nakajima T, et al. Fluctua-tion of extracellular hypocretin-1 (orexin A) levels in the rat in relation to the light-dark cycle and sleep-wake activities. Eur J Neurosci 2001; 14:1075–81.

[58] Zeitzer JM, Buckmaster CL, Parker KJ, et al. Circadian and homeostatic regulation of hypo-cretin in a primate model: implications for the consolidation of wakefulness. J Neurosci 2003; 23:3555–60.

[59] Mileykovskiy BY, Kiyashchenko LI, Siegel JM. Behavioral correlates of activity in identified hypocretin/orexin neurons. Neuron 2005;46: 787–98.

[60] Lee MG, Hassani OK, Jones BE. Discharge of identified orexin/hypocretin neurons across the sleep-waking cycle. J Neurosci 2005;25:6716–20.

[61] Aston-Jones G, Chen S, Zhu Y, et al. A neural circuit for circadian regulation of arousal. Nat Neurosci 2001;4:732–8.

[62] Wu MF, John J, Maidment N, et al. Hypocretin release in normal and narcoleptic dogs after food and sleep deprivation, eating, and movement. Am J Physiol Regul Integr Comp Physiol 2002; 283:R1079–86.

[63] Roehrs T, Zorick F, Wittig R, et al. Alerting effects of naps in patients with narcolepsy. Sleep 1986; 9:194–9.

[64] Thorpy MJ, Goswami M. Treatment of nar-colepsy. In: Thorpy MJ, editor. Handbook of sleep disorders. New York: Marcel Dekker; 1990. p. 235–58.

[65] Mullington J, Broughton R. Scheduled naps in the management of daytime sleepiness in narcolepsy-cataplexy. Sleep 1993;16:444–56.

[66] Rogers AE. Problems and coping strategies iden-tified by narcoleptic patients. J Neurosurg Nurs 1984;16:326–34.

[67] American Narcolepsy Association. Stimulant medication survey. The Eye Opener 1992;1–3.

[68] Mitler MM, Aldrich MS, Koob GF, et al. Narco-lepsy and its treatment with stimulants. Sleep 1994;17:352–71.

[69] Lammers GJ, Arends J, Declerck AC, et al. Gamma-hydroxybutyrate and narcolepsy: a double-blind placebo-controlled study. Sleep 1993;16:216–20.

[70] Scrima L, Hartman PG, Johnson FH, et al. Effi-cacy of gamma-hydroxybutyrate versus placebo in treating narcolepsy-cataplexy: double-blind sub-jective measures. Biol Psychiatry 1989;26:331–43.

[71] Nishino S, Okura M, Mignot E. Narcolepsy: genetic predisposition and neuropharmacologi-cal mechanisms. Sleep Med Rev 2000;4:57–99.

[72] Mignot E. Pathophysiology of narcolepsy. In: Kryger MH, Roth T, Dement WC, et al, editors. Principles and practice of sleep medicine. Phila-delphia: WB Saunders; 2000. p. 663–75.

[73] Nishino S, Mao J, Sampathkumaran R, et al. Increased dopaminergic transmission mediates the wake-promoting effects of CNS stimulants.

Sleep Research Online 1998;1:49–61. Available at: http://www.sro.org/1998/Nishino/49. Accessed December 24, 2005.

[74] Wisor JP, Nishino S, Sora I, et al. Dopaminergic role in stimulant-induced wakefulness. J Neurosci 2001;21:1787–94.

[75] Babcock DA, Narver EL, Dement WC, et al. Effects of imipramine, chlorimipramine, and fluoxetine on cataplexy in dogs. Pharmacol Biochem Behav 1976;5:599–602.

[76] Foutz AS, Delashaw JB, Guilleminault C, et al. Monoaminergic mechanisms and experimental cataplexy. Ann Neurol 1981;10:369–76.

[77] Kiyashchenko LI, Mileykovskiy BY, Lai YY, et al. Increased and decreased muscle tone with orexin (hypocretin) microinjections in the locus coeruleus and pontine inhibitory area. J Neurophysiol 2001;85:2008–16.

[78] Nambu T, Sakurai T, Mizukami K, et al. Distribution of orexin neurons in the adult rat brain. Brain Res 1999;827:243–60.

[79] Hagan JJ, Leslie RA, Patel S, et al. Orexin A activates locus coeruleus cell firing and increases arousal in the rat. Proc Natl Acad Sci U S A 1999; 96:10911–6.

[80] Horvath TL, Peyron C, Diano S, et al. Hypocretin (orexin) activation and synaptic innervation of the locus coeruleus noradrenergic system. J Comp Neurol 1999;415:145–59.

[81] Fujiki N, Ripley B, Yoshida Y, et al. Effects of IV and ICV hypocretin-1 (orexin A) in hypocretin receptor-2 gene mutated narcoleptic dogs and IV hypocretin-1 replacement therapy in a hypocretin ligand deficient narcoleptic dog. Sleep 2003; 6:953–9.

[82] Kanbayashi T, Yano T, Ishiguro H, et al. Hypocretin-1 (orexin-A) levels in human lumbar CSF in different age groups: infants to elderly persons. Sleep 2002;25:337–9.

[83] Kubota H, Kanbayashi T, Tanabe Y, et al. A case of acute disseminated encephalomyelitis presenting hypersomnia with decreased hypocretin level in cerebrospinal fluid. J Child Neurol 2002; 17:537–9.

[84] Hara J, Beuckmann CT, Nambu T, et al. Genetic ablation of orexin neurons in mice results in narcolepsy, hypophagia, and obesity. Neuron 2001; 30:345–54.

[85] Nishino S. The hypocretin/orexin system in health and disease. Biol Psychiatry 2003;54:87–95.

ELSEVIER SAUNDERS

SLEEP
MEDICINE
CLINICS

Sleep Med Clin 1 (2006) 63–78

Excessive Daytime Sleepiness and Obstructive Sleep Apnea Syndrome

Kannan Ramar, MD, Christian Guilleminault, MD, BioID*

- Pathophysiology of excessive daytime sleepiness in obstructive sleep apnea
  Arousals and excessive daytime sleepiness
  Apnea-hypopnea index and excessive daytime sleepiness
  Slow wave activity and excessive daytime sleepiness
  Autonomic activation and excessive daytime sleepiness
  Hypoxemia and excessive daytime sleepiness
  Snoring and excessive daytime sleepiness
  Cyclic alternating pattern
  Respiratory cycle–related EEG change
- Measures of excessive daytime sleepiness
  Objective measures
  Subjective measures
- Consequences of sleepiness
  Quality of life
  Cognitive decline
  Motor vehicle accidents
  Obesity, sleepiness, and obstructive sleep apnea
- Treatment options for excessive daytime sleepiness caused by obstructive sleep apnea syndrome
  Nasal continuous positive airway pressure
  Residual daytime sleepiness
  Modafinil
- References

Excessive daytime sleepiness (EDS) is a common yet very often neglected symptom. Patients may underreport their sleepiness, either because they are not aware of it or because there are social pressures to deny that it is a problem. EDS is increasingly recognized as an important public health problem, affecting at least 12% to 20% of the general adult population [1,2]. EDS is defined as sleepiness (the urge to sleep) that occurs in a situation when an individual is normally expected to be awake and alert. It is important to differentiate true sleepiness from various forms of tiredness, such as lethargy, malaise, or exhaustion.

Obstructive sleep apnea syndrome (OSAS) is the most common cause of EDS among subjects seen

in sleep clinics [3,4]. It is a serious disorder characterized by sleep fragmentation caused by repeated arousals and disruption of normal sleep architecture secondary to partial or complete closure of the upper airway during sleep [5,6]. In patients with OSAS, EDS results in a high rate of accidents in traffic and work. Patients with OSAS are involved in traffic accidents two to three times more often than the general population [7].

Interestingly, not all patients with OSAS, even moderate to severe OSAS, have daytime sleepiness [8]. In the Wisconsin cohort study, only 15.5% of males and 22.6% of females with OSAS (as assessed by apnea-hypopnea index [AHI] at a rate of five events per hour or more) reported sleepiness on

Stanford University Sleep Medicine Program, 401 Quarry Road, Suite 3301, Stanford, CA 94305, USA
* Corresponding author.
E-mail address: cguil@stanford.edu (C. Guilleminault).

1556-407X/06/$ – see front matter © 2006 Elsevier Inc. All rights reserved.
sleep.theclinics.com

doi:10.1016/j.jsmc.2005.11.001

three subjective measures used. A higher percentage of subjects, however, reported sleepiness on at least one of the three measurements used [2]. The complaint of "sleepiness" was the least frequently reported symptom when Chervin [9] conducted an informal questionnaire survey on patients with OSAS; most often patients reported "lack of energy" as the symptom that described their daytime experience. Additionally, a substantial subset of patients who denied the daytime complaints reported a variety of other complaints related to changes in cognitive function, such as impaired short-term memory, reduced capacity to sustain concentration or focus, word-finding difficulties, or a lowered frustration threshold leading to irritability [9].

Pathophysiology of excessive daytime sleepiness in obstructive sleep apnea

Arousals and excessive daytime sleepiness

In normal subjects, brief arousals from sleep produce EDS and impaired daytime performance [10,11]. In subjects with obstructive sleep apnea, arousal from sleep is believed to be an essential mechanism for re-establishing airway patency [12]. The apneic and hypopneic events in OSAS are associated with frequent arousals that lead to sleep fragmentation [12,13], and thereby EDS [14]. Also, arousals can occur without apneas, hypopneas, or hypoxemia, and this leads to the concept of respiratory effort–related arousals. Respiratory effort–related arousals are defined as arousals occurring during and interrupting a succession of loud snores. It has been shown that respiratory effort– related arousals occur mostly in association with a rise in inspiratory effort secondary to increased upper airway resistance, resulting in arousals [6]. Short electroencephalogram (EEG) arousals (defined as detectable lightening of the EEG with alpha and beta waves for 3 seconds or more) were subsequently defined in 1992, as efforts were made to define the minimum degree of sleep disturbance that was needed to result in EDS [15].

Investigators have shown no consistent significant correlations between arousals and EDS [16–19]. A recent study by Goncalves and coworkers [20] showed a stronger correlation between short EEG arousals (as per American Sleep Disorders Association [ASDA] criteria [15]) and severity of OSAS than those previously published, but the polysomnographic measures did not correlate with the subjective measurements of sleepiness. Even when other investigators reduced the length of EEG changes required to define an EEG arousal to 1.5 seconds, it was only minimally better at predicting objective daytime sleepiness [21].

Arousals could be poor correlates of objective EDS for various reasons. First, the reasons for daytime sleepiness could be from many factors other than recurrent arousals, such as sleep deprivation, drugs, xanthines, or cytokines. Second, there is night-to-night variation in sleep apnea severity [22], and a single hospital sleep study may not fully represent what happens normally, because the symptom is a cumulative result of variable sleep fragmentation. Third, approximately 28% of apneas and hypopneas are not terminated by visible cortical arousals [23]. This could be caused by the limitations of visual scoring in detecting all arousals, which might be better appreciated by EEG power spectral analysis [24]; it could be related to the fact that apnea and hypopnea may not necessarily lead to an EEG arousal, but only brain-stem activation without involvement of neuronal network above the thalamus. Further validation is needed to compare this marker with EDS severity. Fourth, integrating EDS with other EEG markers of sleep disruption, like cyclical alternating patterns (CAP) and detection of respiratory cycle–related EEG changes in OSAS subjects [25,26], may improve evaluation of EDS. Finally, subjects may have difficulties recognizing their own degree of sleepiness, as shown in many sleep-deprivation or fragmentation studies, but this is mostly associated with denial of sleepiness.

Apnea-hypopnea index and excessive daytime sleepiness

The severity of OSAS is most frequently gauged by measuring the AHI using the overnight polysomnogram. The AHI is used to reflect the severity of sleep fragmentation, but investigators have not been able consistently to demonstrate an association between AHI and EDS when EDS was assessed by the multiple sleep latency test (MSLT) or other measures [16,17,19,21,27]. Other studies have shown inability to correlate sleep study indices with daytime measures of sleepiness, where the r value rarely rises above 0.4 (ie, less than 20% of symptoms across a sleep clinic population seem explicable on the basis of the sleep study, the primary diagnostic tool).

Slow wave activity and excessive daytime sleepiness

OSAS leads to disruption of normal sleep architecture with deprivation of rapid eye movement (REM) sleep and stages 3 and 4 non–rapid eye movement (NREM) sleep, although their sleep efficiency seems to be unchanged [16,28]. Slow wave activity is considered an objective marker for homeostatic process. It has a broader definition that includes slow wave sleep stage criteria (including slow waves in stage 2 sleep) and a broader frequency distribution (0.75–4.5 Hz). Heinzer and coworkers [29] showed a decrease in slow wave activity across the night with OSAS patients leading to EDS. Slow wave activity increased after nasal continuous positive airway pressure (CPAP) treatment, but there was a lack of correlation with MSLT posttreatment.

Autonomic activation and excessive daytime sleepiness

Autonomic activation has attracted attention as a potential index to quantify sleep disturbance in OSAS [30] because this method identifies even minor disturbing events that occur without visible EEG arousals [31]. There was an increase in EDS in one study, as measured by maintenance of wakefulness test (MWT) in normal subjects when autonomic activations were repeatedly induced in the absence of visible EEG arousals [32]. Subsequently, in OSAS patients, Bennett and coworkers [33] described autonomic activations as predictors of EDS by showing a significant correlation between the autonomic activation index and pretreatment objective sleepiness, and between the autonomic activation index and nasal CPAP responsive objective sleepiness. On the contrary, a recent study [34] showed that activation of brainstem (and thereby autonomic nervous system), without cortical arousal through subthreshold auditory stimulation, did not induce any change in MSLT or subjective sleepiness. Autonomic nervous system changes can be obtained with different types of stimuli; some of them may only involve simple reflexes with relay in medulla and lower brainstem, whereas others are associated with involvement of higher nervous system structures including the cortex. Investigation of autonomic nervous system stimulations, EEG arousal, and importance of autonomic nervous system stimulation necessary to induce sleepiness measured objectively has not been done. To relay only on an autonomic nervous system response to determine cortical arousal is erroneous; some type of EEG analysis is needed.

Hypoxemia and excessive daytime sleepiness

OSAS also leads to repetitive oxygen desaturation, but this variable has not been considered to be of significant importance for EDS [35]. Colt and coworkers [36] showed no change in objective improvement in EDS as measured by MSLT when OSAS patients were treated with nasal CPAP, irrespective of the presence or absence of nocturnal hypoxemia. Their results lend further support to the hypothesis relating EDS to sleep fragmentation. Additionally, many patients with COPD or other

lung diseases who present with chronic hypoxemia, which may tend to be more severe during rapid eye movement sleep, showed no correlation with EDS.

Snoring and excessive daytime sleepiness

Snoring is also associated with EDS, although it could simply be a marker for obstructive sleep apnea. Young and colleagues [2] found that snorers with respiratory disturbance index ≤5 were substantially more likely to report EDS than were nonsnorers with respiratory disturbance index ≤5. Subsequent work by Gottlieb and coworkers [37] showed a significant association between snoring and sleepiness that was independent of the association between AHI and sleepiness. Snoring may be an independent cause of excess sleepiness, through mechanisms that remain to be elucidated [6]. In the recent past studies of snorers were performed with nasal cannula and pressure transducer, and with esophageal pressure. It was shown that these subjects presented with upper airway resistance syndrome when appropriately investigated, but this syndrome is not presented here.

Cyclic alternating pattern

CAP is formed by electrocortical events that recur at regular intervals in the range of seconds during NREM sleep [Table 1] [25]. These events are clearly distinguishable from the background EEG rhythm as abrupt frequency shifts or amplitude changes. Two phases (A and B) are present that are part of a CAP cycle and recur within 2 to 60 seconds [see Table 1]. When neither of the phases (A and B) is identifiable, sleep has reached a new stable state [38]. Phase A is identified by transient events typically observed in NREM sleep. It includes EEG patterns of higher voltage; slower frequency; and faster lower voltage than the background EEG (with an increase in amplitude by at least one third compared with the background EEG). It is an activation phase lasting 2 to 60 seconds. Phase B follows phase A; it is the interval between two phases A with duration of 2 to 60 seconds, and has been defined by decreased EEG amplitude with EEG evidence of stages 1 to 2 NREM. Phase A has been subdivided into three subtypes. Subtype A1 is marked by a predominance of synchronized EEG activity and less than 20% of desynchronization of the EEG (fast frequency and low amplitude), such as delta bursts, K complex sequences, vertex waves, and polyphasic bursts (of slow and fast EEG rhythms). Subtype A2 is scored in the presence of 20% to 50% of desynchronized EEG activity with a predominance of polyphasic bursts. Subtype A3 is scored when at least 50% of the EEG activity is comprised of low amplitude fast rhythms, such

Table 1: **Summary of cyclic alternating pattern phases**

Table 1: **Summary of cyclic alternating pattern phases**

CAP phase	Characteristics
Phase A	2–60 seconds Transient events EEG patterns of higher voltage, slower frequency, and faster-lower voltage than the background EEG (increase in amplitude by at least one third)
Subtype A1	Predominance of synchronized EEG activity <20% desynchronization of EEG activity Delta bursts, K complex sequences, vertex waves, and polyphasic bursts
Subtype A2	20%–50% of desynchronized EEG activity Predominance of polyphasic bursts
Subtype A3	≥50% of desynchronized EEG activity Comprised of low-amplitude fast rhythms K-alpha complexes, ASDA-defined arousals, and polyphasic bursts
Phase B	2–60 seconds Interval between two phases A Decreased EEG amplitude with EEG evidence of stages 1–2 NREM

Abbreviations: ASDA, American Sleep Disorders Association; CAP, cyclic alternating pattern; EEG, electroencephalogram; NREM, non–rapid eye movement.

as K-alpha complexes, ASDA-defined arousals, and polyphasic bursts [25].

The use of ASDA short EEG arousals and CAP scorings is increasingly becoming a popular way to evaluate sleep structure unlike the simple sleep staging evaluation based on at least 15 seconds out of one 30-second epoch that is currently being done using the Rechtschaffen and Kales method of scoring. CAP is a condition of NREM sleep instability [25].

Patients with OSAS have increases in CAP rate (>80% at the expense of non-CAP) with apneas and hypopneas usually occurring during phase B. Sleep fragmentation is associated with a significant enhancement of CAP phase A, especially A3 (that correlates strongly with ASDA EEG arousals), and more than 90% of the respiratory events are noted during CAP [39].

The enhanced resolution offered by the CAP, non-CAP perspective can shed light on the complex interactions between arousal rhythmicity, apneas-hypopnea, sleep disruption, and thereby its role in EDS and the effects of calibrating CPAP to the previously mentioned end points [40]. Further studies are required to explore the advantages of this sleep scoring approach in diagnosis and clinical management of OSAS patients with EDS, including nasal CPAP calibration.

Respiratory cycle–related EEG change

Respiratory cycle-related EEG change is a quantification of computer-based signal analysis that detects subtle cortical responses (otherwise not detected by visual inspection) caused by increased work of breathing in sleep-disordered breathing subjects that might otherwise not be picked up during the nonapneic or hypopneic respiratory cycles. Using this method, Chervin and coworkers [41] showed that in subjects with sleep-disordered breathing the tendency for sigma (13–15 Hz) electroencephalographic power to vary with each respiratory cycle predicted next-day sleepiness as measured by the MSLT. Further investigation is necessary for complete validation of this method.

Measures of excessive daytime sleepiness

Many studies have indicated the difficulty of subjectively recognizing and objectively quantifying sleepiness. Patients and physicians have difficulty recognizing EDS; such terms as "fatigue" and "tiredness" are used interchangeably with EDS by the patients and mistakenly classified by physicians as depression and chronic fatigue syndrome [42]. Table 2 shows a summary of objective and subjective tests currently used in evaluating EDS.

Objective measures

Normally, the initial step in investigating the etiology of EDS is the performance of the overnight polysomnogram test, which can confirm sleep-related breathing disorders. This also helps to rule out other disorders that can potentially cause EDS.

Multiple Sleep Latency Test

As subjective measures of sleep were being formulated, objective measures of sleep were being finalized in 1977 with the advent of the MSLT [43]. This test is administered the day after an all-night polysomnogram to ensure that sleep deprivation does not confound the results. Sleep latency is measured during naps taken at four to five different times during the day. The MSLT is thought to measure physiologic sleep tendency in the absence of alerting factors, with the tendency to fall asleep (decreased sleep latency) increasing as physiologic sleepiness increases. Although the

Table 2: Objective and subjective tests used in assessment of EDS in patients with OSAHS

Objective measures of EDS	
Multiple Sleep Latency Test	Developed in 1977
	Measures sleep latency in the absence of alerting factors
	Measured using EEG during four to five naps taken at different times during the day
	Used as a standard test to evaluate objectively for daytime sleepiness
	May be affected by the amount of sleep before the test
Maintenance of Wakefulness Test	Developed in 1982
	Meant to address shortcomings of MSLT
	Measures ability to function and maintain alertness in common situations of inactivity
	Measured using EEG during four to five set intervals throughout the day
	Has similar shortcomings to MSLT
Oxford Sleep Resistance Test	MWT test without EEG monitoring
	Measures sustained attention and reaction time
	Patients respond to a light-emitting diode device
	Lasts 40 minutes and may be repeated up to four times between the 08.00 and 17.00 hour
	Looks at behavioral lapses, but misses short sleep segments indicated by decreased alertness
	Sensitive to motivation
Psychomotor Vigilance Task	Measures reaction time
	Lasts 10 minutes
	Can be administered at different times of day; there is a circadian modulation of results
	Sensitive to motivation
Subjective measures of EDS	
Epworth Sleepiness Scale	Developed in 1991
	Self-administered questionnaire
	Eight items are rated on a Likert scale from 0 (never) to 3 (high chance), regarding patient's likelihood to doze in sedentary conditions
	The total of the responses is the Epworth score, which can range from 0–24
	Measures patient's perception of sleepiness over time
Stanford sleepiness Scale	Seven-point scale of equal intervals measuring subjective sleepiness from being very alert to excessively sleepy
	Requires collection of many data points during 1 day
	Measures sleepiness at a single point in time
	Investigates the instantaneous degree of sleepiness
Karolinska Sleepiness Scale	9 point scale (1 = very alert to 9 = very sleepy)
	Measures patient's perception of ability to stay awake or fight sleep
	Require collection of many data points during 1 day
	Measure sleepiness at single day in time
	Investigates the instantaneous degree of sleepiness

Abbreviations: EEG, electroencephalogram; MSLT, Multiple Sleep Latency Test; MWT, Maintenance of Wakefulness Test.

MSLT is still used as a standard test to evaluate EDS objectively, the validity of this test was never assessed using a large sample of subjects, and questions have been raised as to whether this test should be considered the gold standard in testing for EDS [44]. Also, it has been shown that the amount of prior sleep affects MSLT [45], and thereby the recommendation of performing actigraphy to ensure that prolonged sleep restriction did not occur before testing has been made, not only for MSLT but for all tests of daytime alertness. Despite its critics, MSLT is still the most documented test of objective daytime alertness, and the only test that can suggest other etiologies for EDS.

When subjects with OSAS were compared with controls, there was significant overlap in mean sleep latency values on the MSLT, but the overall results showed 7.2 ± 6 and 12.8 ± 4.1, respectively, which was about 1 to 1.5 standard deviations less than the mean for normal controls [46,47], indicating that the routine use of MSLT to assess EDS secondary to OSAS may not always contribute significantly in diagnosis or evaluating response to treatment for OSAS. The MSLT showed lower mean sleep latency values in subjects with severe OSAS. EDS secondary to severe OSAS was significantly related to the amount of stage 1 NREM during the night, however, and not to scored sleep fragmentation when using Rechtchaffen and Kales sleep staging [16]. Also, no significant relationship was found between the number of abnormal breathing events (that include more than AHI and has been called respiratory disturbance index) and the results of the MSLT [16,17]. Results were better with the use of short ASDA arousals, and much better with the sigma respiratory cycle–related EEG changes scoring as studied by Chervin and coworkers [41]. Further investigations are needed using the more advanced sleep scoring techniques.

Maintenance of Wakefulness Test
MWT was developed in 1982 [48]. This test measures the ability of the subject to stay awake and thereby their ability to function and maintain alertness in common situations of inactivity; it considers a different function than MSLT. Despite this test being often used currently for medicolegal decisions, it also has shortcomings as the MSLT.

Very few studies have examined the factors associated with MWT sleep latency. Although a recent study of subjects with mild to moderate OSAS found age, previous sleep disorder history, and hypoxemia during the night as independent predictors for MWT sleep latency, respiratory variables (eg, AHI) were not independent predictors [33,49]. The study was vague in showing associations between MWT score and potential predictor variables. Also, there was a discrepancy between the MWT and Epworth Sleepiness Scale (ESS) scores for many of the subjects tested [49,50], but ESS has been shown to explore a different domain than MWT. Although some investigators found that whereas MWT latencies tended to be shorter for patients with severe OSAS, there was only a weak relationship between apnea severity and MWT scores [18,50]. Further studies are needed to assess the reliability of MWT in subjects with OSAS.

The Oxford Sleep Resistance Test is an MWT without EEG monitoring: it uses a light-emitting diode device placed at eye level 2 m away from the subject and asks the subject to respond each time the diode flashes [51]. The test lasts 40 minutes and may be repeated up to four times between the 08:00 and 17:00 hour. As with the following test, it looks at behavioral lapses, but misses short sleep segments indicated by a decrease in alertness. All tests based on lapses have this problem and underscore brief sleep segments. The fact that this test requests motivation to perform from subjects is also a drawback because absence of EEG cannot dissociate real lapses from motivational lapses.

Psychomotor Vigilance Task
Performance tests have also been used frequently to evaluate sleepiness. The most common ones are simple reaction time tests, such as the Psychomotor Vigilance Task, which was standardized to be performed with little training and takes only 10 minutes per session. The test has been administered at different times of day because there is a circadian modulation of results. Different programs perform automatic analysis of the tests and evaluation of the standard deviation of the response time has been indicated as one of the sensitive calculations [52]. No good correlation with the AHI has been shown.

Subjective measures

Epworth Sleepiness Scale
ESS was developed in 1991 as a tool for subjective assessment of EDS [53]. Eight items are rated on a Likert scale from 0 (never) to 3 (high chance) regarding their likelihood to doze in sedentary conditions, and the total of the responses is the Epworth score, which can range from 0 to 24. The validity of the scale was established by correlating it with the gold standard test for EDS, the MSLT; however, the association between the two was weak and the number of subjects was low [53–56]. Additionally, there was no strong association between ESS and OSAS. These associations were measured in studies of smaller sample size. In a study involving a large sample from the Wisconsin Sleep Cohort Study, Punjabi and coworkers [57] described a moderately strong and independent association between ESS and MSLT. Subjects with ESS in the intermediate [6–11] and highest quartiles (≥12) had a 30% and 69% increased risk for sleep onset during MSLT, respectively, compared with the lowest quartiles (≤5). This study also revealed a dose-response relationship between self-reported sleep duration and MSLT, with individuals reporting less than 6.75 hours of sleep having a 73% increased risk of sleep onset during MSLT compared with individuals reporting more than 7.5 hours of sleep.

Bennett and coworkers [58] found that subjective sleepiness (ESS) correlated more closely with health status (quantified with the Short Form-36 questionnaire) than objectively measured sleepiness with either MSLT or MWT. This is probably because the ESS and Short Form-36 are both subjective measures, and both quantify symptoms in the recent past. In contrast, measures of objective sleepiness quantify sleepiness during a single day. Inconsistent and weak correlations between sleepiness and health status emphasize that there is more to the symptom complex of OSAS than just falling asleep.

Stanford Sleepiness Scale

The Stanford Sleepiness Scale is a seven-point scale of equal intervals measuring subjective sleepiness from being very alert to excessively sleepy [59]. This scale was well validated by two studies, again with small sample size [60,61]. It has fallen out of favor, however, because it is harder to administer; requires collection of many data points during one day; measures sleepiness at a single point in time (ie, it only investigates the instantaneous degree of sleepiness in contrast to the ESS, which seems to measure a general longer perception of presence of sleepiness by the patient); and does not always correlate with the MSLT [62].

Other subjective scales, like the Karolinska Sleepiness Scale, are not used regularly because they have problems similar to the Stanford Sleepiness Scale, requiring effort to administer, and measuring instantaneous sleepiness on one particular day.

Although there has been a failure to find consistent evidence of a relation between daytime sleepiness and OSAS, it has been suggested that sleepiness may be related to different factors. Also, important limitations of the existing research should be considered. First, the MSLT and the MWT may not adequately reveal diurnal impairment in sleepy patients and they do not strongly correlate with the subjective estimation. One factor may be that the field covered by each test may be different from the other, and the tests may not ever be comparable, as indicated later. Second, objective tests of sleepiness seem to measure a combination of sleep propensity and underlying arousal and studies are still needed systematically to evaluate motivational and psychologic factors that could affect the objective tests. Third, a decrease in mean sleep latency in the MSLT may occur even when the subjects rated themselves as alert, suggesting that subjective estimation measures different aspects of sleepiness [63–66].

There are other possibilities to consider as to why some OSAS patients have EDS, whereas others do not. First, subjects may not be able readily to perceive their daytime sleep propensity because they may have had slow adaptation. Second, nonsleepy patients may have an innate increased sleep onset threshold or a greater level of brain activation.

Third, a differential, patient-specific detrimental effect on cognitive function may exist and the capacity to elucidate other less obvious deficits with present tests is simply lacking. Neither objective nor subjective measures of alertness currently characterize the phenomenon of sleepiness with complete accuracy.

Consequences of sleepiness

Excessive sleepiness is recognized as an important public health problem. In patients with OSAS, sleepiness can impair social function and can have a major impact on the ability to carry on daily life activities, affecting quality of life (QOL), job performance, and contributing to motor vehicle accidents.

Quality of life

Impaired QOL is common among patients with OSAS [67–70]. These patients may experience moodiness, anxiety, lack of motivation, and compromised performance in social function, all of which may contribute to a lower QOL. EDS is a major symptom of OSAS, and seems to be related to a decreased QOL for patients with OSAS [71]. Although the progression of EDS symptoms and their effect on QOL have not been investigated in detail, and although it has been suggested that QOL is dependent on the patient's depressive status, several studies examining the association between EDS and QOL have shown that EDS, whether measured subjectively or objectively, was associated with decreased QOL [72,73]. Sleep deprivation can also lead to endocrine and metabolic changes associated with diabetes and weight gain; it is not uncommon for obese patients to have lower sleep efficiency and increased daytime sleepiness as measured by ESS [74], but these symptoms get worse when associated with OSAS. A large epidemiologic study of overweight subjects found that those with symptoms of OSAS reported poorer perceived health, lower economic income, increased odds of having had psychiatric care, multiple divorces, and impaired work performance compared with overweight subjects without symptoms of OSAS [75].

Functional impairments are normally mediated by symptom severity. QOL scales, such as the medical outcomes study Short Form-36, have been used to study the effect of OSAS on overall health. The Short Form-36 evaluates physical, emotional, and social functions; pain; general health; vitality; and mental health. This scale has revealed considerable impairments in samples of patients with OSAS, with vitality being most affected indicating a greater affect of OSAS on sleepiness [76].

Cognitive decline

Reports have described an association between OSAS and cognitive decline, and some have implicated EDS as the primary component of this association [77]. Patients with EDS secondary to OSAS can suffer from poor concentration and memory disturbance, making it difficult to function productively and efficiently on a day-to-day basis. A recent study showed two thirds of new patients with OSAS reported difficulties in work efficiency and performing new tasks [78]. Another study of industrial workers described negative effects of EDS on workers' well-being including higher rates of work accidents, less job satisfaction, and higher drug usage [79]. Patients may try to compensate for daytime sleepiness with behavioral adjustments, such as napping or taking stimulants.

Motor vehicle accidents

Also of major concern is sleepiness as an important cause of motor vehicle accidents, which often result in injury and death and cost billions of dollars each year. Habitual sleepiness while driving caused by a chronic condition, such as OSAS, occurs more frequently in middle age, whereas younger drivers more commonly experience sporadic sleepiness caused by sleep deprivation, alcohol, or drug abuse [80]. Drivers with OSAS may be two to seven times more likely to have a motor vehicle accident compared with normal drivers [81,82]. Research using the Psychomotor Vigilance Task to study reaction time and response in subjects with sleep-disordered breathing has shown lapses, slow response time, and variability in response time comparable with actions of sleep-deprived or alcohol-impaired subjects [52]. Interestingly, although drivers may know when they are sleepy, they cannot reliably predict when they have become impaired [83,84].

Previous studies have found that sleepiness measured by the ESS or sleep latency measured by the MSLT does not predict which drivers with OSAS will or will not have a motor vehicle accident [81,85–89]. Additionally, neither of these tests measure sleepiness while driving, making it difficult to measure a possible association of EDS with automobile accident risk. For these reasons it has been suggested that asking about excessive sleepiness while driving rather than asking about overall sleepiness may suggest which breathing-disordered sleepy drivers are at higher risk of having a motor vehicle accident [80]. Currently, there are no clinical methods that identify which drivers with OSAS are at higher or lower risk of causing an accident [90]. The ability subjectively to assess a patient's ability to drive safely may be complicated if the patient is reluctant to admit struggling with daytime sleepiness in fear of losing one's license. This may lead to difficulties with assessment of EDS based on subjective measures. A physician responsible for the care of a patient with OSAS should address the issue of safe driving; however, despite the advice of a physician, patients with excessive sleepiness may often continue to drive in traffic, highlighting the importance of preventive efforts that focus on increasing the awareness of the dangers of sleepiness behind the wheel.

Obesity, sleepiness, and obstructive sleep apnea

Many obese patients suffer from OSAS and EDS. It has even been suggested that there is a continuous interaction between weight increase, OSAS, and sleepiness. Any subject over 25 kg/m^2 is considered overweight, and any small increase in body mass index above 2 standard deviations of the norm (ie, above 25 kg/m^2) increases the chance of abnormal breathing particularly when supine and during REM sleep when weight distribution is android (ie, involving the abdomen). There is also occurrence of disturbances of metabolic and inflammatory factors that may again impact breathing during sleep. Such impairments may have a low key effect on sleep initially, but may have negative feedback on alertness, and may lead to sleep fragmentation and change in normal daytime activity levels with feedback on activity, food intake, and ultimately on weight. Presence of feedback loops with negative impact on both weight and alertness have been suggested; however, further research on these feedback loops with progressive worsening of signs and symptoms is needed.

Treatment options for excessive daytime sleepiness caused by obstructive sleep apnea syndrome

Nasal continuous positive airway pressure

Nasal CPAP therapy has emerged as the primary treatment for OSAS. It works either by increasing the intraluminal pressure in the pharynx, and thereby providing a mechanical pneumatic stent of the upper airway [91,92], or by increasing the lung volume, which then mediates the upper airway stabilizing effect [93] (and probably both factors are active). When used properly and consistently CPAP is the treatment of choice for symptoms of EDS secondary to OSAS. There is still debate, however, regarding the efficacy of this modality in treating symptoms of EDS. Currently, Medicare covers CPAP devices for patients with an AHI of ≥15, or patients with sequelae of OSAS and an AHI of 5 to 14. Such sequelae include

EDS, impaired cognition, hypertension, coronary artery disease, cerebrovascular accident, mood disorders, and insomnia.

Wright and coworkers [94] did a systematic review of the literature in 1997 looking at the treatment of OSAS with CPAP. Although the review consisted of studies that were often poorly designed (except for one randomized controlled trial with a small sample size) with nasal CPAP and control groups often not comparable at baseline, they still strongly suggested that CPAP may be effective in reducing EDS. There have been several randomized controlled trials, including sham CPAP as placebo-control, that consistently show that in patients with symptomatic mild to severe OSAS with daytime sleepiness, CPAP reduced subjective and objective measures of EDS and improved QOL [95–106]. Patients with OSAS who are experiencing EDS may benefit more from treatment with nasal CPAP than patients without EDS. Interestingly, when Barbé and coworkers [8] looked at patients with severe OSAS (with AHI >30 per hour) with no daytime sleepiness, they found 6 weeks of nasal CPAP treatment had no significant effect on objective and subjective measures of daytime sleepiness. The lack of substantial improvement in daytime sleepiness could be related to a "floor effect"; the score was already low at baseline and there is little room for it to decrease further. The results of this study may not be reliable because of the small sample size. A recent meta-analysis was performed by Patel and coworkers [107] looking at all published randomized controlled trials of nasal CPAP in patients with OSAS. They specifically addressed the effects of nasal CPAP on subjective and objective sleepiness, and found that CPAP therapy across diverse populations of patients with OSAS resulted in significant improvement in subjective (decreases ESS by 2.94 points) and objective (increases sleep latency by 0.93 minute) measures of sleepiness. Effectiveness of nasal CPAP for OSAS patients with EDS may be overestimated if negative trials were unpublished and thereby not included in this meta-analysis.

Compliance is an issue in administering nasal CPAP; patients need to maintain long-term use of the treatment for it to be effective. Kribbs and coworkers [108] reported that just one night without treatment was sufficient to reverse improvements, despite a reduced AHI compared with pretreatment levels. Although high success rates with long-term use of nasal CPAP [109] have been reported, most of these studies were subjective, and described rates based on patient self-reports. Later objective studies used time clocks built into CPAP machines to record use and found that rates of CPAP use are actually lower [110,111] and often irregular,

rarely meeting prescribed levels [108,112]. There are few long-term objective studies on nasal CPAP compliance.

There are several reasons for intolerance of nasal CPAP. First, patients using CPAP frequently report nasal discomfort. Often little effort is made to treat the nose, impaired by deviated septum and very commonly enlarged nasal inferior turbinates. Radiofrequency treatment of the nasal turbinates and aggressive treatment of nasal allergies help to decrease nocturnal disruption and residual sleepiness in OSAS patients. Second, problems have been encountered in calibrating nasal CPAP, as described by Thomas [40]. Calibration of nasal CPAP is performed by looking at the nasal flow curve, which does not detect the presence of small sleep disruptions that can only be seen with CAP scoring. Subsequently, inadequate treatment of OSAS with nasal CPAP slowly leads to the reappearance of complaints of tiredness and sleepiness. This is particularly true with autotitrating equipment: this equipment has several drawbacks. First, it is often set up with a very wide range of pressures (eg, 4–20 cm H_2O) and such settings increases the risk of overshoot of pressure and thereby arousals. Second, it reacts slowly to the need for increasing pressures and this fragments sleep. Last but not least, OSAS is associated, at least in a certain number of patients, with permanent neurologic lesions in the upper airways that have been well demonstrated since the early 1990s [113,114]. Treatment with nasal CPAP or bilevel CPAP never cures the permanent lesions. Slow evolution of these lesions over time related to the presence of local neuropathy is expected, and subsequently there is a need to reset pressures at higher levels. This was found in one of the authors' studies exploring patients with clear OSAS at entry (AHI ≥30 events per hour) [115]. This finding indicates the need to recalibrate nasal CPAP on a regular basis (probably every 2 years if no symptom occurs before). Recalibration should be done after interruption of CPAP for 1 night and even more so for 2 or 3 nights. This leads to increased nocturnal sleep disruption, initially demonstrated with CAP scoring during the night, and allows for better recalibration of the machine. Permanent neurologic lesions alone can lead to persistence of EDS, as explained later.

Residual daytime sleepiness

Even with regular use of nasal CPAP, residual daytime sleepiness may persist in patients with OSAS, and reasons for this are not always clear. Many patients who use nasal CPAP regularly may experience insufficient sleep syndrome, which leads to cumulative partial sleep loss and impaired alertness and performance during the day [116].

Interruption of nasal CPAP for 1 night and even more so for 2 or 3 nights before recalibration leads to increased nocturnal sleep disruption and reappearance of sleepiness. Patients using nasal CPAP for only part of the night experience abnormal breathing when CPAP is not being used. Appropriate nocturnal nasal CPAP usage is often described as at least 4 hours per night, but there is no evidence that partial usage of CPAP during the night is sufficient to avoid reappearance of sleepiness in the long run. There is no data supporting the notion of complete treatment of sleepiness with usage of nasal CPAP for only a part of sleep, and thereby recommending a minimum cutoff point of time of usage is speculative.

Persistence of residual EDS despite regular nasal CPAP use and appropriate calibration with monitoring of sleep EEG may also be seen. One study found an association between abdominal obesity and persistence of EDS [117]. Nasal CPAP is a poor treatment of chest bellows syndrome, related to clear abdominal obesity, particularly during rapid eye movement sleep. In this case, bilevel PAP gives a better approach, but residual sleepiness also has been seen with bilevel PAP. Two hypotheses have been raised in this regard. First, the potential association of obesity with EDS: obesity leads to metabolic and inflammatory changes that in themselves have an impact on sleep; however, good studies are lacking to support this plausible hypothesis. Second, the presence of central nervous system lesions that lead to persistence of EDS. Gora and coworkers [118] presented some preliminary data indicative of abnormal evoked potential during the NREM sleep in OSAS patients. A more definitive study was performed by Afifi and coworkers [119], which clearly showed the absence of evoked responses to inspiratory occlusion stimuli during NREM sleep. The absences of these responses may be related to local neuropathy, but secondary neuronal degenerative evolution also could have happened. Another possibility is that repetitive hypoxemia, arousals, and cerebral blood flow changes associated with sleep-disordered breathing for years could account for these permanent central nervous system changes, particularly in an individual with a certain genetic background. For example, the presence of the APOE-4 gene is considered to be a risk factor for neurodegenerative disease, and is currently shown to be present in a series of OSAS patients [120].

Sleepiness may also be indicative of other risk factor associations, such as a coexisting undiagnosed sleep disorder, and antihypertensive or other drug use. Also, as studies are looking at the potential association between obesity and EDS, other causes of EDS apart from sleep disordered breathing should be considered at, such as the association of EDS with mood disorders (eg, depression), metabolic factors like diabetes, and age.

Modafinil

Modafinil, 2-[(diphenylmethyl)-sulfinyl] acetamide, promotes wakefulness and is currently used in treatment of daytime sleepiness in adults suffering from narcolepsy. Use of amphetamine-like drugs for the treatment of EDS secondary to OSAS is limited because of psychiatric disturbances, interference with night sleep, and the addictive nature of these drugs [121]. Alternatively, modafinil is a nonamphetaminic drug that has fewer side effects, does not interfere with night-time sleep, and has lower potential for abuse [122,123].

This drug has no effect on the AHI, but has been shown to reduce objective sleepiness. Six prospective studies report the effects of modafinil on EDS in OSAS patients. Five studies [124–128] have reported the effects of modafinil (200–400 mg/day) on residual sleepiness in subjects with OSAS, despite compliance with CPAP [Table 3]. Across studies, modafinil consistently improved subjective and objective sleepiness, QOL, and vigilance compared with placebo. Dinges and Weaver [129] reported that the frequency of lapses of attention during Psychomotor Vigilance Task performance was significantly decreased, and both the median and slowest reaction times were significantly improved in subjects treated with nasal CPAP and modafinil compared with those treated with nasal CPAP and placebo. It is important to appreciate, however, that most (75%) subjects with severe sleepiness at baseline had multiple sleep latency times of <10 minutes on modafinil, despite effective CPAP and good compliance with therapy. Prescribing modafinil should not lessen the concerns of continued risk for driving-related motor vehicle accidents caused by sleepiness in patients with OSAS.

Adverse events attributed to modafinil include headaches, nervousness, and rhinitis (5%–10% higher likelihood than placebo). A 2-week, placebo-controlled study with one dose (400 mg) of modafinil [124] demonstrated that patients using this stimulant had a modest but significant reduction in their nightly usage of nasal CPAP. This negative effect was not found in two other double-blind studies of longer duration [125–127], or in the open-label continuation study [128].

Acute administration of modafinil increases arterial blood pressure and heart rate [126]. With exercise, modafinil intake (300 mg) results in a

Table 3: Randomized studies showing improved outcomes for treatment with modafinil in patients residual EDS despite compliance with CPAP

Study	No. of subjects	Dose/number of days treated	Outcome measures for modafinil group (compared with placebo group)	P-value
Kingshott et al	32	200 mg × 5 d 400 mg × 9 d	Improved alertness as measured by MWT. No significant improvement with ESS or MSLT. FOSQ showed trend of improved vigilance.	0.02
Pack et al	157	200 mg × 7 d 400 mg × 21d	Improved alertness as measured by MWT. Lower ESS score. Longer sleep latency as measured by MSLT (slightly worsened for placebo).	<.001 0.0001 0.021
Heitmann et al	24	300 mg × 2 d	Shorter mean reaction time as measured by vigilance test. Longer mean sleep latency as measured by MSLT.	0.0023 0.0001
Black et al	305	2 groups 200 mg × 84 d (12wk) 400 mg × 84 d (12wk)	68% patients showed overall clinical improvement in both treated groups. Improved alertness as measured by MWT. Lower ESS score. Improved FOSQ score.	<.001 ≤.0001 <.0001 <.001
Schwartz et al	125	(12wk) 200 mg week 1 400 mg week 2 By week 12, 17% of patients were on 200 mg, 19% on 300 mg, and 64% on 400 mg	73% patients showed overall clinical improvement. Improved FOSQ score. Lower ESS score.	0.001 <.0001 <.001

Abbreviations: ESS, Epworth Sleepiness Scale; FOSQ, Functional Outcomes of Sleep Questionnaire; MSLT, Multiple Sleep Latence Test; MWT, Maintenance of Wakefulness Test.

significant increase in mean, systolic, and diastolic pressures and heart rate, compared with placebo. No long-term investigation of cardiovascular outcomes with the use of modafinil has been reported.

In summary, the double-blind, placebo-controlled clinical trials that examined the effectiveness of modafinil in patients compliant with nasal CPAP in treating residual sleepiness found that modafinil subjectively and objectively improved vigilance and sleepiness for as long as 12 weeks. Modafinil, however, does not fully reverse severe baseline sleepiness. It seems that 200 mg daily is as efficacious as 400 mg. There is concern that compliance with nasal CPAP may decrease with modafinil usage [124], and this requires further study. In the interim, patients must be advised of the importance to continue CPAP therapies and physicians must carefully monitor CPAP compliance in this group. The question of the long-term effect of modafinil on the hemodynamic status of OSA patients treated with nasal CPAP remains unresolved. Nevertheless, findings from one study measuring cardiovascular responses to modafinil raise the possibility that modafinil use may increase blood pressure [126]. Careful consideration of an individual patient's

health risks (the risk of motor vehicle accidents compared with the risk of cardiovascular morbidities) is required before prescribing modafinil.

Modafinil may also prove useful in patients with mild OSAS, who often go untreated because of the relatively inconvenient nature of current treatments [129,130]. Although modafinil does seem to enhance alertness, it does not treat the underlying pathophysiology of airway collapse in OSAS and may not be of therapeutic benefit for patients who are not receiving adequate prophylactic treatment for apneas and hypopneas, and may result in serious complications because of long-term OSAS that has gone untreated.

References

[1] Klink M, Quan SF. Prevalence of reported sleep disturbances in a general adult population and their relationship to obstructive airways diseases. Chest 1987;91:540–6.

[2] Young T, Palta M, Dempsey J, et al. The occurrence of sleep disordered breathing among middle-aged adults. N Engl J Med 1993;328: 1230–5.

[3] National Commission on Sleep Disorders Research. Wake up America: a national sleep alert. Washington: Government Printing Office; 1993.

[4] Dement W, Carskadon M, Richardson G. (1978) Excessive daytime sleepiness in the sleep apnea syndrome. In: Guilleminault C, Dement WC, editors. Sleep apnea syndromes. New York: Alan R Liss; 1978. p. 23–46.

[5] McNamara SG, Grunstein RR, Sullivan E. Obstructive sleep apnoea. Thorax 1993;48:754–64.

[6] Guilleminault C, Stoohs R, Duncan S. Snoring (I): daytime sleepiness in regular heavy snorers. Chest 1991;99:40–8.

[7] Findley LJ, Fabizio M, Thommi G, et al. Severity of sleep apnea and automobile crashes. N Engl J Med 1989;320:868–9.

[8] Barbé F, Mayoralas LR, Duran J, et al. Treatment with continuous positive airway pressure is not effective in patients with sleep apnea but no daytime sleepiness: a randomized, controlled trial. Ann Intern Med 2001;134:1015–23.

[9] Chervin RD. Sleepiness, fatigue, tiredness, and lack of energy in obstructive sleep apnea. Chest 2000;118:372–9.

[10] Martin SE, Engleman HM, Deary IJ, et al. The effect of sleep fragmentation on daytime function. Am J Respir Crit Care Med 1996;153: 1328–32.

[11] Philip P, Stoohs R, Guilleminault C. Sleep fragmentation in normals: a model for sleepiness associated with upper airway resistance syndrome. Sleep 1994;17:242–7.

[12] Remmers JE, deGroot WJ, Sauerland EK, et al. Pathogenesis of upper airway occlusion during sleep. J Appl Physiol 1978;44:931–8.

[13] Stepanski E, Lamphere J, Badia P, et al. Sleep fragmentation and daytime sleepiness. Sleep 1984;7:18–26.

[14] Younes M. Role of arousals in the pathogenesis of obstructive sleep apnea. Am J Respir Crit Care Med 2004;169:623–33.

[15] Bonnet M, Carley D, Carskadon M, et al. EEG arousals: scoring rules and examples: a preliminary report from the Sleep Disorders Atlas Task Force of the American Sleep Disorders Association. Sleep 1992;15:173–84.

[16] Guilleminault C, Partinen M, Quera-Salva MA, et al. Determinants of daytime sleepiness in obstructive sleep apnea. Chest 1988;94:32–7.

[17] Roth T, Hartse KM, Zorik F, et al. Multiple naps and the evaluation of daytime sleepiness in patients with upper airway sleep apnea. Sleep 1980;3:425–40.

[18] Kingshott RN, Engleman HM, Deary IJ, et al. Does arousal frequency predict daytime function? Eur Respir J 1998;12:1264–70.

[19] Partinen M, Guilleminault C. Daytime sleepiness and vascular morbidity at seven-year follow-up in obstructive sleep apnea patients. Chest 1990;97:27–32.

[20] Goncalves MA, Paiva T, Ramos E, et al. Obstructive sleep apnea syndrome, sleepiness, and quality of life. Chest 2004;125:2091–6.

[21] Cheshire K, Engleman H, Deary I, et al. Factors impairing daytime performance in patients with the sleep apnoea/hypopnoea syndrome. Arch Intern Med 1992;152:538–41.

[22] Mosko SS, Dickel MJ, Ashurst J. Night-to-night variability in sleep apnea and sleep-related periodic leg movements in the elderly. Sleep 1988; 11:340–8.

[23] Rees K, Spence DPS, Earis JE, et al. Arousal responses from apneic events during NREM sleep. Am J Respir Crit Care Med 1995;152: 1016–21.

[24] Svanborg E, Guilleminault C. EEG frequency changes during sleep apneas. Sleep 1996;19: 248–54.

[25] Terzano MG, Parrino L, Shierieri A, et al. Atlas, rules and recording techniques for the scoring of cyclic alternating pattern (CAP) in human sleep. Sleep Med 2001;2:537–54.

[26] Chervin RD, Burns JW, Subotic NS, et al. Method for detection of respiratory cycle-related EEG changes in sleep disordered breathing. Sleep 2004;27:105–9.

[27] Chervin RD, Guilleminault C. Assessment of sleepiness in clinical practice. Nat Med 1995;1: 1252–3.

[28] Reimao R, Lemni H, Belluomini J. Obstructive apnea during sleep: clinical and polygraphic evaluation of 150 cases. Arq Neuropsiquiatr 1985; 43:140–6.

[29] Heinzer R, Gaudreau H, Decary A, et al. Slow-wave activity in sleep apnea patients before and after continuous positive airway pressure treatment: contribution to daytime sleepiness. Chest 2001;119:1807–13.

[30] Pitson D, Chhina N, Knijn S, et al. Changes in pulse transit time and pulse rate as markers of arousal from sleep in normal subjects. Clin Sci Colch 1994;87:269–73.

[31] Davies RJO, Belt PJ, Robert SJ, et al. Arterial blood pressure responses to graded transient arousal from sleep in normal humans. J Appl Physiol 1993;74:1123–30.

[32] Martin SE, Wraith PK, Deary IJ, et al. The effect of nonvisible sleep fragmentation on daytime function. Am J Respir Crit Care Med 1995;155: 1596–601.

[33] Bennett LS, Langford BA, Stradling JR, et al. Sleep fragmentation indices as predictors of daytime sleepiness and nCPAP response in obstructive sleep apnea. Am J Respir Crit Care Med 1998;158:778–86.

[34] Guilleminault C, Abad V, Stoohs R. Effects of CNS activation versus EEG arousal during sleep on heart rate response and daytime tests. Clin Neurophysiol, in press.

[35] Roehrs T, Zorick F, Wittig R, et al. Predictors of objective level of daytime sleepiness in patients with sleep-related breathing disorders. Chest 1989;95:1202–6.

[36] Colt HG, Haas H, Rich GB. Hypoxemia vs. sleep fragmentation as cause of excessive daytime sleepiness in obstructive sleep apnea. Chest 1991; 100:1542–8.

[37] Gottlieb DJ, Yao Q, Redline S, et al. Does snoring predict sleepiness independently of apnea and hypopnea frequency? Am J Respir Crit Care Med 2000;162:1512–7.

[38] Ferrillo F, Gabarra M, Nobili L, et al. Comparison between visual scoring of cyclic alternating pattern (CAP) and computerized assessment of slow EEG oscillations in the transition from light to deep non-REM sleep. J Clin Neurophysiol 1997;14:210–6.

[39] Terzano MG, Parrino L, Boselli M, et al. Polysomnographic analysis of arousal responses in obstructive sleep apnea syndrome by means of the cyclic alternating pattern. J Clin Neurophysiol 1996;13:145–55.

[40] Thomas RJ. Cyclic alternating pattern and positive airway pressure titration. Sleep Med 2002;3: 315–22.

[41] Chervin RD, Burns JW, Ruzicka DL. Electroencephalographic changes during respiratory cycles predict sleepiness in sleep apnea. Am J Respir Crit Care Med 2005;171:652–8.

[42] Guilleminault C, Stoohs R, Kim Y, et al. Sleep-related upper airway disordered breathing in women. Ann Intern Med 1995;122:493–501.

[43] Carskadon MA, Dement WC. Sleep tendency: an objective measure of sleep loss. Sleep Res 1977;6:200.

[44] Johns MW. Sensitivity and specificity of the multiple sleep latency test (MSLT), the maintenance of wakefulness test and the Epworth sleepiness scale: failure of the MSLT as a gold standard. J Sleep Res 2000;9:5–11.

[45] Devoto A, Lucidi F, Violani C, et al. Effects of different sleep reductions on daytime sleepiness. Sleep 1999;22:336–43.

[46] George CF, Boudreau AC, Smiley A. Comparison of simulated driving performance in narcolepsy and sleep apnea patients. Sleep 1996;19: 711–7.

[47] George CF, Boudreau AC, Smiley A. Effects of nasal CPAP on simulated driving performance in patients with obstructive sleep apnoea. Thorax 1997;52:648–53.

[48] Mitler MM, Gujavarty KS, Browman CP. Maintenance of Wakefulness test: a polysomnographic technique for evaluation treatment efficacy in patients with excessive somnolence. Electeroencephalogr Clin Neurophysiol 1982; 53:658–61.

[49] Banks S, Barnes M, Tarquinio N, et al. Factors associated with maintenance of wakefulness test mean sleep latency in patients with mild to moderate obstructive sleep apnoea and normal subjects. J Sleep Res 2004;13:71–8.

[50] Sauter C, Asenbaum S, Popovic R, et al. Excessive daytime sleepiness in patients suffering from different levels of obstructive sleep apnoea syndrome. J Sleep Res 2000;9: 293–301.

[51] Bennett LS, Stradling JR, Davies RJ. A behavioral test to assess daytime sleepiness in obstructive sleep apnoea. J Sleep Res 1997;6:142–5.

[52] Dinges DF, Powell JW. Microcomputer analyses of performance on a portable simple visual RT task during sustained operations. Behav Res Methods Instrum Comput 1985;17: 652–5.

[53] John MW. A new method for measuring daytime sleepiness: the Epworth Sleepiness Scale. Sleep 1991;14:540–5.

[54] John MW. Sleepiness in different situations measured by the Epworth Sleepiness Scale. Sleep 1994;17:703–10.

[55] Chervin RD, Aldrich MS, Pickett R, et al. Comparison of the results of the Epworth Sleepiness Scale and the Multiple Sleep Latency Test. J Psychosom Res 1997;42:145–55.

[56] Chervin RD, Aldrich MS. The Epworth Sleepiness Scale may not reflect objective measures of sleepiness or sleep apnea. Neurology 1999;52: 125–31.

[57] Punjabi NM, Bandeen-Roche K, Young T. Predictors of objective sleep tendency in the general population. Sleep 2003;26:678–83.

[58] Bennett LS, Langford BA, Stradling JR, et al. Health status in obstructive sleep apnea: relationship with sleep fragmentation and daytime sleepiness, and effects of continuous positive airway pressure treatment. Am J Respir Crit Care Med 1999;159:1884–90.

[59] Hoddes E, Dement WC, Zarcone V. The development and use of the Stanford Sleepiness Scale (SSS). Psychophysiology 1972;9:150.

[60] Hoddes E, Zarcone V, Smythe H, et al. Quantification of sleepiness: a new approach. Psychophysiology 1973;10:431–6.

[61] Herscovitch J, Broughton R. Sensitivity of the Stanford Sleepiness Scale to the effects of cumulative partial sleep deprivation and recovery oversleeping. Sleep 1981;4:83–92.

[62] Cook Y, Schmitt F, Berry D, et al. The effects of nocturnal sleep, sleep disordered breathing and periodic movements of sleep on the objective and subjective assessment of daytime somnolence in healthy aged adults. Sleep Res 1988; 17:95.

[63] Chervin RD, Kraemer HC, Guilleminault C. Correlates of sleep latency on the multiple sleep latency test in a clinical population. Electroencephalogr Clin Neurophysiol 1995;95:147–53.

[64] Poceta JS, Timms RM, Jeong DO, et al. Maintenance of wakefulness test in obstructive sleep apnea syndrome. Chest 1992;101:893–7.

[65] Sangal RB, Thomas L, Mitler MM. Maintenance of wakefulness test and multiple sleep latency test: measurement of different abilities in patients with sleep disorders. Chest 1992; 101:898–902.

[66] Johns MW. Sensitivity and specificity of the

multiple sleep latency test (MSLT), the maintenance of wakefulness test and the Epworth Sleepiness Scale: failure of the MSLT as a gold standard. J Sleep Res 2000;9:5–11.

[67] Smith IE, Shneerson JM. Is the SF-36 sensitive to sleep disruption? A study in subjects with sleep apnea. J Sleep Res 1995;4:183–8.

[68] Jenkinson C, Stradling J, Petersen S. Comparison of three measures of quality of life outcome in the evaluation of continuous positive airways pressure therapy for sleep apnoea. J Sleep Res 1997;6:199–204.

[69] Flemons WW, Reimer MA. Development of a disease-specific health-related quality of life questionnaire for sleep apnea. Am J Respir Crit Care Med 1998;158:494–503.

[70] Weaver TE, Laizner AM, Evans LK, et al. An instrument to measure functional status outcomes for disorders of excessive sleepiness. Sleep 1997;20:835–43.

[71] Briones B, Adams N, Strauss M, et al. Relationship between sleepiness and general health status. Sleep 1996;19:583–8.

[72] Bennet LS, Barbour C, Langford B, et al. Health status in obstructive sleep apnea: relationship with sleep fragmentation and daytime sleepiness, and effects of continuous positive airway pressure. Am J Respir Crit Care Med 1999;159:1884–90.

[73] Baldwin CM, Griffith MPH, Neito J, et al. The association of sleep symptoms with quality of life in the sleep heart health study. Sleep 2001;24:96–105.

[74] Resta O, Foschino Barbaro MP, et al. Low sleep quality and daytime sleepiness in obese patients without sleep apnea syndrome. J Intern Med 2003;253:536–43.

[75] Grunstein RR, Stenlöf JA, Hedner JA, et al. Impact of self-reported breathing disturbances on psychosocial performance in the Swedish obese subjects (SOS) study. Sleep 1995;18:635–43.

[76] Engleman HM, Davis NJ. Sleep 4: Sleepiness, cognitive function, and quality of life in obstructive sleep apoena/hypopnoea syndrome. Thorax 2004;59:618–22.

[77] Cohen-Zion M, Stepnowsky C, Marler M, et al. Changes in cognitive function associated with sleep-disordered breathing in older people. J Am Geriatr Soc 2004;49:1622–7.

[78] Ulfberg J, Carter N, Talback M, et al. Excessive daytime sleepiness at work and subjective work performance in the general population and among heavy snorers and patients with obstructive sleep apnea. Chest 1996;110:659–63.

[79] Lavie P. Sleep habits and sleep disturbances in industrial workers in Israel: main findings and some characteristics of workers complaining of excessive daytime sleepiness. Sleep 1981;4:147–58.

[80] Masa JF, Rubio M, Findley LJ, et al. Habitually sleepy drivers have a high frequency of automobile crashes associated with respiratory disorders during sleep. Am J Respir Crit Care Med 2000;162:1407–12.

[81] Young T, Blustein J, Finn L, et al. Sleep-disordered breathing and motor vehicle accidents in a population-based sample of employed adults. Sleep 1997;20:608–13.

[82] Teran-Santos J, Jimenez-Gomez A, Cordero-Guevara J. The association between sleep apnea and the risk of traffic accidents. N Engl J Med 1999;340:847–51.

[83] Powell NB, Schechtman KB, Riley RW, et al. The road to danger: the comparative risks of driving while sleepy. Laryngoscope 2001;111:887–93.

[84] Dinges DF. The nature of sleepiness: causes, contexts, and consequences. In: Stunkard AJ, Baum A, editors. Eating, sleeping, and sex. Hillsdale (NJ): Lawrence Erlbaum Associates; 1989. p. 147–79.

[85] Findley LJ, Unverzagt ME, Suratt PM. Automobile accidents involving patients with obstructive sleep apnea. Am Rev Respir Dis 1988;138:337–40.

[86] Krieger J, Meslier N, Lebrun T, et al. Accidents in obstructive sleep apnea patients treated with nasal continuous positive airway pressure. Chest 1997;112:1561–6.

[87] Barbé F, Pericás J, Muñoz A, et al. Automobile accidents in patients with sleep apnea syndrome. Am J Respir Crit Care Med 1998;158:18–22.

[88] Terán J, Jiménez A, Cordero J. The association between sleep apnea and the risk of traffic accidents. N Engl J Med 1999;340:847–51.

[89] Stoohs RA, Bingham L, Itoi A, et al. Sleep and sleep-disordered breathing in commercial long-haul truck drivers. Chest 1995;107:1275–82.

[90] George CF, Findley LJ, Hack MA, et al. Across-country viewpoints on sleepiness during driving. Am J Respir Crit Care Med 2002;165:746–9.

[91] Sullivan CE, Issa FG, Berthon-Jones M, et al. Reversal of obstructive sleep apnoea by continuous positive airway pressure applied through the nares. Lancet 1981;1:862–5.

[92] Alex CG, Aronson RM, Onal E, et al. Effects of continuous positive airway pressure on upper airway and respiratory muscle activity. J Appl Physiol 1987;62:2026–30.

[93] Begle RL, Badr S, Skatrud JB, et al. Effect of lung inflation on pulmonary resistance during NREM sleep. Am Rev Respir Dis 1990;141:854–60.

[94] Wright J, Johns R, Watt I, et al. Health effects of obstructive sleep apnoea and the effectiveness of continuous positive airway pressure: a systematic review of the research evidence. BMJ 1997;314:851–60.

[95] Engleman HM, Cheshire KE, Deary IJ, et al. Daytime sleepiness, cognitive performance and mood after continuous positive airway pressure for the sleep apnoea/hypopnoea syndrome. Thorax 1993;48:911–4.

[96] Engleman HM, Martin SE, Deary IJ, et al. Effect of continuous positive airway pressure treatment on daytime function in sleep apnoea/hypopnoea syndrome. Lancet 1994;343:572–5.

[97] Engleman HM, Martin SE, Kingshott RN, et al. Randomised placebo controlled trial of daytime function after continuous positive airway pressure (CPAP) therapy for the sleep apnoea/hypopnoea syndrome. Thorax 1998;53:341–5.

[98] Munoz A, Mayoralas LR, Barbé F, et al. Long-term effects of CPAP on daytime functioning in patients with sleep apnoea syndrome. Eur Respir J 2000;15:676–81.

[99] Derderian SS, Bridenbaugh RH, Rajagopal KR. Neuropsychologic symptoms in obstructive sleep apnea improve after treatment with nasal continuous positive airway pressure. Chest 1988;94: 1023–7.

[100] Lamphere J, Roehrs T, Wittig R, et al. Recovery of alertness after CPAP in apnea. Chest 1989; 96:1364–7.

[101] Monasterio C, Vidal S, Duran J, et al. Effectiveness of continuous positive airway pressure in mild sleep apnea-hypopnea syndrome. Am J Respir Crit Care Med 2001;164:939–43.

[102] Ballester E, Badia JR, Hernandez L, et al. Evidence of the effectiveness of continuous positive airway pressure in the treatment of sleep apnea/hypopnea syndrome. Am J Respir Crit Care Med 1999;159:495–501.

[103] Engleman HM, Kingshott RN, Wraith PK, et al. Randomized placebo-controlled crossover trial of continuous positive airway pressure for mild sleep apnea/hypopnea syndrome. Am J Respir Crit Care Med 1999;159:461–7.

[104] Stradling JR, Davies RJ. Is more NCPAP better? Sleep 2000;23(Suppl 4):S150–3.

[105] Jenkinson C, Davies RJ, Mullins R, et al. Comparison of therapeutic and sub therapeutic nasal continuous positive airway pressure for obstructive sleep apnoea: a randomised prospective parallel trial. Lancet 1999;353:2100–5.

[106] Montserrat JM, Ferrer M, Hernandez L, et al. Effectiveness of CPAP treatment in daytime function in sleep apnea syndrome: a randomized controlled study with an optimized placebo. Am J Respir Crit Care Med 2001;164: 608–13.

[107] Patel SR, White DP, Malhotra A, et al. Continuous positive airway pressure therapy for treating sleepiness in a diverse population with obstructive sleep apnea: results of a meta-analysis. Arch Intern Med 2003;163:565–71.

[108] Kribbs NB, Pack AI, Kline LR, et al. Objective measurement of patterns of nasal CPAP use by patients with obstructive sleep apnea. Am Rev Respir Dis 1993;147:887–95.

[109] Sanders MH, Gruendl CA, Rogers RM. Patient compliance with nasal CPAP therapy for sleep apnea. Chest 1986;90:330–3.

[110] Engleman HM, Martin SE, Douglas NJ. Compliance with CPAP therapy in patients with the sleep apnea/hypopnea syndrome. Thorax 1994; 49:263–6.

[111] Meurice J, Dore P, Paquereau J, et al. Predictive factors of long-term compliance with nasal continuous positive airway pressure treatment in sleep apnea syndrome. Chest 1994;105:429–33.

[112] Reeves-Hoche MK, Meek R, Zwillich CW. Nasal CPAP: an objective evaluation of patient compliance. Am J Respir Crit Care Med 1994;149: 149–54.

[113] Edstrom L, Larsson H, Larsson L. Neurogenic efforts on the palatopharyngeal muscle in patients with obstructive sleep apnea: a muscle biopsy study. J Neurol Neurosurg Psychiatry 1992;55:916–20.

[114] Friberg D, Ansved T, Borg K, et al. Histological indications of a progressive snorers disease in an upper-airway muscle. Am J Respir Crit Care Med 1998;157:586–93.

[115] Guilleminault C, Huang YS, Kirisoglu C, et al. OSAS a neurological disorder? A follow-up nasal CPAP study. Ann Neurol 2005;58:880–7.

[116] Bonnet MH, Arand DL. Clinical effects of sleep fragmentation versus sleep deprivation. Sleep Med Rev 2003;7:293–5.

[117] Guilleminault C, Philip P. Tiredness and somnolence despite initial treatment of obstructive sleep apnea syndrome (what to do when an OSAS patient stays hyper somnolent despite treatment). Sleep 1996;19(9 Suppl):S117–22.

[118] Gora J, Trinder J, Pierce R, et al. Respiratory evoked potentials in moderate obstructive sleep apnea syndrome: evidence of a sleep specific blunted cortical response. Am J Respir Crit Care Med 2002;166:1225–34.

[119] Afifi L, Guilleminault C, Colrain I. Sleep and respiratory stimulus specific dampening of cortical responsiveness in OSAS patients. Respir Physiol Neurobiol 2003;136:221–34.

[120] Kadotani H, Kadotani T, Young T, et al. Association between apolipoprotein E epsilon4 and sleep-disordered breathing in adults. JAMA 2001;285:2888–90.

[121] Parkes JD, Baraitser M, Marsden CD, et al. Natural history, symptoms, and treatment of the narcoleptic syndrome. Acta Neurol Scand 1975;52:337–53.

[122] Saletu B, Frey R, Krupka M, et al. Differential effects of a new central adrenergic agonist-modafinil-and D-amphetamine on sleep and early morning behavior in young healthy volunteers. Int J Clin Pharmacol Res 1989;9:183–95.

[123] Billiard M, Besset A, Montplaisir J, et al. Modafinil: a double-blind multicentric study. Sleep 1994;17:S107–12.

[124] Kingshott R, Venelle M, Coleman E, et al. Randomized, double-blind, placebo-controlled crossover trial of modafinil in the treatment of residual excessive daytime sleepiness in the sleep apnea-hypopnea syndrome. Am J Respir Crit Care Med 2001;163:918–23.

[125] Pack A, Black J, Schwartz J, et al. Modafinil as

an adjunct therapy for daytime sleepiness in obstructive sleep apnea. Am J Respir Crit Care Med 2001;164:1675–81.

[126] Heitmann J, Cassel W, Grote L, et al. Does short-term treatment with modafinil affect blood pressure in patients with obstructive sleep apnea? Clin Pharmacol Ther 1999;65:328–35.

[127] Black J, Hirshkowitz M. Modafinil for treatment of residual excessive sleepiness in nasal continuous positive airway pressure-treated obstructive sleep apnea-hypopnea syndrome. Sleep 2005;28:464–71.

[128] Schwartz J, Hirshkowitz M, Erman MK, et al.

Modafinil as adjunct therapy for daytime sleepiness in obstructive sleep apnea: a 12 week open-label study. Chest 2003;124:2192–9.

[129] Dinges DF, Weaver TE. Effects of modafinil on sustained attention performance and quality of life in OSA patients with residual sleepiness while being treated with nCPAP. Sleep Med 2003;4:393–402.

[130] Newcombe JP, Desai A, Joffe D, et al. Modafinil improves alertness and driving simulator performance in sleep-deprived mild obstructive sleep apnoea (OSA) patients. J Sleep Res 2004; 13(Suppl 1):443J.

ELSEVIER SAUNDERS

SLEEP
MEDICINE
CLINICS

Sleep Med Clin 1 (2006) 79–88

Chronic Hypersomnia

Yves Dauvilliers, MD, PhD[a,b,*], Michel Billiard, MD[c]

Chronic hypersomnias correspond to numerous etiologies of patients with a complaint of excessive daytime sleepiness. The identification of specific phenotypes of hypersomnia is useful to classify patients into different clinical diagnosis. Idiopathic hypersomnia remains a relatively poorly defined and rare condition, and the final diagnosis rests on the exclusion of other causes of hypersomnias. Although considerable progress has been made in understanding hypersomnias in the last few years with the discovery of the hypocretin system, the pathophysiology of idiopathic hypersomnia is still totally unknown. There is a definite need to further develop sleep laboratory investigations to assess the correct diagnosis. Studies at the genetic and biological levels are needed also to further our understanding of the pathophysiology of IH and to develop specific treatment.

Idiopathic hypersomnia

Idiopathic hypersomnia (IH) is a rare condition of excessive daytime sleepiness. IH remains a rela- tively poorly defined condition because of the ab- sence of specific symptoms, such as cataplexy or sleep apnea. The recent International Classifica- tion of Sleep Disorders (ICSD) classifies IH in two forms: IH with long sleep time and IH without long sleep time [1]. Differential diagnosis is fre- quent and insufficiently recognized. Pathophysiol- ogy is almost totally unknown and more studies are needed to recognize IH as an independent disorder in terms of clinical and biologic processes.

History

IH is a rare condition, 5 to 10 times less frequent than narcolepsy, which has been confused with narcolepsy for a long time. Roth et al [2–4] was the first in the late 1950s to describe this disorder characterized by excessive daytime sleepiness, pro- longed nocturnal sleep, sleep drunkenness, and the absence of irresistible sleep episodes and cataplexy. Two clinical forms of IH were distinguished by Roth: the monosymptomatic form characterized by excessive daytime sleepiness only, and the poly- symptomatic form characterized by excessive day-

[a] Service de Neurologie B, Hôpital Gui-de-Chauliac, 80 Avenue Augustin Fliche, 34295 Montpellier Cedex 5, France
[b] INSERM E0361, Hôpital La Colombière, Montpellier, France
[c] Faculté de Médecine, Hôpital Gui-de-Chauliac, 80 Avenue Augustin Fliche, 34295 Montpellier Cedex 5, France
* Corresponding author. Service de Neurologie B, Hôpital Gui-de-Chauliac, 80 Avenue Augustin Fliche, 34295 Montpellier Cedex 5, France.
E-mail address: y-dauvilliers@chu-montpellier.fr (Y. Dauvilliers).

doi:10.1016/j.jsmc.2005.11.007

time sleepiness, abnormally long nocturnal and diurnal sleep, and sleep drunkenness on awakening. In contrast to narcolepsy, diurnal sleep is not irrepressible and does not restore normal alertness. Nocturnal sleep remains undisturbed but with a delayed morning awakening.

Several terms were used to define this hypersomnia: hypersomnia with sleep drunkenness, essential narcolepsy, non–rapid eye movement (NREM) sleep narcolepsy, idiopathic central nervous system hypersomnia. The term "idiopathic hypersomnia" was finally approved and included in the ICSD in 1990 [5] and defined as "a disorder of presumed central nervous system cause that is associated with a normal or prolonged major sleep episode and excessive sleepiness consisting of prolonged (1–2 hours) sleep episodes of non-REM sleep." A possible overlap between narcolepsy without cataplexy and monosymptomatic IH can exist, however, with similar clinical features between the two conditions [6,7]. Recently, the revised version of the ICSD [1] proposes two forms of IH: IH with long sleep time, which corresponds to the polysymptomatic form; and IH without long sleep time, which corresponds to the monosymptomatic form. Although called "idiopathic," this hypersomnia must not correspond to all diagnosis of hypersomnia that do not have well-defined origin [1,8].

IH is individualized based on clinical features and polysomnography (PSG) followed by a Multiple Sleep Latency Test (MSLT), which confirms the objective hypersomnia. PSG shows a sleep of normal quality with few awakenings, a normal proportion of the different sleep stages, and normal sleep efficiency [1]. Sleep apnea, periodic leg movements, and crescendo (by monitoring of esophageal pressure) must not be present. In that sense, the upper airway resistance syndrome [9], first described in 1993, revealed that many patients with previous IH diagnosis may actually have the upper airway resistance syndrome diagnosis.

Although important advances have been made in the clinical description of IH, no clear biologic or genetic markers are available. The normality of cerebrospinal fluid (CSF) hypocretin-1 level and the absence of association with HLA DQB1*0602 reinforce the possible overlap between patients affected with IH without long sleep time and those affected with narcolepsy without cataplexy [10–13].

Epidemiology

The diagnosis of IH, especially IH without long sleep time, is often overestimated; however, the prevalence of IH in the general population is unknown. The nosologic uncertainty and the rarity of the condition may explain the absence of any epidemiologic study. Recent sleep center reports revealed a ratio of one patient with IH for 10 with narcolepsy with cataplexy [6,14].

In contrast to narcolepsy, the age at onset is not always easy to pinpoint because of the insidious development of the condition. In most patients, however, the disease starts before 30 years of age [8,14].

There is no indication of gender predominance. The familial aspect of patients with IH is frequent and known since the first description of the disease [15]. In the authors' experience of 28 well-defined IH cases with long sleep time, 67.85% of patients have at least one relative affected with hypersomnia with a possible autosomal-dominant mode of transmission.

Clinical signs

In both forms of IH with and without long sleep time, patients have a complaint of excessive daytime sleepiness occurring almost daily for at least 3 months. Clinical diagnosis of IH also requires that hypersomnia is not better explained by another sleep disorder, medical or mental disorder, medication use, or substance use disorder [1].

IH with long sleep time is a well-defined clinical entity. Patients tend to complain of constant excessive daytime sleepiness with the Epworth Sleepiness Scale above 11. This daytime sleepiness leads to long (more than 1 hour) and unrefreshing naps, less irresistible than in narcolepsy. The nocturnal sleep is also long (more than 10 hours) and uninterrupted, but does not restore normal alertness. Awakening after nighttime or daytime sleep is difficult. These patients may be confused and unable to react adequately to external stimuli on awakening for up to 1 to 3 hours, a state referred to as "sleep drunkenness" or "sleep inertia." Episodes of automatic behavior can occur during this drowsy state especially in the morning, with frequent amnesia postepisodes [4]. Total sleep time, whenever made possible, mainly during holidays and weekends, is always above 12 hours.

In contrast, patients affected with IH without long sleep time never report "sleep inertia." This condition is characterized by isolated excessive daytime sleepiness. Patients complain of recurrent daytime naps more irresistible and more refreshing than in IH with long sleep time. Nocturnal sleep is normal, sometimes prolonged (more than 6 hours but less than 10 hours) but always refreshing [1]. A clinical overlap between IH without long sleep time and narcolepsy without cataplexy may be hypothesized. The presence of both conditions within the same family has also been reported [6].

Although cataplexy is always absent in IH, sleep paralysis and hypnagogic or hypnopompic hallucinations may be present as in other sleep disorders or in the general population. Other symptoms have been reported, such as headache (mainly migraine or tension-type headache), and manifestations of neurovegetative impairment with cold hands and feet, orthostatic hypotension, or syncope. Those symptoms are nonspecific, however, and may be found within same proportion in other sleep disorders and in the general population. Mood changes are also frequently reported in IH, probably as in other chronic sleep disorders impeding quality of life, such as narcolepsy with cataplexy. Mood changes must not reach the point of major depression, however, psychiatric hypersomnia being a main clinical differential diagnosis of IH [16].

Evolution of IH over time is not well known but seems to be stable in severity without any spontaneous disappearance of the symptoms. The psychosocial and professional consequences are similar to those found in narcolepsy [17].

Polysomnography and other laboratory findings

Polysomnography

PSG is required to ascertain the diagnosis and to exclude other etiologies of hypersomnia. PSG demonstrates short sleep latency and a normal sleep of prolonged duration (at least 10 hours) in the case of IH with long sleep time. In IH without long sleep time, PSG shows normal sleep or sleep of slightly prolonged duration, always between 6 and 10 hours [1].

NREM and REM sleep are usually in normal proportions. An increased amount of NREM sleep can be found, however, as is the case for sleep spindles [18,19]. Sleep efficiency is above 90% in the authors' experience and 85% in the new ICSD criteria [1]; microarousal index is less than 10 per hour. The presence of important nighttime sleep disruption cannot fit the diagnosis of IH and PSG needs to exclude other causes of daytime sleepiness. Sleep-onset REM period is not reported in IH. Obstructive sleep apnea (index >5 per hour) and periodic limb movements (index >5 per hour) are exclusion criteria; however, in rare cases of an early onset of IH and their late occurrence the diagnosis of IH is still possible. Systematic monitoring of the esophageal pressure during sleep, to exclude upper airway resistance syndrome that may fragment sleep and induce daytime sleepiness, is still subject to debate. Nevertheless the authors recommend the procedure.

Multiple Sleep Latency Test

The most widely used procedure is an all-night PSG recording followed by a MSLT. MSLT is always necessary to confirm the objective hypersomnia and to exclude other causes of hypersomnia, especially narcolepsy without cataplexy. A mean sleep latency of less than 8 minutes with less than two sleep onset rapid eye movement period (SOREMPs) is necessary for the positive diagnosis [1]. Mean sleep latency is at 6.2 ± 3 minutes in IH with or without long sleep time, higher than in narcolepsy [1]. MSLT is of limited diagnostic value, however, in IH with long sleep time. The first reason is the usual difficulty to keep the patient awake before the test and between sessions of the test. The second one is the obligation to wake up the patient in the morning to perform MSLT, precluding the recording of the prolonged nighttime sleep, a typical symptom of IH with long sleep time. Regarding these limits, several patients may have normal mean sleep latency on the MSLT, being above 8 but less than 10 minutes [6,8].

Other polysomnographic protocols

Because of the previously listed limits of the PSG-MSLT procedure, a 24-hour continuous PSG on an ad libitum sleep-wake protocol may be proposed [8]. This protocol is of potential interest, especially for the diagnosis of IH with long sleep time, in recording a major sleep episode (more than 10 hours) and at least one daytime sleep episode

---

Box 1: Sleep-wake Montpellier protocol in idiopathic hypersomnia with long sleep time

Day 1-Night 1-Day 2

Overnight PSG recording (after 16 hours sleep deprived) and MSLT (9 AM, 11 AM, 1 PM, 3 PM, and 5 PM) were performed. After 1 minute of sleep on the MSLT, subjects were awakened in order not to interfere with the homeostatic process. Batteries of neuropsychologic tests (including vigilance and cognitive tests) were performed during Day 2 between each nap. Three cognitive evoked potential recording (auditory P 300) sessions took place on Day 1 at 7 PM and on Day 2 at 7 AM and 11 AM

Night 2-Day 3-Night 3

A 32-hour continuous PSG on an ad libitum sleep-wake protocol is performed. After a 16-hour sleep deprivation (Day 2), a PSG recording is performed during 32 hours in the bed rest protocol from 11 PM to 7 AM 2 days after. Conditions are as follows: sound attenuated; dim light (10 lux); interdiction to get up or to listen to music or radio; possibility to ask for food and drink (without alcohol). The choice of the bed rest condition has been made to increase sleepiness, to decrease wakefulness, and to reduce sleep propensity at the end of the study.

of more than 1 hour duration. Spontaneous sleep periods of up to 19.4 hours have been previously reported in that condition, with normal MSLT latency [20]. That procedure still waits for standardization and validation, however, especially regarding the level of physical activity allowed during the recording. At present the authors perform a bed rest 32-hour continuous PSG (a bed rest is always on an ad libitum sleep-wake protocol) on an ad libitum sleep-wake protocol to ascertain the diagnosis and to assess abnormalities of the sleep-wake regulation [Box 1, Fig. 1]. Because of financial cost, this protocol is not recommended to ascertain the diagnosis of IH patients.

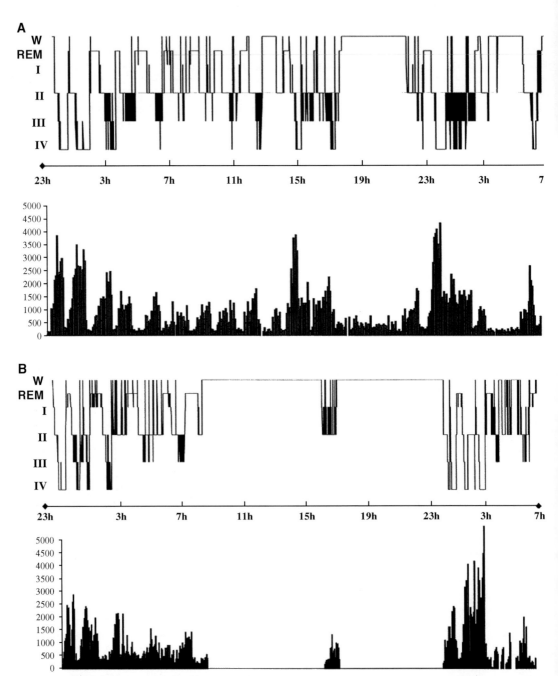

Fig. 1. Hypnogram and slow wave activity (SWA) in a 32-hour bed rest protocol. (*A*) A 26-year-old woman affected with IH with long sleep time. (*B*) A 28-year-old control. An increase in total sleep time and in level of SWA was noted, with a slow exponential decay of SWA during the first night when compared with the control. Also noted was a longer duration of the nap during the day in IH patient with an increase in SWA around 3 PM.

Other tests

Several authors recommend ambulatory actigraphy monitoring over several days to demonstrate prolonged nighttime and daytime sleep episodes that are typical of IH with long sleep time [13]. Actigraphy cannot differentiate sleep and wake periods while resting, although this is extremely important for the diagnosis of IH. In addition, as is the case for 24-hour PSG, the actigraphy protocol still needs standardization and validation in IH.

Cognitive evoked potentials (auditory or visual P 300) are also of interest to measure sleep inertia objectively [21–23]. This result is of no practical value, however, in the diagnosis of a single patient. In contrast to narcolepsy, HLA typing is of no help in the positive diagnosis of IH, given the lack of any consistent association with HLA. In addition, CSF hypocretin-1 levels are normal in most cases and especially in all cases of IH with long sleep time [10–12].

Neurologic and psychologic evaluations are necessary. They have to be normal to exclude the possibility of hypersomnia associated with neurologic or psychiatric disorders. Finally, brain CT or MRI is of value to rule out an underlying brain lesion.

Pathophysiology

Pathophysiology of IH is almost totally unknown and still speculative. Because of clinical feature differences between the two conditions (IH with and without long sleep time) one may hypothesize a different pathophysiology mechanism. Another hypothesis may be drawn for continuum in the pathophysiology of IH without long sleep time and narcolepsy without cataplexy [12].

There is no available natural model of IH comparable with the narcoleptic dog. The central nervous system changes that lead to the symptoms of IH are unknown, although altered central nervous system monoaminergic activity may be involved. In the cat, destruction of noradrenergic neurons of the rostral third of the locus coeruleus complex or of the norepinephrine bundle at the level of the isthmus leads to hypersomnia with normal NREM and REM cycles, mimicking IH [24]. This state is accompanied by a decrease of diencephalic norepinephrine. In IH subjects, Montplaisir and coworkers [25] found a significant decrease in dopamine and indoleacetic acid (a tryptamine metabolite) in the CSF of both IH and narcoleptics in comparison with controls. In addition, Faull and coworkers [26] found a desynchronization of the dopamine system with the diencephalic norepinephrine and serotonin (5-HT) systems in narcolepsy and a desynchronization of the diencephalic norepinephrine system with the dopamine and 5-HT systems in IH.

In the context of the recently discovered CSF hypocretin-1 deficiency in narcolepsy with cataplexy, CSF hypocretin-1 has been assessed in IH by several groups. None of the investigations done so far, however, has evidenced a clear decreased CSF hypocretin-1 level [10–12]. This is of particular interest in view of the possible relationship between IH and narcolepsy without cataplexy, both characterized by a normal level of CSF hypocretin-1.

Familial aggregation of IH patients is frequent, suggesting a genetic component for IH. The limited number of family studies has not clearly determined any mode of inheritance [6,8,15]. Because of the association of narcolepsy with HLA subtype, immunogenetic studies have also been performed with no consistent result [27,28].

An impaired sleep-wake regulation could be hypothesized in IH with long sleep time. In contrast to narcolepsy, nighttime awakenings are rare, but daytime sleep episodes are also frequent in IH. The difficulty in achieving normal morning or afternoon awakening could be the result of any combination of abnormal homeostatic, circadian, or inertia processes.

From a homeostatic point of view, the difficulty in morning awakening could be related to an abnormal high level of slow wave activity toward the end of the night, caused by either an abnormally slow decay of slow wave activity or by a normal decay of an enhanced level of slow wave activity, as it is the case following sleep deprivation. In the latter case, IH patients could be considered as sleep deprived long sleepers. In contrast with this hypothesis, a recent study by Sforza and coworkers [18] reported a lower level of slow wave activity in IH subjects without any modification of the exponential decay. No behavioral control of wakefulness was performed the day before PSG, however, to enforce the necessary 16-hour sleep deprivation; no wake-up time was indicated and no analysis of sleep spindles and their relation to slow wave activity was reported in this study. Given the inverse relationship between slow wave activity and sleep spindles, another possibility could be an alteration of the time course of activity in the spindle frequency range in IH patients, such as a lesser increase toward the end of the night. A higher sleep spindle density in both cerebral hemispheres at the beginning and at the end of nocturnal sleep has been documented in a few IH patients [19], suggesting a weakened awakening mechanism. These results warrant replication.

A second possibility could be an alteration of the circadian process. In line with this hypothesis, a tendency to a delayed evening melatonin rise and a delayed morning decline has been reported in IH patients, without significant difference with controls [29,30]. In addition, no body temperature recording has been performed in IH patients to date.

Finally, sleep inertia, the most common feature of IH with long sleep time, could be enhanced in subjects with IH. One study revealed that patients with IH had longer visual P300 latency and smaller amplitude than in normals and narcoleptics. This result was in favor of cognitive dysfunction and not simply of impaired attention [22]. Only one morning P300 was been recorded in this study, however, and no distinction between IH with or without long sleep time was available [22]. The authors perform the recording of auditory P300 at three different times (7 PM, 7 AM, and 11 AM) in patients with IH with long sleep time, and show a clear decrease in amplitude especially at 7 AM immediately after provoked awakening [23].

Differential diagnosis

IH is frequently overdiagnosed, especially the form without long sleep time [6,8]. IH is frequently diagnosed in cases of hypersomnia just after excluding narcolepsy and sleep apnea or hypopnea syndrome.

Sleep-deprived long sleepers

A long sleeper sleeps more than the amount of sleep of their normal age group. In the condition of behaviorally induced insufficient sleep, the individual starts suffering from excessive sleepiness in the afternoon, in the evening, or after meals [31]. Patients report that they sleep 5 to 6 hours nightly on week days, and 9 hours during weekends. They have difficulty rising in the morning and sometimes experience sleep drunkenness–like episodes. Work and cognitive performance, and decision making may be impaired. The patient may also complain about increasing levels of fatigue, mood deterioration, muscular pain, gastrointestinal unrest, and visual disturbances. Symptoms disappear on weekends and during the holidays. A detailed history of the subject's current sleep schedule is needed for the diagnosis. The diagnosis is mainly done by interview. In the case of suspected associated pathology, however, such as respiratory disturbances during sleep, PSG may be indicated. In the insufficient sleep syndrome, this recording usually shows good sleep efficiency (>90%) and short sleep latency, indicative of a sleep rebound [31]. It has been suggested that IH with long sleep time may represent the extreme in the distribution of habitual sleep time and that subjects with IH may be long sleepers in a permanent state of sleep deprivation [8]. Subjects with IH with long sleep time do not report any improvement of their excessive daytime sleepiness, however, after prolonged sleeping for days.

Upper airway resistance syndrome

Before ascertaining the diagnosis of IH, sleep-disordered breathing syndromes need to be excluded. Sleep apnea-hypopnea syndrome is easily diagnosed by classical procedures. The upper airway resistance syndrome needs complex investigation. Patients affected are nonobese men or women with a complaint of excessive daytime sleepiness; snoring (especially in men); with frequent fatigue on awakening [9]. Clinical examination often reports a triangular face, a small chin, an arched palate, a class II malocclusion, and a retroposition of the mandible. The diagnosis is ascertained during PSG associated with esophageal pressure monitoring, by the presence of repetitive increase of esophageal pressure that leads to transient arousals without any changes in respiratory disturbance index (index of apnea-hypopnea <5 per hour) and in oxygen saturation [9].

Narcolepsy without cataplexy

This clinical variant of narcolepsy is rare when compared with narcolepsy with cataplexy with a ratio from 1 to 10. In clinical terms, it is almost impossible to differentiate patients affected with IH without long sleep time and those with narcolepsy without cataplexy [6,8]. Associated REM abnormalities, however, such as hypnagogic hallucinations and sleep paralysis, are less frequent and severe in IH patients. The final diagnosis is easy to determine with the MSLT procedure, which demonstrates the presence of two or more SOREMPs only in cases of narcolepsy without cataplexy. The presence of HLA DQB1*0602 or low CSF hypocretin-1 levels also argues in favor of narcolepsy without cataplexy. Most of these patients have normal CSF hypocretin-1 level, however, as in IH patients. A continuum between narcolepsy without cataplexy and IH without long sleep time is also possible in terms of physiopathologic mechanisms [12,13].

Periodic limb movement disorder

This disorder associates a sleep complaint (insomnia or hypersomnia) or daytime fatigue, and polysomnographic demonstration of periodic highly stereotyped limb movements during sleep, exceeding more than five per hour in adults [1]. The periodic highly stereotyped limb movements during sleep must be interpreted in the context of a patient's related complaint with an important overlap between symptomatic and asymptomatic subjects according to the index of periodic highly stereotyped limb movements during sleep.

Hypersomnia caused by medical condition
This includes several different conditions that may mimic IH (see later).

Hypersomnia caused by drug or substance
Hypersomnia secondary to the abuse of sedative-hypnotic drugs or to abrupt cessation of stimulant drugs are easily recognized by clinical interview.

Nonorganic hypersomnia
This condition should be considered as an important differential diagnosis of IH and it is always difficult to rule out hypersomnia associated with depression (see later). Patients may have mood changes that do not qualify for the diagnosis of affective disorders (*Diagnostic and Statistical Manual-IV*). In contrast, patients may have had excessive daytime sleepiness before the appearance of mood changes and clinical manifestations may evolve independently [30].

Pain or other medical symptoms
Pain or other medical symptoms (eg, tumors, migraine, rheumatoid arthritis) responsible for fragmented night sleep may result in excessive daytime sleepiness. A detailed medical history of the patient clarifies the cause of EDS.

Chronic fatigue syndrome
Chronic fatigue syndrome is characterized by persistent or relapsing fatigue that does not resolve with sleep or rest [32]. In addition to fatigue, patients report complaints of myalgia, anxiety, fever, headaches, and cognitive alterations. Chronic fatigue syndrome is not a cause of chronic hypersomnia but a differential diagnosis. Patients have frequent difficulties in clearly distinguishing excessive sleepiness from fatigue. PSG in chronic fatigue syndrome shows reduced sleep efficiency and may document alpha intrusion into sleep electroencephalogram.

Treatment
The lack of understanding of the IH pathophysiology leads to the fact that treatment can only be symptomatic. Treatment does not differ in narcolepsy and IH, and modafinil has become the first-line treatment. Modafinil, 200 to 400 mg per day, seems effective in the management of daytime symptoms [6,8,33]. No double-blind, randomized, controlled study has been performed, however, in IH. Other stimulant drugs including methylphenidate, mazindol, dextroamphetamine, and methamphetamine may be of interest in cases resistant to modafinil. Adverse effects with stimulant drugs include headache, tachycardia, hypertension, irritability, and insomnia. They are less frequent with modafinil than with other stimulants. Real success on daytime sleepiness could be noted with stimulants, but prolonged nighttime sleep and difficulty in morning awakening still persist in IH with long sleep time. Actually, no treatment clearly improves sleep inertia, a consistent complaint of IH patients with long sleep time.

An alternative treatment with melatonin (2 mg of slow release at bedtime) has been proposed in 10 IH patients with long sleep time, with a tendency to a decrease in sleep drunkenness and excessive daytime sleepiness with shorter nocturnal melatonin duration in half of the patients [30]. Several authors have also proposed tricyclic antidepressants, monoamine oxidase inhibitors, or selective serotonin reuptake inhibitors in the management of IH but without clear positive effect, except in cases of mood alteration associated symptoms [6].

Behavioral treatments and sleep hygiene also can be proposed but are of limited effect in IH with long sleep time. Naps are always long and nonrestorative. They are not advisable in these patients.

Hypersomnia caused by medical condition
A variety of neurologic disorders including Parkinson's disease, head trauma, stroke (in the thalamic or mesencephalic levels), encephalitis, and genetic disorders (eg, Niemann-Pick type C disease, Norrie's disease, Prader-Willi syndrome, myotonic dystrophy) may lead to chronic hypersomnia [1] and in some cases may mimic IH. Most of these hypersomnia disorders are discussed elsewhere in this issue. Posttraumatic and postviral hypersomnia, however, are detailed next.

Posttraumatic hypersomnia
Posttraumatic hypersomnia is a common diagnosis of chronic hypersomnia. It occurs mainly in cases of initial coma after head trauma with hypersomnia occurring 6 to 18 months after the trauma. An important study focused on a systematic evaluation of 184 hypersomnia patients with a history of head trauma [34]. Posttraumatic complaint of somnolence was associated with variable degrees of impaired daytime functioning and patients who had been in a coma for 24 hours, who had a head fracture, or who had undergone an immediate neurosurgical procedure had higher scores on the Epworth Sleepiness Scale and decreased sleep latencies on the MSLT. Another study performed on 71 adults with brain injuries revealed that objective hypersomnia was common (47%) in this population, with a relatively high prevalence of sleep apnea-hypopnea syndrome, periodic limb move-

ment disorder, and posttraumatic hypersomnia alone (30%) [35]. Subjects with objectively measured sleepiness were not identified on self-reporting questionnaires, suggesting their inability to perceive their hypersomnolence. No significant differences between hypersomnia and nonhypersomnia groups were present in the Glasgow Coma Scale score and in the length of coma, gender, or time since brain injury. A recent study prospectively assessed CSF hypocretin-1 levels in patients with acute trauma brain injury [36]. Hypocretin-1 deficiency was found in 95% of patients with moderate to severe trauma and in 97% of patients with posttrauma brain CT abnormalities, a result that may reflect hypothalamic damage and lead to hypersomnia. Finally, a head injury in previously asymptomatic individuals may rarely trigger narcolepsy [37].

Hypersomnia following infection

Several patients affected with infectious mononucleosis, Guillain-Barré syndrome, pneumonia, hepatitis, or Whipple's disease may develop, several months after the acute infection, a hypersomnia syndrome that may mimic IH [38,39]. An encephalitic process or an elevation of inflammatory cytokines (tumor necrosis factor-α, interferon-β, and interleukin-1) may play a pathogenic role [40]. In bacterial and viral diseases sleep modifications are coupled with immune reactions with unclear mechanisms. Polysomnographic examinations in infectious diseases are still scarce, except for the Gambian form of human African trypanosomiasis, which is caused by the transmission of trypanosomes by tsetse flies [41].

Nonorganic hypersomnia

This condition, also referred to as "hypersomnia not caused by a substance or known physiologic condition" in the currently revised version of the ICSD [1], includes several different types of hypersomnia with abnormal personality traits, major depressive episode, seasonal affective disorder, or with conversion episode.

The complaint of daytime sleepiness in nonorganic hypersomnia may mimic symptoms in IH patients. In nonorganic hypersomnia, however, symptoms often vary from day to day and are often associated with poor sleep at night [8]. In that sense, insomnia and excessive daytime sleepiness are frequently associated, especially in cases of depression. There are several relationships between sleep difficulties and depression. Chronic insomnia may be a precursor, symptom, residual symptom, or adverse effect of depression or its treatment. Excessive daytime sleepiness may be a precursor,

symptom, or adverse effect of depression [42]. In addition, physicians need to resolve both insomnia and excessive daytime sleepiness because of the risk of depression onset, worsening of depressive symptoms, and relapse of depression after response to antidepressant treatment.

Polysomnographic studies in hypersomnia with mood disorders are rare. In all studies, however, MSLT does not demonstrate shortened mean sleep latency when compared with normal controls [16, 43,44]. In addition, REM sleep is totally absent during daytime naps in depressed patients. A 24-hour continuous PSG revealed a lowered total sleep time, an increased sleep stage 1, and decreased stages 3 and 4 in patients with a complaint of hypersomnia associated with mood disorder in comparison with IH patient [43]. The complaint of hypersomnia in patients associated with mood disorders is rarely objective. The complaint of sleepiness seems to be related to the lack of interest, withdrawal, and decreased energy inherent in the depressed condition, rather than to an increase in sleep propensity or REM sleep propensity. A diagnosis of fatigue seems more likely in that condition, although no objective criteria of fatigue are currently available.

Seasonal affective disorder characterizes the fall and winter recurrence of depressive episodes, with remission of symptoms in spring and summer [45]. Patients with winter depression report hypersomnia, fatigue, loss of energy, carbohydrate craving, appetite, and weight gain. Sleep recordings in seasonal affective disorder patients confirm the presence of hypersomnia and show reduced slow wave sleep during symptomatic episodes. Many hypotheses exist regarding the pathogenic mechanisms of seasonal affective disorder, including circadian phase shifting, abnormal pineal melatonin secretion, and abnormal serotonin synthesis. Light therapy is a natural, noninvasive, effective method of treatment of choice. Light therapy for 14 days every morning seems an effective and interesting treatment in seasonal affective disorder with a significant mood improvement (57%), increased sleep efficiency, decreased sleep latency, decreased slow wave sleep latency, and increased sleep spindles in the first hour of sleep [46]. Light treatment, although a safe and satisfactory treatment for many patients, may be insufficient for more severely ill patients.

Summary

In contrast to narcolepsy, the diagnosis of IH is difficult, still being an exclusion diagnosis of other hypersomnia. IH does not correspond, however, to all patients affected with hypersomnia of unclear origin. Recent important progress has been made in clarifying the phenotype of IH with two forms in the last revised ICSD: IH with long sleep time and without long sleep time. Although IH with long sleep time is a quite well-characterized clinical entity, IH without long sleep time still needs clarification and new methods of investigation of hypersomnia are needed to make accurate diagnosis of IH. No advance has been made regarding the pathophysiology of both IH conditions. In contrast to narcolepsy with cataplexy, neither HLA typing nor CSF hypocretin-1 measurements have helped in understanding the disease. Much evidence leads to a continuum between IH without long sleep time and narcolepsy without cataplexy with also unclear origin. Further studies at biologic, genetic, neuroanatomic, and pharmacologic levels are highly necessary in IH disorders. Finally, several other causes of chronic hypersomnia exist, mostly insufficiently recognized and with pathophysiology mechanism almost totally unknown.

References

[1] American Academy of Sleep Medecine. International classification of sleep disorders. 2nd edition. Diagnostic and coding manual. Westchester (IL): American Academy of Sleep Medicine; 2005.

[2] Roth B. Narkolepsie a hypersomnie s hlediska fysiologie spanku. Praha: Statni Zdravonické Nakladatelstvi; 1957.

[3] Rechtschaffen A, Roth B. Nocturnal sleep of hypersomniacs. Acti Nevr Sup (Praha) 1969;11: 229–33.

[4] Roth B, Nevsimalova S, Rechtschaffen A. Hypersomnia with sleep drunkenness. Arch Gen Psychiatry 1972;26:456–62.

[5] ICSD. International classification of sleep disorders: diagnostic and coding manual. Diagnostic Classification Steering Committee. Rochester (MN): American Sleep Disorders Association; 1990.

[6] Bassetti C, Aldrich MS. Idiopathic hypersomnia: a series of 42 patients. Brain 1997;120:1423–35.

[7] Aldrich MS. The clinical spectrum of narcolepsy and idiopathic hypersomnia. Neurology 1996;46: 393–401.

[8] Billiard M, Dauvilliers Y. Idiopathic hypersomnia. Sleep Med Rev 2001;5:349–58.

[9] Guilleminault C, Stoohs R, Clerk A, et al. A cause of excessive daytime sleepiness: the upper airway resistance syndrome. Chest 1993;104:781–7.

[10] Kanbayashi T, Inoue Y, Chiba S, et al. CSF hypocretin-1 (orexin-A) concentrations in narcolepsy with and without cataplexy and idiopathic hypersomnia. J Sleep Res 2002;11:91–3.

[11] Mignot E, Lammers GJ, Ripley B, et al. The role of cerebrospinal fluid hypocretin in the diagnosis of narcolepsy and other hypersomnias. Arch Neurol 2002;59:1553–62.

[12] Dauvilliers Y, Baumann CR, Carlander B, et al. CSF hypocretin-1 levels in narcolepsy, Kleine-Levin syndrome, and others hypersomnias and neurological conditions. J Neurol Neurosurg Psychiatry 2003;74:1667–73.

[13] Bassetti C, Gugger M, Bischof M, et al. The narcoleptic borderland: a multimodal diagnostic approach including cerebrospinal fluid levels of hypocretin-1 (orexin A). Sleep Med 2003;4: 7–12.

[14] Billiard M, Besset A. Idiopathic hypersomnia. In: Billiard M, editor. Physiology, investigations and medicine. New York: Kluver Academic / Plenum Publishers; 2003. p. 429–35.

[15] Nevsimalova-Bruhova S, Roth B. Heredofamilial aspects of narcolepsy and hypersomnia. Schweiz Neurol Neurochir Psychiatry 1972;110:45–54.

[16] Billiard M, Dolenc L, Aldaz C, et al. Hypersomnia associated with mood disorders: a new perspective. J Psychosom Res 1994;38(Suppl 1): 41–7.

[17] Broughton R, Nevsimalova S, Roth B. The socioeconomic effects (including work, education, recreation and accidents) of idiopathic hypersomnia. Sleep Res 1978;7:217.

[18] Sforza E, Gaudreau H, Petit D, et al. Homeostatic sleep regulation in patients with idiopathic hypersomnia. Clin Neurophysiol 2000;111:277–82.

[19] Bove A, Culebras A, Moore JT, et al. Relationship between sleep spindles and hypersomnia. Sleep 1994;17:449–55.

[20] Voderholzer U, Backhaus J, Hornyak M, et al. 19-h spontaneous sleep period in idiopathic central nervous system hypersomnia. J Sleep Res 1998; 7:101–3.

[21] Bastuji H, Perrin F, Garcia-Larrea L. Event-related potentials during forced awakening: a tool for the study of acute sleep inertia. J Sleep Res 2003; 12:189–206.

[22] Sangal RB, Sangal JM. P300 latency: abnormal in sleep apnea with somnolence and idiopathic hypersomnia, but normal in narcolepsy. Clin Electroencephalogr 1995;26:146–53.

[23] Billiard M, Rondouin G, Espa F, et al. Pathophysiology of idiopathic hypersomnia. Rev Neurol (Paris) 2001;157:5S101–6.

[24] Petitjean F, Jouvet M. Hypersomnie et augmentation de l'acide 5-hydroxy-indolacétique cérébral par lésion isthmique chez le chat. C R hebd Séanc Acad Sci (Paris) 1970;164:2288–93.

[25] Montplaisir J, de Champlain J, Young SN, et al. Narcolepsy and idiopathic hypersomnia: biogenic amines and related compounds in CSF. Neurology 1982;32:1299–302.

[26] Faull KF, Thiemann S, King RJ, et al. Monoamine interactions in narcolepsy and hypersomnia: a preliminary report. Sleep 1986;9:246–9.

[27] Harada S, Matsuki K, Honda Y, et al. Disorders of excessive daytime sleepiness without cataplexy, and their relationship with HLA in Japan. In: Honda Y, Juji T, editors. HLA in narcolepsy. Berlin: Springer-Verlag; 1988. p. 172–85.

[28] Montplaisir J, Poirier G. HLA in disorders of excessive daytime sleepiness without cataplexy in Canada. In: Honda Y, Juji T, editors. HLA in narcolepsy. Berlin: Springer-Verlag; 1988. p. 186–90.

[29] Nevsimalova S, Blazejova K, Illnerova H, et al. A contribution to pathophysiology of idiopathic hypersomnia. Clin Neurophysiol 2000;53:366–70.

[30] Montplaisir J, Fantini L. Idiopathic hypersomnia: a diagnostic dilemma. Sleep Med Rev 2001;5: 361–2.

[31] Roehrs T, Roth T. Chronic insufficient sleep and its recovery. Sleep Med 2003;4:5–6.

[32] Fukuda K, Straus SE, Hickie I, et al. The chronic fatigue syndrome: a comprehensive approach to its definition and study. International Chronic Fatigue Syndrome Study Group. Ann Intern Med 1994;121:953–9.

[33] Bastuji H, Jouvet M. Successful treatment of idiopathic hypersomnia and narcolepsy with modafinil. Prog Neuropsychopharmacol Biol Psychiatry 1988;12:695–700.

[34] Guilleminault C, Yuen KM, Gulevich MG, et al. Hypersomnia after head-neck trauma: a medicolegal dilemma. Neurology 2000;54:653–9.

[35] Masel BE, Scheibel RS, Kimbark T, et al. Excessive daytime sleepiness in adults with brain injuries. Arch Phys Med Rehabil 2001;82:1526–32.

[36] Baumann CR, Stocker R, Imhof HG, et al. Hypocretin-1 (orexin A) deficiency in acute traumatic brain injury. Neurology 2005;65:147–9.

[37] Lankford DA, Wellman JJ, O'Hara C. Posttraumatic narcolepsy in mild to moderate closed head injury. Sleep 1994;17(8 Suppl):S25–8.

[38] Guilleminault C, Mondini S. Mononucleosis and chronic daytime sleepiness: a long-term follow-up study. Arch Intern Med 1986;146:1333–5.

[39] Voderholzer U, Riemann D, Gann H, et al. Transient total sleep loss in cerebral Whipple's disease: a longitudinal study. J Sleep Res 2002;11: 321–9.

[40] Opp MR, Toth LA. Neural-immune interactions in the regulation of sleep. Front Biosci 2003;8: 768–79.

[41] Buguet A, Bourdon L, Bouteille B, et al. The duality of sleeping sickness: focusing on sleep. Sleep Med Rev 2001;5:139–53.

[42] Fava M. Daytime sleepiness and insomnia as correlates of depression. J Clin Psychiatry 2004; 65(Suppl 16):27–32.

[43] Dolenc L, Besset A, Billiard M. Hypersomnia in association with dysthymia in comparison with idiopathic hypersomnia and normal controls. Pflugers Arch 1996;431:303–4.

[44] Nofzinger EA, Thase ME, Reynolds III CF, et al. Hypersomnia in bipolar depression: a comparison with narcolepsy using the multiple sleep latency test. Am J Psychiatry 1991;148:1177–81.

[45] Rosenthal NE, Sack DA, Gillin JC, et al. Seasonal affective disorder: a description of the syndrome and preliminary findings with light therapy. Arch Gen Psychiatry 1984;41:72–80.

[46] Ibatoullina E, Praschak-Rieder N, Kasper S. Severe atypical symptoms without depression in SAD: effects of bright light therapy. J Clin Psychiatry 1997;58:495.

SLEEP
MEDICINE
CLINICS

Sleep Med Clin 1 (2006) 89–103

The Kleine-Levin Syndrome

Yu-Shu Huang, MD[a,c], Isabelle Arnulf, MD, PhD[b,c],*

- Diagnostic criteria
- Epidemiology
- Triggering factors and recurrences
- Burden of the disease
- Clinical presentation
  Hypersomnia
  Cognitive disturbances
  *Derealization, hallucination, and
    delusion*
  Eating behavior disorders
  Hypersexuality
  Other compulsive behaviors
  Mood disorders and irritability
  *Clinical examination and signs of
    autonomic dysfunction*
- Pathophysiology of Kleine-Levin syndrome
  Blood tests
  Hormonal tests
  Cerebrospinal fluid analysis
  Electroencephalograms
  CT and MRI brain imaging
  SPECT
  Genetics
  Human leucocyte antigens (HLA)
  Neuropathologic findings
- Secondary Kleine-Levin syndrome cases
- Treatment
- Summary
- References

In 1862, Dr. Wilson, from Middlesex, observed an intriguing case of "double mind" in a child [1]:

> This patient was defiant, timid, and modest; he ate with moderation; in his usual state, he showed by his acts that he had an honest and scrupulous nature. But, as soon as the disease reoccurred, he lost all these qualities. He slept a lot, was difficult to arouse, and as soon as he was awakened, he extemporaneously sang, recited, and acted with great ardor and aplomb. When he was not asleep, he ate ravenously. As soon as he got out of his bed, he would go close to another patient's bed, and overtly seize without any scruple all the food he could find. Apart from this intriguing disease, he was intelligent and skilful.

Kleine [2] was the first to report on a case series of nine patients with recurrent hypersomnias (two with increased food intake) in 1925 in the Professor Kleist hospital in Frankfurt and to propose the existence of a novel disease entity. Less known is the fact his case series included a young woman with menstruation-linked hypersomnia, a syndrome now considered as a distinct type of recurrent hypersomnia [3]. Levin [4,5], a New York psychiatrist, emphasized the association of periodic somnolence with morbid hunger (a symptom subsequently called megaphagia) in 1929 and 1936. Critchley [6], in 1962, reviewed 15 genuine cases published by various authors, added 11 of his own personal cases (notably young marines in the Brit-

a Departments of Child Psychiatry and Sleep Medicine, Chang Gung Memorial Hospital, 5 Fu-Shing Street, kwei-shan, Taoyaung, Taipei 33300, Taiwan
b Fédération des Pathologies du Sommeil, Hôpital Pitié-Salpêtrière, Assistance Publique–Hôpitaux de Paris, 47-83 Boulevard de l'Hôpital, Paris 75013, France
c Sleep Disorders Center, Stanford University School of Medicine, 401 Quarry Road, Suite 3301, Stanford, CA 94305–5730, USA
* Corresponding author. Fédération des Pathologies du Sommeil, Hôpital Pitié-Salpêtrière, 47-83 Boulevard de l'Hôpital, Paris 75013, France.
E-mail address: isabelle.arnulf@psl.aphp.fr (I. Arnulf).

1556-407X/06/$ – see front matter © 2006 Elsevier Inc. All rights reserved.
sleep.theclinics.com

doi:10.1016/j.jsmc.2005.11.011

ish Royal Navy where Critchley had served during World War II) [7], and gave the eponymous name of the disease, "Kleine-Levin Syndrome (KLS)." He pointed out the recurrent aspect of hypersomnia, the male predominance, the onset during adolescence, the compulsive rather than bulimic nature of the eating disorder, and the trend of the disease to spontaneously disappear.

Diagnostic criteria

According to the International Classification of Sleep Disorders, it belongs to the category of recurrent hypersomnia [8], defined as episodes of excessive sleepiness lasting more than 2 days and less than 4 weeks, intermixed with long intervals of normal alertness lasting usually months to years, recurring at least every year, and not better explained by a sleep disorder; a neurologic disorder (eg, idiopathic recurrent stupor, epilepsy); a mental disorder (eg, bipolar disorder, psychiatric hypersomnia, depression); or the use of drugs (eg, benzodiazepines, alcohol). The essential clinical criterion of KLS is recurrent episodes of hypersomnia. Moreover, patients have to experience at least one of these symptoms only during the episodes: (1) cognitive or mood disturbances (confusion, irritability, mutism, aggressiveness, derealization, hallucinations, delusion), which is almost always present; (2) megaphagia with compulsive eating;

(3) hypersexuality with inappropriate or odd behavior; and (4) abnormal behavior such as irritability, aggression and odd behavior.

Epidemiology

The exact prevalence of KLS is unknown, but it is considered a very rare disease, possibly affecting one in a million. The authors recently collected all cases published in the literature and indexed in PubMed between 1962 and 2004, in English and non-English languages, and found 186 cases [9]. The patients were reported worldwide, as shown in Fig. 1. If most cases were reported in Western countries, one sixth of patients were found in Israel [10], suggesting that Jewish heritage could provide a vulnerability for the disease. Men were more frequently affected than women, with a gender ratio of 2:1. The disease primes mostly teenagers: in our meta-analysis, the median age at disease onset was 15 years (range, 4–80 years), with 81% of the cases beginning during the second decade. Cases starting before puberty were rare, as were the six cases with an onset after 35 years [11–17]. Most cases are sporadic, but four multiplex KLS families have been reported [18–20]. When defining as secondary the KLS patients having neurologic symptoms before disease onset that persisted during the intervals free of KLS symptoms, the authors found that 18 KLS cases were secondary and 168 were primary.

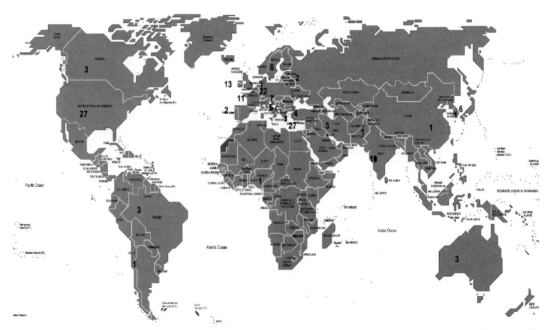

Fig. 1. Distribution of the 186 primary KLS cases of the 1962 to 2004 literature in the world. *Data from* Arnulf I, Zeitzer JM, File J, et al. Kleine-Levin syndrome: a systematic review of 186 cases in the literature. Brain 2005; 128(3):2763–76.

Triggering factors and recurrences

An intriguing aspect of KLS is the presence of an infection 3 to 5 days before disease onset in 43% patients [Table 1] [11,14,17,19–51]. In most cases, it is a trivial, flu-like fever, or a winter upper airway infection, more rarely summer gastroenteritis. The infectious agent, identified in only a few cases, can be either a virus (chicken pox, mononucleosis, Asian influenza, and enterovirus) or bacteria (*Streptococcus*). More rarely, the first or important use of alcohol, a head trauma, physical exertion, stress, and anesthesia trigger the disease.

The major characteristic of KLS is the recurrence of symptoms during episodes that lasted, in the authors' analysis, a median of 10 days, and were separated by periods of normal sleep and behavior lasting a median of 3.5 months [Fig. 2]. Episodes as long as 80 days, although they are rare, unfortunately may happen [20]. Similarly, severe forms of KLS may contain one episode per month. The intervals do not follow, however, a specific periodicity in a given patient, but rather an unpredictable course. Rarely, patients can identify various factors triggering relapses, such as infections, tonsillitis, the use of alcohol or marijuana, sleep deprivation, head trauma [see Table 1]. Frequently, the disease abates with time, the episodes being less frequent, less long, and less severe, with reduced sleepiness. It is also possible to observe relapses occurring up to 7 years after the last episode [see Fig. 2].

Burden of the disease

It is frequently assumed that KLS is benign because it is not associated with mortality and is self-limited. In teenager and young adult cases, however, the frequent occurrence of attacks and severe behavioral-emotional disturbances cause enormous stress for the patients and their families. Indeed, two patients attempted suicide during an episode [11,52]. The aggressive or odd behavior was severe enough to require the intervention of the police in some patients [21,53,54]; besides, the condition causes disturbances in study, work, and social interaction for teenagers and young adults. Some adolescents cannot return to normal psychosocial and academic functioning between episodes because of repetition of symptoms or social and school demands, such as seen in Asian countries, even if their intelligence quotient test has not significantly changed in a 5-year follow-up investigation. There have been rare cases of death caused indirectly by the KLS symptoms, such as a 6-year-old girl having broken a leg during a restless episode (and having died from subsequent pulmonary embolism) [55], or a 46-year-old man choking on meat during an episode of megaphagia [13].

The median disease course, estimated with a Kaplan-Meier type analysis (half of the cases were not cured at time of publication), was 8 years in the authors' meta-analysis [Fig. 3]. It is also important to note that as many as one third of the patients were still not cured 15 years after the onset of KLS, suggesting again that the disease is not that

Table 1: Precipitating factors reported at KLS onset and before recurrences in 168 patients

Event at KLS onset	No. of patients	% Frequency at KLS onset	% Frequency before KLS recurrences
None reported	66	39	84
Infection or fever	72	42.8	8.9
Unspecific fever, flu-like fever [20,30,33,40,41,46–48]	42		
Upper respiratory tract infection, tonsillitis, sore throat, cough [17,21,25,28,32,33,38–40,42,43,49]	20		
Gastroenteritis [11,31,45,50]	5		
Identified virus or bacteria	5		
Septicemia with streptococcus [24], scarlet [14], Asian influenza, [35] chicken pox and mononucleosis [39], enterovirus [43] post-typhoid vaccine fever [14]			
Alcohol or marijuana [19,23,27,34,44,51]	7	4.2	0.6
Head trauma [14,19,37]	4	2.4	0
Sleep deprivation, Mental effort, stress [22,26,36]	5	3	0
Menses [19,29,30,48,49] or lactation [50]	6	2.7	0.6
Miscellaneous: local or general anesthesia, physical exertion [51], clavicle fracture	6	3.6	4.8

From Arnulf I, Zeitzer JM, File J, et al. Kleine-Levin syndrome: a systematic review of 186 cases in the literature. Brain 2005;128(3):2763–76; with permission.

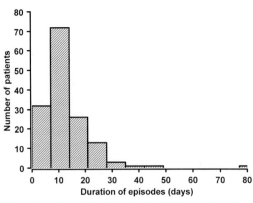 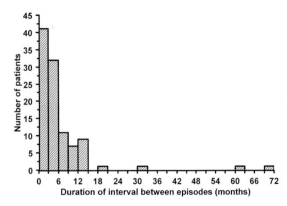

Fig. 2. Duration of each episode (*left panel*) and of symptom-free interval (*right panel*) in 168 patients with primary KLS. *From* Arnulf I, Zeitzer JM, File J, et al. Kleine-Levin syndrome: a systematic review of 186 cases in literature. Brain 2005;128(3):2763–76; with permission.

benign. Women had a longer disease course (median, 13 years) than men (median, 6 years; logrank test, $P = .02$) in the published cases.

Although KLS is defined by normal sleep, cognition, and behavior between the episodes, eight patients with persistent memory disturbances and academic decline between the episodes have been reported [14,22,23,56,57]. The possibility of residual dysfunction after KLS termination was also reported in three cases [14,23]. A recent imaging study during nonsymptomatic phase supports this possibility in subjects with long evolution of the syndrome [58]. A long-lasting disease that affects young patients, causes severe symptoms, and possibly permanent damage should motivate early intervention and further treatment studies.

Clinical presentation

The symptoms of KLS were extremely diverse, including sleep, eating, mood, behavioral, visual, or

cognitive disturbances [Table 2]. The core symptoms, present in almost all the patients, were hypersomnia, cognitive disturbances, and irritability, whereas megaphagia and hypersexuality were described in only half of the patients. Even within a class of symptoms, manifestation could be variable with somnolence being described as a narcolepsy-like or idiopathic hypersomnia-like sleepiness or a generalized apathy without a true increase in sleep amounts. Similarly, eating disorders varied from megaphagia in typical cases to reduced appetite or even weight loss in others. Such variations could also be observed in the same patient over the episodes. Several symptoms, such as food use, verbal

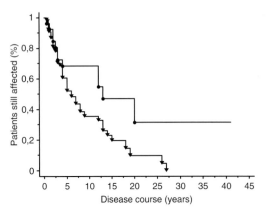

Fig. 3. Disease course in 110 primary KLS cases. A total of 45.5% of the data are censored (ie, were not cured at time of publication). Women (*plain circles*) had twice longer disease course than men (*plain triangles*).

Table 2: **Frequency of symptoms during episodes of Kleine-Levin syndrome**

Symptoms	Percentage
Hypersomnia	100
Cognitive disorders	96
Abnormal speech	60
Confusion	51
Amnesia	48
Derealization	24
Hallucinations	14
Delusions	16
Eating behavior disorders	80
Megaphagia	62
Craving for sweet	9.5
Increased drinking	6.4
Binge eating	4.4
Decreased appetite	3.8
Food use behavior	3.2
Other behavioral disorders	
Hypersexuality	43
Compulsions to sing, write, pace	29
Depression	48
Irritability	92
Autonomic dysfunction	6

perseverations, withdrawal, and deinhibition behavior, are reminiscent of frontal lobe syndrome, whereas the association of megaphagia and hypersexuality has also been described in the syndrome of Klüver-Bucy associated with bitemporal lesions [59] and in orbitofrontal lesions [60]. Of note, KLS patients had no parkinsonism and no dysfunction of upper motor neurons, cerebellar system, and cranial nerves.

Hypersomnia

Hypersomnia, a major clinical symptom of KLS, is mandatory for diagnosis and was present in all cases selected for the authors' meta-analysis. When reported, usual sleep duration during episodes ranged from 12 to 24 hours per day (mean, 18 ± 2 hours). A sudden, overwhelming tiredness was reported as prodroma. The patients remained arousable, waking up spontaneously to void and eat, but were irritable or even aggressive when awakened or prevented from sleep. The need for sleep was so intense that a male teenager "was found sleeping under a neighbor's porch" [54], another "left his classroom during a lesson, lay down on the floor of the corridor and fell asleep" [61], whereas an adult patient was "found asleep on the pavement of the street" [53]. At the end of an episode, a short-lasting insomnia was noted in three cases [24,62,63]. Sleep symptoms changed from frank hypersomnia during the first KLS episodes to a heavy fatigue accompanied by a feeling of "as if in twilight between sleep and waking" during later episodes, with apathetic patients staying in their bed during the day even without sleeping.

Polysomnographic findings in 40 KLS patients in the meta-analysis were variable and highly dependant on the delay between the onset of the episode and the laboratory test. Recordings included daytime nap (N = 5) or multiple sleep latency tests (N = 7); nighttime sleep (N = 18); and 24 to 72 hours continuous recordings (N = 10). These results, with comparison with two other analyses of large samples [10,64], are summarized in Table 3. Rapid eye movement sleep was commonly reported during daytime sleep recordings. Six (21%) of 19 patients had a narcolepsy-like pattern (≥2 sleep onset in rapid eye movement periods). In other cases, the duration of sleep stages during daytime sleep contained an excess of stage 1 to 2, as observed in some idiopathic hypersomnias. Of interest, a 3-day long continuous sleep monitoring could be performed since the first day of an episode in a patient; it showed a continuous undisturbed 24-hour long sleep time during Day 1, with an almost 100% sleep efficiency and an excess in stages 1 and 2, followed by a progressive decrease in sleep amount, particularly during the night hours during the following days [65]. Two patients had moderately decreased nocturnal sleep efficiency [66,67],

Table 3: Polysomnography in Kleine-Levin Syndrome patients

Period	Gadoth et al, 2001 During episodes	Gadoth et al, 2001 Between episodes	Dauvilliers et al, 2002 During episodes	Arnulf et al, 2005 During episodes	Huang et al 2005 During episodes
Overnight polysomnography					
No. patients	14	14	18	19	9
TST (min)	568 ± 204	384 ± 59	MD[a]	445 ± 122 (284–678)	391 ± 77
Stage 1 (%)	0.7 ± 0.8	1.4 ± 2.5	9 ± 8	6 ± 4	9 ± 7
Stage 2 (%)	52 ± 9	49 ± 7	53 ± 8	56 ± 9	61 ± 9
Stages 3–4 (%)	13 ± 9	24 ± 8	16 ± 8	19 ± 11	15 ± 9
REM sleep (%)	18.5 ± 7	17.5 ± 5	17 ± 6	19 ± 6	15 ± 6
REM sleep latency	85 ± 47	82 ± 52	133 ± 93	88 ± 53	128 ± 78
Continuous 24-h polysomnography					
No. patients	MD	MD	18	10	7
TST (min)	MD	MD	701 ± 270	838 ± 288	
Multiple Sleep Latency Tests					
No. patients	MD	MD	MD	7	7
Sleep onset latency		MD	MD	3.6 ± 1.1	7.5 ± 1
Sleep onset in REM periods ≥2		MD	MD	2/7 (28.6%)	0/7

Abbreviations: MD, missing data; REM, rapid eye movement; TST, total sleep time.
[a] Percentage given for 24-h sleep recordings.

but were not monitored during the daytime. In another study covering seven patients daytime electroencephalogram (EEG) analysis of 24-hour study emphasized the absence of slow wave sleep during daytime sleep episode and the dominance of stage 1 non–rapid eye movement sleep.

Cognitive disturbances

Almost all patients had cognitive disturbances, such as attention, confusion, concentration, and memory defects [see Table 2]. Two thirds of the patients had an abnormal speech. They were mute; uncommunicative with no spontaneous speech; used monosyllabic or short sentences with limited vocabulary; had slurred, muddled, incoherent, or childish stereotypical language; were slow to speak and to comprehend; with verbal perseverations (eg, answering with the time at each question) or echoing questions. This state of "mental viscosity" or slowness was qualitatively described by some patients as a "struggle to follow a thought" [25], requiring "too much energy with racing thoughts," while "everything was going fast" [21]. A 13-year-old girl found multiple simultaneous stimuli "overwhelming," whereas her brother compared his way of thinking during an episode to "a single-channel television versus a 100-channel television between episodes" [20]. Many patients reported amnesia of the events that occurred during an attack.

Derealization, hallucination, and delusion

A feeling of unreality (surroundings seemed wrong, distorted, or unreal, as in a dream), or of disconnected thinking during episodes was reported by most patients and believed to be the most specific symptom. Five patients discussing together agreed that it was the most important and disabling symptom in KLS [23]. Altered perception was expressed qualitatively as a "strange," "detached," or "different" feeling [18,26,68]. Objects were perceived to be a long way off and voices to be distant (one patient's own voice appearing strange to himself) [22,27,69] with an "unpleasant perception, bizarre and wrong," "with a nightmarish sense of the surroundings" [20], or "with the feeling of being almost in a dream" [70,71]. This feeling also included depersonalization, anguish, a belief of splitting between mind and body [71], and "a persistent sense of unreality and disconnection" from the environment, like being "underwater" [20]. Some of the depersonalization and presentation were similar to those seen during an acute psychotic episode. Other more unusual changes included a blurred vision, tubular vision [72], and the eyes being "dull" or "glassy" [73].

Aside from this feeling of unreality, some patients experienced visual or auditory hallucinations, and paranoid or paranoiac delusions. Patients reported seeing "scary snakes on television and tried to break it" [28]; seeing "the dead bodies of her parents" [29]; seeing ghosts and famous television actors, and believing he was being pursued by armed attackers [74]. Another girl believed that someone was trying to eat her, and that she was being filmed during the night [75]. One teenager was afraid of people trying to kill him; heard threatening voices (mostly at night); and brought his razor to the nurses' desk to prevent people from killing him [54]. Grandiosity delusion was also observed, with a patient saying "I am the Chance" [76].

Eating behavior disorders

Three quarters of the patients had changes in eating behaviors during episodes [see Table 2]. Most (62%) typically ate larger amounts of food (megaphagia), ranging from a mild increase to "three times his usual diet" [30], or "six to eight meals a day" [77], with a 7- to 30-lb weight gain. A patient was hospitalized for breathlessness caused by a distended abdomen, caused by recent enormous meals [53]. Increased drinking of water and juice was also occasionally present, but was never observed alone. A minority of patients had an aversion to food or ate less during one or several episodes, but would overeat during other episodes [17,31,32,69]. Several authors noted that the symptoms were distinct from bulimia, because patients never alternated with periods of self-induced vomiting and voluntary fasting. Some patients stole food in shops or off the plates of other patients in the hospital [25,33,53], searched for food in dust bins [22], and stuffed food in their mouths with both hands [29]. One "would wake in the morning and be the first to go to the cafeteria, where he took a big helping. If objected to, he would raise his voice, yell and swear" [13]. Five other patients had an inability to restrain themselves from eating in the presence of food, a behavior that shares similarities with the behavior of use described in frontal lobe syndrome. One patient "ate anything within her reach" [15], another patient "was several times offered another meal shortly after he had eaten, which he also finished" [78], two patients would "grab any food in sight" [57], whereas another would "eat mechanically, finishing whatever amount was given" [20]. The food craving was mainly directed toward sweets. For example, a patient added 8 teaspoons of sugar in his cereal [34], ate "six bowls of desserts, six chocolate bars in a semi-automatic manner" [63], or drank several bottles per day of pure chocolate syrup [79] or blackberry syrup [35]. Interestingly, some patients ate things they would have refused in the past, such as watermelon rinds by a Turkish girl [71], or non-vegetarian food by a vegetarian Indian [36].

Hypersexuality

One third of the patients had symptoms consistent with hypersexuality during episodes, whereas 67.5% did not report these symptoms and a single patient had decreased libido during his episodes [17]. Hypersexuality was briefly described in the second KLS patient of Kleine [2], in 1925. A 19-year-old officer-cadet "indecently exposed himself in the ward, and while lying unclothed on the bed he masturbated, grinning broadly. Lewd remarks were made to the nursing staff. Once he urinated in the garden in the presence of a sister" [6]. The changes in sexual behavior shared some similarities with the disturbed eating behavior, such as increased quantities (increased frequency of masturbation or of sexual intercourse, demanding several intercourses per day [14]); compulsions (with active and uncontrolled research of sex); lack of judgment in the choice of sexual partner (sexual advances were made to religious sisters, to the patient's daughter [12] or sister [22,37,80], to a nurse "who is said to have been old enough to be his grandmother" [6], and in three cases to other males by otherwise nonhomosexual male patients [12,35,56]); inattention to the environment (eg, masturbating in public); and absence of self-awareness of the inappropriateness of the behavior. A typical example of the compulsive component of KLS was observed a 39-year-old man who, during his third episode of KLS, attacked two women sexually, and the same day attacked his daughter sexually. He would show exhibitionistic behavior and would run naked in the ward, threatening to attack the nurses sexually, and would fondle the female patients. During the sixth episode, he undressed himself, exposing himself to other patients, made advances to the nurses and patients, and threatened to sleep with them. During the seventh episode he was confined to a male-only, locked psychiatric ward for 5 months, where he approached a male patient to have relations with him [12]. A young father in India had a severe fever for 13 days, and "after the fever subsided, he had an increased sexual urge and began using profanity. He would drag away his wife, and would start undressing her in the presence of everybody, unconcerned and completely oblivious of their great horror and embarrassment. Not only that, he made amorous advances to other females too" [30]. In contrast, certain behaviors were frankly just disruptive. For example, a school boy went to a neighbor's house, masturbated into his neighbor's underwear, stole football tickets, and set fire to the drapes [54].

In contrast with other symptoms that were equally frequent in both genders, hypersexuality was twice as more frequent in men (51%) than in women (24%; odds-ratio, 3.4; $P = .002$). One young lady was hospitalized because she was somnolent and had been, during the last 2 days, "scratching her genital in public, lifting her clothes over her head to warm her buttocks at the fire" [29]. The symptoms of sexual disinhibition were also reported in three prepubescent children [38, 39,57]. Interestingly, the plasma levels of sex hormones (testosterone, luteinizing hormone, follicle-stimulating hormone) were normal in 14 patients and mildly decreased in two patients.

Other compulsive behaviors

Other compulsions that occurred during the episodes included inappropriate and compulsive singing in eight patients [34,35,40,81–83], body rocking [70,84], chewing lips [18], compulsive writing on walls or on the sole of the patient's foot in three patients [37,85,86], stripping down wallpaper in two patients [37,85], continuously switching lights on and off [41], pacing, wringing hands and tearing out hair [29], nail-biting, hair pulling, scratching skin, laughing and crying, walking along straight lines [87], and the compulsion to set fire in one patient [54].

Mood disorders and irritability

Half of the patients had a depressive mood during the hypersomnia episodes [see Table 2]. Fifteen percent of the patients reported suicidal thoughts and two attempted suicide [11,52]. In most cases, the depressed mood resolved at the end of each episode, although in rare cases it persisted longer. A few cases (8%) reported to be hypomanic for a couple of days at the end of a KLS episode [42,66]. Another 8% had a flattened affect, and 7% were anxious, with two of them panicking when left alone. Some patients cried without being able to stop [81]. Contrasting with the high frequency of siblings affected in patients with bipolar disorders, a familial history of severe depression was found in only six KLS patients, parental alcoholism in seven patients, and parental schizophrenia in only two patients.

Irritability was present in almost all patients, especially when sleep, sexual, or food drive were prohibited. It culminated in rare but severe aggressive behavior. A child beat his grandmother [54], an adult patient beat his dog [12], another child bit his father [88], one teenager spat in the face of his physician [85], one young man threw stones and was caught by the police [53], while another teenager had such an anger outburst at school that the police evacuated the classroom [21].

Clinical examination and signs of autonomic dysfunction

Clinical examination was unremarkable in all cases with primary KLS. In particular, the absence of neurologic signs indicative of a focal lesion or of meningitis was notable, despite headaches reported at episode onset in one fourth of the patients. Signs of autonomic dysfunction were rare and included a flushed face [63], thermoregulatory change [14], hyperventilation [89], 10-minute long episodes of flushes, profuse sweating, excessive salivation, hypertension and tachycardia [15], and hypotension and bradycardia [17,72,83,90,91]. One patient died of cardiorespiratory arrest following an ataxic respiratory pattern. There was no evidence of neuronal damage in his hypothalamus.

Pathophysiology of Kleine-Levin syndrome

No specific marker for KLS is yet available. Numerous tests were performed in KLS patients to find a cause for the disease. Results were generally negative or poorly informative, except for the functional tests (single-photon emission CT [SPECT], EEG) frequently showing evidences of cortical and subcortical dysfunction during the episodes, which could partly persist in between. Brain neuropathologic analysis of four cases yielded inhomogeneous results. Finally, an association between HLA DQB1*201 genotype and KLS was recently evidenced. If confirmed in larger samples, such an association suggests an immune mediation for the disease.

Blood tests

Numerous blood biologic tests have been performed in patients: there was no evidence of porphyria (a disease that also associates recurrent behavioral disturbances) [35,42,70,92]; metabolic diseases (except in one patient, who had elevated leucine-enkephalin levels and absent free cysteine levels in plasma that normalized between episodes) [62]; drug ingestion; or infectious or inflammatory signs. A slight G-immunoglobulin deficiency was reported in one patient [23].

Hormonal tests

In contrast with the frequent assumption that KLS is associated with hypothalamic dysfunction, changes in levels of pituitary hormones were only rarely found in KLS patients. These hormones were normal in 40 patients, whereas two patients had increased [33] or decreased [25] growth hormone levels. The diurnal profiles of secretion of growth hormone, melatonin, thyroid-stimulating hormone, and cortisol were unchanged during and after episodes in five of five patients, suggesting that circadian systems were basically intact [27]. The dynamic testing of hypothalamic functioning was rarely done (three patients) and yielded inconsistent results. The thyroid-stimulating hormone response to thyroid-releasing hormone and cortisol and adrenocorticotropic hormone responses to hypoglycemic stimulation were abolished [93] or blunted [82] during an episode and normalized thereafter in two patients. A patient had a paradoxical growth hormone response to thyroid-releasing hormone [67], whereas another had a normal growth hormone in response to hypoglycemia [82].

Cerebrospinal fluid analysis

Basic cerebrospinal fluid analysis were negative, with no increased white blood cell or protein levels, except for a single secondary case of KLS associated with an acute viral meningoencephalitis and high cerebrospinal fluid lymphocytes counts [74]. Immunoelectrophoresis of the cerebrospinal fluid was performed and found to be normal in four patients. This excludes the possibility of frequent oligoclonal secretion of antibodies as observed in multiple sclerosis, another remittent neurologic disease [38,45,54,94]. Cerebrospinal fluid levels of serotonin and a serotonin metabolite were increased in one patient [90] but not in four other patients, as were dopamine and norepinephrine metabolite levels [13,31,95–97]. The cerebrospinal fluid levels of hypocretin-1, a hypothalamic peptide that has been shown to be deficient in narcolepsy, were found within normal ranges in nine KLS patients, including three of the authors' (Huang-Nishino, personal communication, 2005) but slightly decreased (111 and 134 $pmol \cdot L^{-1}$) in two patients during an episode [20,43,98].

Electroencephalograms

EEG was the most frequently abnormal test in KLS. It was routinely performed to rule out complex partial epilepsy in the patients with recurrent confusion, decreased alertness, or odd behavior, generally during the first episodes, and was normal in only one fourth of them. In 70% of the patients, a nonspecific diffuse slowing of background EEG activity, such as the alpha frequency band being slowed toward 7 to 8 Hz (versus 10–11 Hz in between) [70,78,84,99], was observed. Less frequently, low-frequency high-amplitude hypersynchronous waves (delta or theta) occurred in isolation or in sequence, and could be either lateralized or bilateral, in the temporal or frontal areas. These findings, however, can be related to presence of drowsiness and intrusion of sleep during the EEG recording. A remarkable finding was the ubiquitous absence of epileptic activity, even in the rare patients who had a personal history of seizures [22]; an intracerebral sphenoid electrode was even recorded in five patients. Rarely, isolated spike discharges [78], self-limited photoparoxysmal response [26], and sharp waves [82] were observed but were considered of no clinical significance.

CT and MRI brain imaging

Brain imaging using CT or MRI was normal in all patients with primary KLS. In 18 secondary cases, lesions of various mechanisms and locations were found. They included a multi-infarct dementia [100]; a thalamic ischemic stroke [101]; traumatic hemorrhages of the right hemisphere [44,102,103]; a hypodense suprasellar lesion on CT suggestive of infundibulum lipoma [104]; multiple MRI hypersignals of periventricular, supraventricular, brainstem, and cerebellum white matter in KLS associated with multiple sclerosis [105]; hydrocephalus [106]; and a cortical dysplasia. But these secondary cases had commonly associated neurologic symptoms and signs.

SPECT

SPECT has been performed usually initially on individual cases. Cerebral blood flow was normal in one patient [107] and reduced in five patients. The reduction occurred in the temporal or temporofrontal areas of either or both sides [23,32,37,100, 107–109] and in the basal ganglia [108]. Recently seven KLS subjects, the largest successively studied group, underwent an imaging investigation [58]. After routine blood and urine tests, each subject had an awake and asleep clinical EEG, a brain CT scan, brain MRI, and Tc-99m ethyl cysteinate dimer SPECT. Subtraction was performed. The quantitative analysis of SPECT was done based on the level of cerebellum and analyzed by using the mean concentration on ECD (25 mCi Tc-99m ECD). Two of seven subjects who underwent SPECT during the asymptomatic period withdrew consent for further imaging study during the symptomatic period. The last five patients showed a hypoperfusion covering both thalami in all cases (five of five). The thalamus was the only brain structure that was consistently affected during the symptomatic period.

Furthermore, hypoperfusion was seen in the basal ganglia (four of five cases) and cortex (three of five cases), specifically the temporal cortex (three of five cases); occipital cortex (three of five cases); and frontal cortex (three of five cases). At a follow-up SPECT study at least 1 month after the end of the symptomatic period, complete resolution of the perfusion problems involving the thalami was seen in all five cases, and the thalami of the last two subjects who had refused imaging during the symptomatic period showed normal perfusion. A more than 30% difference in thalamic perfusion was seen in all SPECT when comparing the two studies. Similarly, decrement was noted in the basal ganglia in four of five subjects, but it was completely absent in one subject, and was limited in two patients. The consistent finding during the symptomatic period in all subjects was the presence of thalamic hypoperfusion. This hypoperfusion was always more marked on the left thalamus when a right-left difference was noted in these right-handed subjects. Thalamic involvement has been the most consistent finding during symptomatic period.

A patient with the longest syndromic evolution, with symptoms present over 13 years, had decreased cerebral perfusion over the temporal lobe, the right posterior frontal lobe, bilateral parietal and occipital lobes, and the left basal ganglia during the asymptomatic period [58].

Genetics

Most KLS cases were sporadic, with the exception of four familial cases: an uncle and nephew [18], a brother and a sister [20], two first-degree cousins [19], and a mother and son [64]. In contrast, a homozygous twin sister of a KLS patient was not affected [96]. Seven patients with genetic disease and secondary KLS were reported, in association with mosaicism of Roberts' syndrome, phocomelia, mild mental retardation, optic atrophy, and bilateral facial palsy (N = 1) [45]; Asperger's syndrome (N = 2), with cortical dysplasia and retinitis pigmentosa in one of them [110]; Prader-Willi syndrome (N = 2) [44,86]; an unidentified disease with mental retardation and bilateral pyramidal syndrome [111]; and a complex case of consanguinity, mental retardation, ectodermal disorder (incontinentia pigmenti), acanthosis nigricans, and hereditary exostosis [96].

There was no association between KLS and gene polymorphism of tryptophan hydroxylase (an enzyme of the serotonin synthesis) or catechol O-methyltransferase (an enzyme of dopamine degradation) in 30 patients [64].

Human leucocyte antigens (HLA)

In the hypothesis of an immune mediation of KLS, the HLA phenotypes or genotypes were determined in 43 patients. In 13 case reports, the DR2 phenotype (which is strongly associated with narcolepsy-cataplexy) was positive in four cases [20,83,85,112] and negative in nine other patients [17,32,45,100]. In a controlled series of 30 European patients, the DQB1*0201 genotypic allele was twice more frequent in the KLS patients than in controls matched for ethnicity ($P < .03$) [64]. But this finding was not replicated in eight of nine Taiwanese cases (Huang

Table 4: Neuropathologic findings in four cases with Kleine-Levin syndrome

	Primary KLS		Secondary KLS	
	Carpenter et al, 1982	*Koerber et al, 1984*	*Takrani and Cronin, 1976*	*Fenzi et al, 1993*
Patient	Male, 46 y	Male, 17 y	Female, 50 y	Female, 6 y
Typical signs	Hypersomnia, megaphagia, hypersexuality, seven attacks	Hypersomnia, megaphagia, masturbation, several attacks	Hypersomnia, megaphagia, aggressiveness, four attacks	Hypersomnia, megaphagia, agitation, two attacks
Atypical signs	Late onset, some attacks lasted 3 months	Autonomic dysfunction, muscle weakness	Late onset, uterine carcinoma	Upward-gaze palsy, mild ptosis
Cause of death	Aspiration pneumonia (caused by megaphagia)	Cardiopulmonary arrest	Complications of cancer	Pulmonary embolism after a bone fracture when agitated during an episode
Lesions				
Cortex	Normal	Normal	Perivascular temporal infiltrate	Normal
Amygdala	Normal	Normal	Perivascular infiltrate	Normal
Thalamus (medial and intralaminar)	Major new and old lesions of the thalamus: abundant infiltrates of inflammatory cells, with microglial proliferation; cuffing of veins with monocytes and lymphocytes	Normal	Normal	Perivascular lymphomonocyte infiltrate in the thalamus: scattered foci of cellular infiltrates with parenchymal nodular-microglial proliferation
Hypothalamus	Very mild proliferation of subependymal astrocytes on the third ventricle wall, small amounts of lymphocytic cuffing in the lateral hypothalamus	Normal	Perivascular infiltrate	Perivascular lymphomonocyte infiltrate in the hypothalamus, and floor of the third ventricle
Brainstem	Normal	Mildly depigmented substantia nigra and locus coeruleus, no Lewy bodies or tangles		Microglial nodule in the periacqueductal gray region and in the oculomotor nerve nuclei

Abbreviation: KLS, Kleine-Levin syndrome.
From Arnulf I, Zeitzer JM, File J, et al. Kleine-Levin syndrome: a systematic review of 186 cases in the literature. Brain 2005;128(3):2763–76; with permission.

et al, personal communication, 2005). Of note, this DQB1*0201 HLA belongs to the extended haplotype DRB1*0301-DQA1*0501-DQB1*0201 that is associated with many autoimmune disorders. Because DQB1*0201 is part of not one but two major haplotypes, DR3 and DR7, further DQA1 and DRB1 typings are needed to establish the predisposing haplotype.

Neuropathologic findings

Brain neuropathologic examinations [Table 4] were performed in two patients with primary KLS [13,90] and in two patients with secondary KLS [55,113]. The cortex was intact in all but one patient (a patient with paraneoplastic syndrome). There were intense signs of inflammatory encephalitis within the hypothalamus in two patients, mild inflammation in one patient, and none in the last patient and in the thalamus in two patients.

Secondary Kleine-Levin syndrome cases

The authors collected 18 patients with KLS-like symptoms observed in association with stroke or posttraumatic brain hematoma (N = 5); genetic or developmental diseases (N = 6); multiple sclerosis (N = 1); hydrocephalus (N = 1); paraneoplasia in the context of a carcinoma of the cervix utero (N = 1); an autoimmune encephalitis (N = 1); or a severe infectious encephalitis (N = 3). The clinical spectrum of the secondary KLS cases was similar to primary KLS, with the exception of an older age at onset, and longer and more frequent episodes [Table 5]. The older age was probably caused by the presence of stroke as a cause in five patients, a disease that affects preferentially older subjects. Because symptoms were similar in nature and fre-

quency to those with primary KLS, as were responses to treatment and disease duration, one can hypothesize that secondary cases were not actually "secondary," but rather primary cases incidentally coexisting with genetic, vascular, or inflammatory neural lesions. These lesions would only facilitate KLS, causing longer and more frequent episodes. One has, however to be cautious because many of the patients presented other neurologic symptoms and signs, and disorganization of brain organization because of the other lesions may be responsible for the reported presentations.

Treatment

The evaluation of treatment, based on case-reports, was hard to assess because of the unpredictable spontaneous course of the disease and of the absence of double-blind, placebo-controlled studies. In 75 patients, one or several drug therapies were attempted, constituting a total of 213 open-labeled trials. As generally predicted, results were extremely disappointing. The effects of drugs were compared with natural evolution, as reported in a group of 32 patients who did not receive drug treatment (because the patients, parents, or doctors decided not to treat the disease); 16% of them had a spontaneous cessation of relapse. Amphetamine-stimulants (71% of 17 patients) but not methylphenidate (20% of 15 patients) nor modafinil (four of four), significantly improved sleepiness, but not the other more serious symptoms, suggesting a very imperfect therapeutic relief. Importantly, none of these drugs improved the more troublesome behavioral and cognitive disturbances. In two patients, flumazenil, a benzodiazepine receptor antagonist, failed to elicit wakefulness. Neurolep-

Table 5: Differences between patients with primary and secondary Kleine-Levin syndrome

	Primary KLS	Secondary KLS	*P* value
No. of patients	168	18	
Sex ratio (% men)	69	67	.83
Age of onset (years)	18.9 ± 72.3	26.1 ± 17.5[a]	.0002
Disease course (years) median ± SE	8 ± 2	10 ± 2	.24
Episode duration (days)	11.7 ± 8.9	31.4 ± 56.5[a]	.0001
Interval duration (months)	5.9 ± 9.6	6.8 ± 9.3	.73
Number of episodes	11.9 ± 14.5	38.3 ± 72.6[a]	.0005
Time incapacitated (days)	135.5 ± 168.5	673.5 ± 1245[a]	<.0001
% Megaphagia	80	83	.95
% Hallucinations, delusions	26	44	.10
% Hypersexuality	43	28	.2

Data are mean ± SD, unless specified.
Abbreviation: KLS, Kleine-Levin syndrome.
[a] Significant difference with primary KLS, Student *t* test, except for disease course (log-rank test in Kaplan-Meier analysis), and for % of symptoms (chi-square test).
From Arnulf I, Zeitzer JM, File J, et al. Kleine-Levin syndrome: a systematic review of 186 cases in the literature. Brain 2005;128(3):2763–76; with permission.

tics (including chlorpromazine, levomepromazine, trifluoperazine, haloperidol, thioridazine, clozapine, and risperidone) were notably ineffective against derealization, psychotic, and behavioral symptoms in 25 cases, and beneficial in only three cases. Numerous antidepressants including tricyclic and serotonin-acting drugs were tried in 23 cases but had no effect on preventing relapses, except for one isolated reported case of recovery with the use of the monoamine oxidase inhibitor moclobemide [114]. Electroconvulsive therapy [11,12,52,74,79] and insulin coma therapy had no effect on KLS symptoms (and even worsened confusion in the case of electroconvulsive therapy).

Because KLS shares some similarities with bipolar disorder (eg, recurrence of episodes and sudden changes from a depressed mood during an episode to hypomania at the end of an episode in some patients), various mood stabilizers, such as lithium, carbamazepine, valproate, phenytoin, and phenobarbital, were tried. Of these treatments, only lithium had a reported response rate significantly higher than medical abstention (odds ratio, 3.8; $P = .02$) by some authors [14,27,33]. It was effective at preventing relapses in 41% of cases, but was only administered in 29 cases, making the results tentative. Recovery was imputable to lithium in three cases, with KLS episodes stopping when the drug was introduced, KLS relapsing soon after stopping the drug, and recovering again when lithium was reintroduced [14,27,33]. A systematic trial in five of the seven teenagers submitted to SPECT, however, had no beneficial effect; it did not lead to remission or reduced length of symptomatic period. The results are very variable, and indicate the difficulties of performing drug trials because placebos were never used in the reported positive cases. The potential benefit of lithium, if confirmed, should be balanced against its known difficulty of use and unfavorable side effect profile. The authors also noted that antiepileptic mood stabilizers (especially carbamazepine) were commonly prescribed, probably based on the possible efficacy of lithium, but results were similar to no drug treatment (21% response in 29 patients versus 16% in 32 cases). No clear justification for initiating these treatments (and particularly an impressive absence of epileptic signs, which is surprising in a disease affecting the cortex) or antidepressant therapies were found from this meta-analysis. In one of the authors' centers that received many teenagers suspect of KLS from the entire state, and where a systematic diagnosis and follow-up protocol is in place, none of the therapeutic trials that involved all the previously mentioned drugs, but also trials with acetazolamide, flu vaccination, and anti-inflammatory drugs eliminated recurrences. Some of the antipsychotics may have helped in no more than three of nine cases of relief of some of the psychiatric symptoms during episodes, and modafinil may have shortened episodes in three of nine cases, but the variability of the duration of each episode may be the reason for this decrease. The authors believe that additional therapeutic trials using other medications, such as immunosuppressive or novel antiviral agents, with double-blind, placebo-controlled, multicenter design, are warranted.

Summary

KLS is an intriguing, severe, homogenous disease, known for more than a century, with no clear cause or treatment. Recent methods of investigation, such as SPECT, indicate that the brain dysfunction could be larger than expected, and encompass both cortical and subcortical (and especially thalamus and hypothalamus) areas. In addition, persistent post-KLS memory and SPECT defects recently observed in a few cases raise the possibility of long-term brain damage in a disease that was usually assumed to be benign. The finding of a possible Jewish predisposition, occasional familial clustering, and the association with infectious triggering factors suggest that KLS is caused by environmental factors acting on a vulnerable genetic background. This general picture and the fluctuating symptomatology in KLS are consistent with the recent report of an HLA association in KLS and the possibility of an autoimmune mediation of the disorder.

References

[1] Brierre de Boismont A. Des hallucinations ou histoire raisonnée des apparitions, des visions, des songes, de l'extase, des rêves, du magnétisme et du somnambulisme. Paris: Germer Baillière; 1862.

[2] Kleine W. Periodische schlafsucht. Monatsschrift fur Psychiatrie und Neurologie 1925;57: 285–320.

[3] Billiard M, Guilleminault C, Dement WC. A menstruation-linked periodic hypersomnia: Kleine-Levin syndrome or new clinical entity? Neurology 1975;25:436–43.

[4] Levin M. Narcolepsy (Gelineau's syndrome) and other varieties of morbid somnolence. Arch Neurol Psychiat 1929;22:1172–200.

[5] Levin M. Periodic somnolence and morbid hunger: a new syndrome. Brain 1936;59:494–504.

[6] Critchley M. Periodic hypersomnia and megaphagia in adolescent males. Brain 1962;85: 627–56.

[7] Critchley M, Hoffman H. The syndrome of periodic somnolence and morbid hunger (Kleine-Levin syndrome). BMJ 1942;1:137–9.

[8] American Academy of Sleep Medicine. The international classification of sleep disorders-revised. Westchester (IL): American Academy of Sleep Medicine; 2005.

[9] Arnulf I, Zeitzer J, File J, et al. Kleine-Levin syndrome: a systematic review of 186 cases in the literature. Brain 2005;128:2763–76.

[10] Gadoth N, Kesler A, Vainstein G, et al. Clinical and polysomnographic characteristics of 34 patients with Kleine-Levin syndrome. J Sleep Res 2001;10:337–41.

[11] Gallinek A. The Kleine-Levin syndrome: hypersomnia, bulimia, and abnormal mental states. World Neurol 1962;3:235–43.

[12] Yassa R, Nair NP. The Kleine-Levine syndrome: a variant? J Clin Psychiatry 1978;39:254–9.

[13] Carpenter S, Yassa R, Ochs R. A pathologic basis for Kleine-Levin syndrome. Arch Neurol 1982;39:25–8.

[14] Smolik P, Roth B. Kleine-Levin syndrome ethiopathogenesis and treatment. Acta Univ Carol Med Monogr 1988;128:5–94.

[15] Hegarty A, Merriam AE. Autonomic events in Kleine-Levin syndrome. Am J Psychiatry 1990;147:951–2.

[16] Badino R, Caja A, Del Conte I, et al. Kleine-Levin syndrome in an 82 year old man. Ital J Neurol Sci 1992;13:355–6.

[17] Manni R, Martinetti M, Ratti MT, et al. Electrophysiological and immunogenetic findings in recurrent monosymptomatic-type hypersomnia: a study of two unrelated Italian cases. Acta Neurol Scand 1993;88:293–5.

[18] Thacore VR, Ahmed M, Oswald I. The EEG in a case of periodic hypersomnia. Electroencephalogr Clin Neurophysiol 1969;27:605–6.

[19] Janicki S, Franco K, Zarko R. A case report of Kleine-Levin syndrome in an adolescent girl. Psychosomatics 2001;42:350–2.

[20] Katz JD, Ropper AH. Familial Kleine-Levin syndrome: two siblings with unusually long hypersomnic spells. Arch Neurol 2002;59:1959–61.

[21] Crumley FE. Valproic acid for Kleine-Levin syndrome. J Am Acad Child Adolesc Psychiatry 1997;36:868–9.

[22] Masi G, Favilla L, Millepiedi S. The Kleine-Levin syndrome as a neuropsychiatric disorder: a case report. Psychiatry 2000;63:93–100.

[23] Landtblom AM, Dige N, Schwerdt K, et al. Short-term memory dysfunction in Kleine-Levin syndrome. Acta Neurol Scand 2003;108:363–7.

[24] Gallinek A. The Kleine-Levin syndrome. Dis Nerv Syst 1967;28(7 Pt 1):448–51.

[25] Chesson Jr AL, Levine SN, Kong LS, et al. Neuroendocrine evaluation in Kleine-Levin syndrome: evidence of reduced dopaminergic tone during periods of hypersomnolence. Sleep 1991;14:226–32.

[26] Papacostas SS. Photosensitivity during the hypersomnic phase in a patient with Kleine-Levin syndrome. J Child Neurol 2003;18:432–3.

[27] Mayer G, Leonhard E, Krieg J, et al. Endocrinological and polysomnographic findings in Kleine-Levin syndrome: no evidence for hypothalamic and circadian dysfunction. Sleep 1998;21:278–84.

[28] Fresco R, Giudicelli S, Poinso Y, et al. Kleine-Levin syndrome (recurrent hypersomnia of male adolescents). Ann Med Psychol (Paris) 1971;1:625–68.

[29] Duffy JP, Davison K. A female case of the Kleine-Levin syndrome. Br J Psychiatry 1968;114:77–84.

[30] Shukla G, Bajpai H, Mishra D. Kleine-Levin syndrome: a case-report from India. Br J Psychiatry 1982;141:97–104.

[31] Portilla P, Durand E, Chalvon A, et al. SPECT-identified hypoperfusion of the left temporo-mesial structures in a Kleine-Levin syndrome. Rev Neurol (Paris) 2002;158(5 Pt 1):593–5.

[32] Poppe M, Friebel D, Reuner U, et al. The Kleine-Levin syndrome: effects of treatment with lithium. Neuropediatrics 2003;34:113–9.

[33] Rosenow F, Kotagal P, Cohen BH, et al. Multiple sleep latency test and polysomnography in diagnosing Kleine-Levin syndrome and periodic hypersomnia. J Clin Neurophysiol 2000;17:519–22.

[34] Chiles JA, Wilkus RJ. Behavioral manifestations of the Kleine-Levin syndrome. Dis Nerv Syst 1976;37:646–8.

[35] Garland H, Sumner D, Fourman P. The Kleine-Levin syndrome: some further observations. Neurology 1965;15:1161–7.

[36] Shukla GD, Bajpai HS, Mishra DN. Kleine-levin syndrome: a case report from India. Br J Psychiatry 1982;141:97–8.

[37] Will RG, Young JP, Thomas DJ. Kleine-Levin syndrome: report of two cases with onset of symptoms precipitated by head trauma. Br J Psychiatry 1988;152:410–2.

[38] Pike M, Stores G. Kleine-Levin syndrome: a cause of diagnostic confusion. Arch Dis Child 1994;71:355–7.

[39] Salter MS, White PD. A variant of the Kleine-Levin syndrome precipitated by both Epstein-Barr and varicella-zoster virus infections. Biol Psychiatry 1993;33:388–90.

[40] Sadeghu M. Kleine-Levin syndrome: a report of three adolescent female patients. Arch Iran Med 1999;2:1–3.

[41] Jensen J. The Kleine-Levin syndrome: periodic hypersomnia and hyperphagia with abnormal behavior. Ugeskr Laeger 1985;147:709–10.

[42] Goldberg MA. The treatment of Kleine-Levin syndrome with lithium. Can J Psychiatry 1983;28:491–3.

[43] Mignot E, Lammers GJ, Ripley B, et al. The role of cerebrospinal fluid hypocretin measurement in the diagnosis of narcolepsy and other hypersomnias. Arch Neurol 2002;59:1553–62.

[44] Chiu HF, Li SW, Lee S. Kleine-Levin syndrome 15 years later. Aust N Z J Psychiatry 1989;23:425–7.

[45] Billard C, Ponsot G, Lyon G, et al. Kleine-Levin syndrome: apropos of a case. Arch Fr Pediatr 1978;35:424–31.

[46] Reimao R, Shimizu MH. Kleine-Levin syndrome: clinical course, polysomnography and multiple sleep latency test. Case report. Arq Neuropsiquiatr 1998;56:650–4.

[47] Wilkus RJ, Chiles JA. Electrophysiological changes during episodes of the Kleine-Levin syndrome. J Neurol Neurosurg Psychiatry 1975; 38:1225–31.

[48] Gilbert GJ. Periodic hypersomnia and bulimia: the Kleine-Levin syndrome. Neurology 1964;14: 844–50.

[49] Papy JJ, Conte-Devolx B, Sormani J, et al. The periodic hypersomnia and megaphagia syndrome in a young female, correlated with menstrual cycle [author's translation]. Rev Electroencephalogr Neurophysiol Clin 1982;12: 54–61.

[50] Ledic P, Milohanovic S, Willheim K. Kleine-Levin syndrome. Neuropsihijatrija 1972;20: 335–40.

[51] Lavie P, Klein E, Gadoth N, et al. Further observations on sleep abnormalities in Kleine-Levin syndrome: abnormal breathing pattern during sleep. Electroencephalogr Clin Neurophysiol 1981;52:98–101.

[52] Vlach V. Periodical somnolence, bulimia and mental changes (Kleine-Levin syndrome). Cesk Neurol 1962;25:401–5.

[53] Prabhakaran N, Murthy GK, Mallya UL. A case of Kleine-Levin syndrome in India. Br J Psychiatry 1970;117:517–9.

[54] Powers PS, Gunderman R. Kleine-Levin syndrome associated with fire setting. Am J Dis Child 1978;132:786–9.

[55] Fenzi F, Simonati A, Crosato F, et al. Clinical features of Kleine-Levin syndrome with localized encephalitis. Neuropediatrics 1993;24: 292–5.

[56] Fresco R, Blumen G, Tatossian A, et al. Two cases of Kleine-Levin syndrome. Rev Neuropsychiatr Infant 1970;1:55–9.

[57] Sagar RS, Khandelwal SK, Gupta S. Interepisodic morbidity in Kleine-Levin syndrome. Br J Psychiatry 1990;157:139–41.

[58] Huang YS, Guilleminault C, Kao PF, et al. SPECT findings in Kleine-Levin syndrome. Sleep 2005;28:955–60.

[59] Terzian H, Dalle-Ore P. Syndrome of Kluver and Bucy reproduced in man by bilateral removal of the temporal lobes. Neurology 1955;5:373–80.

[60] Murad A. Orbitofrontal syndrome in psychiatry. Encephale 1999;25:634–7.

[61] Frank Y, Braham J, Cohen BE. The Kleine-Levin syndrome: case report and review of the literature. Am J Dis Child 1974;127:412–3.

[62] Frösher W, Maier V, Fritschni T. Periodic hypersomnia: case-report with biochemical and EEG findings. Sleep 1991;14:460–3.

[63] Russell J, Grunstein R. Kleine-Levin syndrome:

[64] Dauvilliers Y, Mayer G, Lecendreux M, et al. Kleine-Levin syndrome: an autoimmune hypothesis based on clinical and genetic analyses. Neurology 2002;59:1739–45.

[65] Ugoljew A, Kurella B, Nickel B. Sleep polygraphic studies as an objective method for assessing the therapeutic result in a case of periodic hypersomnia (Kleine-Levin syndrome). Nervenarzt 1991;62:292–7.

[66] Reynolds III CF, Black RS, Coble P, et al. Similarities in EEG sleep findings for Kleine-Levin syndrome and unipolar depression. Am J Psychiatry 1980;137:116–8.

[67] Gadoth N, Dickerman Z, Bechar M, et al. Episodic hormone secretion during sleep in Kleine-Levin syndrome: evidence for hypothalamic dysfunction. Brain Dev 1987;9:309–15.

[68] George HR. A case of the Kleine-Levin syndrome of long duration. Br J Psychiatry 1970; 117:521–3.

[69] Kellett J. Lithium prophylaxis of periodic hypersomnia. Br J Psychiatry 1977;130:312–6.

[70] Green LN, Cracco RQ. Kleine-Levin syndrome: a case with EEG evidence of periodic brain dysfunction. Arch Neurol 1970;22:166–75.

[71] Mukaddes NM, Alyanak B, Kora ME, et al. The psychiatric symptomatology in Kleine-Levin syndrome. Child Psychiatry Hum Dev 1999;29:253–8.

[72] Domzal-Stryga A, Emeryk-Szajewska B, Kowalski J. A case of hypersomnia resembling Kleine-Levin syndrome. Neurol Neurochir Pol 1986; 20:158–60.

[73] Roth B, Smolik P, Soucek K. Kleine-Levin syndrome: lithium prophylaxis. Cesk Psychiatr 1980; 76:156–62.

[74] Merriam AE. Kleine-Levin syndrome following acute viral encephalitis. Biol Psychiatry 1986; 21:1301–4.

[75] Overweg J. Lethargy and gluttony as an organic syndrome (Kleine-Levin syndrome). Ned Tijdschr Geneeskd 1971;115:556–8.

[76] Lemire I. Review of Kleine-Levin syndrome: toward an integrated approach. Can J Psychiatry 1993;38:277–84.

[77] Hart EJ. Kleine-Levin syndrome: normal CSF monoamines and response to lithium therapy. Neurology 1985;35:1395–6.

[78] Elian M. Periodic hypersomnia. Electroencephalogr Clin Neurophysiol 1968;24:192–3.

[79] Haberland C, Weissman S. The Kleine-Levin syndrome: a case study with a psychopathologic approach. Acta Psychiatr Scand 1968;44:1–10.

[80] Arias M, Crespo Iglesias JM, Perez J, et al. Kleine-Levin syndrome: contribution of brain SPECT in diagnosis. Rev Neurol 2002;35:531–3.

[81] Ferguson BG. Kleine-Levin syndrome: a case report. J Child Psychol Psychiatry 1986;27:275–8.

[82] Malhotra S, Das MK, Gupta N, et al. A clinical study of Kleine-Levin syndrome with evidence

for hypothalamic-pituitary axis dysfunction. Biol Psychiatry 1997;42:299–301.

[83] Muratori F, Bertini N, Masi G. Efficacy of lithium treatment in Kleine-Levin syndrome. Eur Psychiatry 2002;17:232–3.

[84] Papacostas SS, Hadjivasilis V. The Kleine-Levin syndrome: report of a case and review of the literature. Eur Psychiatry 2000;15:231–5.

[85] Mukaddes NM, Kora ME, Bilge S. Carbamazepine for Kleine-Levin syndrome. J Am Acad Child Adolesc Psychiatry 1999;38:791–2.

[86] Gau SF, Soong WT, Liu HM, et al. Kleine-Levin syndrome in a boy with Prader-Willi syndrome. Sleep 1996;19:13–7.

[87] Wilder J. A case of atypical Kleine-Levin syndrome: 30 years' observation. J Nerv Ment Dis 1972;154:69–72.

[88] Bouchard C, Levasseur M. Kleine-Levin syndrome. Rev Neurol (Paris) 2001;157:344–5.

[89] Fukunishi I, Hosokawa K. A female case with the Kleine-Levin syndrome and its physiopathologic aspects. Jpn J Psychiatry Neurol 1989;43:45–9.

[90] Koerber RK, Torkelson R, Haven G, et al. Increased cerebrospinal fluid 5-hydroxytryptamine and 5-hydroxyindoleacetic acid in Kleine-Levin syndrome. Neurology 1984;34:1597–600.

[91] Gillberg C. Kleine-Levin syndrome: unrecognized diagnosis in adolescent psychiatry. J Am Acad Child Adolesc Psychiatry 1987;26:793–4.

[92] Wenzel U. Kleine-Levin syndrome: female cases and catamneses. Fortschr Neurol Psychiatr Grenzgeb 1976;44:137–50.

[93] Fernandez JM, Lara I, Gila L, et al. Disturbed hypothalamic-pituitary axis in idiopathic recurring hypersomnia syndrome. Acta Neurol Scand 1990;82:361–3.

[94] Da Silveira Neto O, Da Silveira OA. Kleine-Levin syndrome: report of a case. Arq Neuropsiquiatr 1991;49:330–2.

[95] Livrea P, Puca F, Barnaba A, et al. Abnormal central monoamine metabolism in humans with true hypersomnia and subawkefulness. Eur Neurol 1977;15:71–6.

[96] Hasegawa Y, Morishita M, Suzumura A. Novel chromosomal aberration in a patient with a unique sleep disorder. J Neurol Neurosurg Psychiatry 1998;64:113–6.

[97] Landtblom AM, Dige N, Schwerdt K, et al. A case of Kleine-Levin syndrome examined with SPECT and neuropsychological testing. Acta Neurol Scand 2002;105:318–21.

[98] Dauvilliers Y, Baumann CR, Carlander B, et al. CSF hypocretin-1 levels in narcolepsy, Kleine-Levin syndrome, and other hypersomnias and neurological conditions. J Neurol Neurosurg Psychiatry 2003;74:1667–73.

[99] Servan J, Marchand F, Garma L, et al. Two new cases of Kleine-Levin syndrome associated with CT scan abnormalities. Can J Neurol Sci 1993; 20(Suppl 4):A5137.

[100] Drake Jr ME. Kleine-Levin syndrome after multiple cerebral infarctions. Psychosomatics 1987; 28:329–30.

[101] McGilchrist I, Goldstein LH, Jadresic D, et al. Thalamo-frontal psychosis. Br J Psychiatry 1993;163:113–5.

[102] Kostic VS, Stefanova E, Svetel M, et al. A variant of the Kleine-Levin syndrome following head trauma. Behav Neurol 1998;11:105–8.

[103] Pelin Z, Ozturk L, Bozluolcay M. Posttraumatic Kleine-Levin syndrome: a case report. Eur Psychiatry 2004;19:521–2.

[104] Testa S, Opportuno A, Gallo P, et al. A case of multiple sclerosis with an onset mimicking the Kleine-Levin syndrome. Ital J Neurol Sci 1987; 8:151–5.

[105] Lobzin VS, Shamrei RK, Churilov Iu K. Pathophysiologic mechanisms of periodic sleep and the Kleine-Levin syndrome. Zh Nevrol Psikhiatr Im S S Korsakova 1973;73:1719–24.

[106] Pfeiffer E. Kleine-Levin syndrome: diagnostic and therapeutic problems. Z Kinder Jugendpsychiatr Psychother 1997;25:117–21.

[107] Arias M, Crespo Iglesias JM, Perez J, et al. Kleine- Levin syndrome: contribution of brain SPECT in diagnosis. Rev Neurol 2002;35:531.

[108] Portilla P, Durand E, Chalvon A, et al. SPECT-identified hypoperfusion of the left temporomesial structures in a Kleine-Levin syndrome. Rev Neurol 2002;158:593–5.

[109] Landtblom AM, Dige N, Schwerdtk K, et al. A case of Kleine-Levin syndrome examined with SPECT and neuropsychological testing. Acta Neurol Scand 2002;150:318–21.

[110] Berthier ML, Santamaria J, Encabo H, et al. Recurrent hypersomnia in two adolescent males with Asperger's syndrome. J Am Acad Child Adolesc Psychiatry 1992;31:735–8.

[111] Lu ML, Liu HC, Chen CH, et al. Kleine-Levin syndrome and psychosis: observation from an unusual case. Neuropsychiatry Neuropsychol Behav Neurol 2000;13:140–2.

[112] Visscher F, van der Horst AR, Smit LM. HLA-DR antigens in Kleine-Levin syndrome. Ann Neurol 1990;28:195.

[113] Takrani LB, Cronin D. Kleine-Levin syndrome in a female patient. Can Psychiatr Assoc J 1976; 21:315–8.

[114] Chaudhry HR. Clinical use of moclobemide in Kleine-Levin syndrome. Br J Psychiatry 1992; 161:720.

SLEEP
MEDICINE
CLINICS

Sleep Med Clin 1 (2006) 105–118

Sleepiness in Children

Sarah Blunden, PhD[a],*, Timothy F. Hoban, MD[b,c],
Ronald D. Chervin, MD, MS[c]

Excessive daytime sleepiness (EDS) represents a common but often underrecognized phenomenon in children. The condition accompanies a variety of intrinsic and extrinsic sleep disorders or can arise from other medical or psychiatric pathologies. Insufficient sleep is probably the most frequent cause of EDS [1]. The precise prevalence of EDS in children is unknown. Questionnaire-based estimates suggest that up to 40% of children and adolescents report sleep problems that either restrict or disrupt sleep [2,3], whereas daytime sleepiness has been more specifically reported in 17% to 21% of school-aged children and adolescents [4].

What constitutes daytime sleepiness in children and adolescents, and what defines it as excessive? When does daytime sleepiness become detrimental to daytime function, and how does one identify when this level of sleepiness is attained? Can it be prevented or treated? This article defines EDS, discusses its measurement and contributors, and focuses on consequences and treatment options.

[a] Centre for Sleep Research, University of South Australia, Level 7, Playford Building, City East Campus, Frome Road, Adelaide SA 5000, Australia
[b] Department of Pediatrics, Pediatric Sleep Medicine Program, University of Michigan, L3227 Women's Hospital, 200 East Hospital Drive, Ann Arbor, MI 48109, USA
[c] Department of Neurology, Sleep Disorders Center, University of Michigan, Box 0117, 8D 8702 Medical Center Drive, Ann Arbor, MI 48109, USA
* Corresponding author.
E-mail address: sarah.blunden@unisa.edu.au (S. Blunden).

1556-407X/06/$ – see front matter © 2006 Elsevier Inc. All rights reserved.
sleep.theclinics.com

doi:10.1016/j.jsmc.2005.11.006

What is sleepiness?

Defining sleepiness

Sleepiness and alertness are thought to reflect functions of the anatomy, physiology, and neurochemistry that control sleep and wakefulness. Sleepiness has been defined as "an awake condition that is associated with an increased tendency…to fall asleep" [5]. Sleepiness is often regarded as the opposite of alertness.

Daytime sleepiness is generally a direct result of sleep loss from either insufficient sleep (reduced sleep quantity) or disrupted sleep (reduced sleep quality), although it is possible (but less common) to experience EDS even in the context of normal nighttime sleep quantity (eg, in idiopathic hypersomnia). Daytime sleepiness resulting from these phenomena has been studied in both primary sleep disorders and experimental paradigms. Results can be affected by individual differences, age, and variable parental awareness of sleep patterns and sleep problems. All these factors can affect the severity, expression, or perception of sleepiness.

Daytime sleepiness can be described as excessive when it interferes with daytime work, school, or social activities in a significant manner. Quantification of sleepiness remains complex, however, and specific criteria that define excessive sleepiness have not been studied systematically across childhood and adolescence. Sleepiness can be measured, however, with either objective physiologic measurements or subjective assessment of behavioral symptoms.

Measuring sleepiness

Assessment of sleepiness is covered in detail elsewhere in this issue and in previous articles [6,7]. In children, daytime sleepiness is sometimes readily apparent on observation of yawning, reduced activity, difficulty concentrating, and rubbing or closing the eyes. There is considerable between-subject variability in the manifestation of the behaviors attributable to sleepiness in children, however, and these behaviors differ substantially from those exhibited in sleepy adults. Overt somnolence is sometimes only evident intermittently in children, often during sedentary activities, such as reading, watching television, or travelling in a vehicle. Instead, sleepy children, especially before puberty, may demonstrate inattention, hyperactivity, or behavioral problems that seem to be the opposite of sleepiness (see below). By contrast, adolescents are more likely to display symptoms of sleepiness that resemble those seen in adults.

A thorough clinical history is of paramount importance in the initial evaluation of a child with EDS. A detailed review of sleep-wake patterns, the child's typical daytime and bedtime behavior, sleep hygiene, and sleep schedule often permit either a provisional diagnosis or identification of what testing may be helpful. Sleep diaries should be obtained to confirm the history provided by parents or the child and to permit more effective screening of insufficient sleep. Overt somnolence inappropriate for a child's age is strongly suggestive of either sleep deprivation or an underlying sleep disorder particularly because less overt manifestations of sleepiness, such as hyperactive behaviors, are more common [8]. The physical examination is often unremarkable in children with EDS.

In addition to a sleep diary, subjective instruments may be used to assess the complaint of sleepiness in a standardized manner. Brief, widely used, and inexpensive self-report questionnaires for adults include the Stanford Sleepiness Scale [9] and the Epworth Sleepiness Scale [10]. The Stanford Sleepiness Scale should be readily applicable for older teenagers, but has not been validated in this age group or younger children. The Epworth Sleepiness Scale was recently modified and used effectively in children [11]. Subjective sleepiness can be quantified using diagrams of faces that show different levels of subjective sleepiness [6] if children are developmentally able to interpret the scales. A range of neurobehavioral self-report or parental measures of sleep problems (which contain subscales of sleepiness) are the most commonly used method of assessing (although not diagnosing) sleep problems in children and adolescents. These include the Pediatric Sleep Questionnaire [12], The Children's Sleep Habits Questionnaire [13], the Sleep Disturbance Scale for Children [14], and the Pediatric Daytime Sleepiness Scale [15]. Although these provide appropriate cost- effective screening tools that are sensitive to the broad range of behavioral symptoms that may accompany daytime sleepiness, they should be used in the context of a thorough clinical evaluation. Despite the informative value of subjective questionnaires such as these, they may be limited by the restricted knowledge or biased reporting of sleep issues in some parents and children and the fact that respondents may not be fully aware of intermittently presenting symptoms.

When necessary, some of the objective methods used in adults may be used to assess sleepiness in children. The Multiple Sleep Latency Test (MSLT) measures time taken to fall asleep during four to five daytime nap opportunities, based on the premise that sleepy children fall asleep more quickly. Healthy children deprived of sleep show decreased mean sleep latency on the MSLT, indicating increased sleepiness [16–18]. The MSLT has been

Table 1: Normative values for children and adolescents on the Multiple Sleep Latency Test

Developmental age	Mean sleep latency in minutes (SD)
Stage I	19 (1.6)
Stage II	18.5 (1.9)
Stage III	16.1 (3.8)
Stage IV	15.8 (3.4)
Stage V	16.6 (2.2)
Older adolescents	15.7 (3.4)

Adapted from Carskadon MA. The second decade. In: Guilleminault C, editor. Sleeping and waking: indications and techniques. Menlo Park (CA): Addison Wesley; 1982. p. 112.

particularly helpful for the diagnosis of narcolepsy in adolescents [19]. The test may be useful when a child presents with EDS but clinical history, self-report or parental report, or polysomnography are inconsistent when measuring the severity of sleepiness or a response to treatment. Because children typically have longer mean sleep latencies than adults, the use of a 30-minute nap rather than the 20-minute nap opportunities used in adults may make the test more discriminatory [20]. Normative data for children exist [Table 1] but are limited. The MSLT is not recommended for children <6 years for whom some degree of daytime napping may still be normal [21,22]. MSLT is time consuming, expensive, and labor intensive and may be vulnerable to changes in a child's mood, activity level, and ability to cooperate with instructions.

A variation of the MSLT, the Maintenance of Wakefulness Test, is often used in adults. This test requires the subject to try and stay awake rather than to fall asleep and has some face validity as a measure of the subject's sleepiness. The Maintenance of Wakefulness Test, however, has not been validated for use in children.

Contributors to sleepiness in children

Although EDS may occur rarely as a primary problem in the context of sufficient nighttime sleep, in general sleepiness arises from either reduced quantity or quality of sleep. Sleep quantity and quality can be affected by biologic rhythms (including homeostatic and circadian influences); environmental, psychosocial, and psychologic factors; or particular medical and psychiatric conditions (central nervous system pathology, syndromes, and sleep disorders). Medications can produce sleepiness directly or by interface with nocturnal sleep [5].

Homeostatic influences

Largely understood through the analyses of MSLT studies and discussed in detail elsewhere in this issue, homeostatic influences on sleepiness in children include the amount of prior sleep, time awake since the last the sleep period, and the amount of sleep debt incurred over time.

Circadian influences

Innate circadian rhythms influence daily fluctuations in sleepiness and alertness; in particular, they reduce alertness during nocturnal and midday hours. Regardless of homeostatic influences a child is likely to feel sleepier during a circadian "dip." For example, these dips may contribute to sleepiness during classes after lunch.

The circadian system is probably functional at birth even if it is not initially apparent [23]. The circadian system is increasingly entrained by environmental cues or "zeitgebers" as the child develops a consolidated major nocturnal sleep period. During puberty, a shift or lengthening in circadian rhythm is thought to cause the observed biologic tendency to later sleep onset and subsequent, difficulty waking in the morning [24].

Environmental influences

The environment in which the child sleeps and the circumstances present during sleep can significantly affect sleep quality or quantity. Although age dependent, a child's ability to ignore disturbing influences (temperature, comfort, noise) is limited [25]. Although many of environmental problems can be modified, some, such as cramped bedrooms, remain a challenge.

Social and psychosocial influences

A child's developing sleep patterns are subject to social, cultural, and psychosocial influences. For example, during preadolescence and adolescence, there are increasing demands on a child's evening activities that compete for sleep time. These demands include social activities, part-time employment, increased computer or mobile telephone activity at night, sports, and academic workloads [26]. These evening activities not only delay sleep onset directly because of their time-consuming nature but also because they may be stimulating enough (eg, vigorous exercise, video games) to increase alertness, interfering with natural sleep onset at the regular bedtime. This sleepiness is further aggravated in children who must wake early to attend school. As a result, adolescents are commonly sleep deprived. The effects of early school start times and late sleep onset on sleepiness levels have been demonstrated where American students from the ninth and tenth grades with early school starts showed significant levels of sleepiness on MSLT [26]. The significance of this problem has been recognized by some education systems in the United States with the introduction of delayed school starts during the adolescent years [26].

One of the most important factors affecting the development of pediatric sleep problems is parent-child interactions. Inadequate limit setting by parents and bedtime fears or resistance by children can result in behavioral sleep problems, insufficient sleep, and daytime sleepiness. Similarly, voluntary sleep restriction in older children (eg, late night television viewing) is also strongly related to parent-child interactions. These interactions are equally related to sleep problems through such factors as child temperament (eg, high persistence, adaptability); number of siblings; and parenting style (eg, authoritarian, permissive, authoritative) [27].

Sleep has been shown to be sensitive to family dynamics and family stress. Sadeh and coworkers [28] report that not only did family stress measures correlate increased arousals but also, as reported in other studies [29,30], the higher the parent's education level, the better the child's sleep quality. Perhaps poorer health, which is prevalent among lower socioeconomic groups [30], negatively impacts sleep quantity and quality [29]. Parents of a higher education level may have broader strategies for limit setting or increased awareness of issues relating to sleep.

Finally, some research suggests that maternal mental health, although influencing childhood development in general, may especially impact the sleep behavior of young children. Maternal depression and pediatric sleep problems have shown strong associations [31,32], although causal relationships have not been determined [33].

Physiologic contributors

The developmental processes of sleep involve the combination of psychosocial mechanisms described previously with physiologic mechanisms that lead to the consolidation of sleep. These include but are not restricted to age, primary sleep disorders, and sleepiness secondary to other illnesses and syndromes.

Age is a major factor in sleepiness and how it is manifested. In infants and toddlers where sleep consolidation is directly linked to night wakings [28], residual daytime sleepiness is usually alleviated by daytime napping. EDS does not usually become apparent until after the shift to the monophasic sleep pattern of school-aged children [28]. In prepubescent and pubescent children, daytime sleepiness is frequently the result of sleep-onset insomnia, early wake times, and insufficient sleep, sometimes developing into the clinical phenomena of delayed phase syndrome (discussed later).

Changes in sleep patterns with age have been studied in a comprehensive series of longitudinal studies [24,26,34]. Sleepiness was measured (MSLT) in 24 children for 6 to 7 years [34] through several stages of development [35]. Findings suggested that from prepuberty to postpuberty, there was no increased need for sleep, but compared with prepuberty, sleepiness increased even though participants slept the same amount each night. More recently, this biobehavioral change in sleepiness was observed at an earlier age (8–9 years of age) [28]. These findings suggest that pubertal development is associated with increased physiologic levels of sleepiness. Adolescent sleep patterns, additionally influenced by lifestyle factors, may not be in accordance with their physiologic needs. In fact, adolescents may need more sleep to maintain prepubertal levels of alertness. Adolescents are commonly at risk of chronic sleep deprivation.

Sleep disorders

Sleepiness can be the result of a primary or secondary sleep disorder. The daytime sleepiness from primary sleep disorders in adults is discussed elsewhere in this issue. Although many sleep disorders have similar underlying physiology in children and adults, their manifestations often differ.

Sleep-disordered breathing

It is well documented and extensively reviewed both externally and elsewhere in this issue that adults with sleep-disordered breathing (SDB) experience EDS and that this is associated with decreased daytime performance [36,37]. By contrast, identification of sleepiness in children with SDB is more difficult [38] because sleepy children may manifest restless, inattentive, and hyperactive behavior [39] to stay alert. Despite this, sleepiness is reported in 36% to 42% of children with SDB [40–42] even though polysomnography shows sleep architecture changes less severe than those seen in adults [43]. Three studies have used MSLT to confirm sleepiness in children with SDB. One reported that shortened sleep latencies were more likely to occur in children with more severe disease [20], another noted that shortened sleep latencies returned to normal levels following treatment [44], and a third reported that sleep latency in children with sleep apnea was similar to those for children whose sleep was restricted to 4 hours for one night [18].

Narcolepsy

Daytime sleepiness is a fundamental characteristic of narcolepsy. Specific patterns of nocturnal sleep disruption have been reported in children with narcolepsy, although it is unclear whether daytime sleepiness in narcoleptic children is in part caused by this disturbed sleep architecture as opposed to central nervous system changes associated with the sleep disorder per se. The few studies of narcolepsy in children and adolescents have confirmed decreased sleep efficiency [45–47], fragmented sleep with increased arousals [45], and increased time awake after sleep onset compared with controls [47]. Although a considerable proportion of adults consider that their disorders originated before the age of 15 years [48], narcolepsy in children and adolescents often goes unnoticed. As a result, sleepiness is often misattributed to laziness or insufficient sleep and narcolepsy is often erroneously diagnosed and treated.

Restless legs

Clinical and epidemiologic research into childhood restless leg syndrome is limited [49]. Symptoms of restless leg syndrome can begin in childhood [50] but are often misdiagnosed as growing pains with subjective descriptions, such as "creeping" or "crawling" feelings in the legs. Although diagnostic criteria have recently been published [51] and despite several studies [39,50,52], only one study has established that children with growing pains may have restless leg syndrome [53]. To the authors' knowledge no studies have measured the level of daytime sleepiness in children with restless leg syndrome. Restless leg syndrome in children can result in sleep onset and sleep maintenance insomnia, however, potentially leading to significant EDS.

Parasomnias

Parasomnias are common sleep disorders that can disrupt sleep. They may result in daytime sleepiness [54], and although this is unlikely, no studies have to date specifically assessed sleepiness in children with chronic parasomnias. It has been suggested that sleepy children may be more prone to parasomnias, for which insufficient sleep may act as a trigger [55]. Chronic sleep walking and night terrors are often associated with subtle SDB and are responsive to treatment by adenotonsillectomy [56].

Behavioral sleep disorders

Behavioral sleep problems, reported in up to 37% of school-aged children [3,57], include poor sleep hygiene (eg, late night television viewing or exercise too close to bedtime); poor sleep habits (eg, irregular bed and wake times); and limit-setting sleep disorder (inconsistent or inadequate parental responses to demands of children at sleep time). Although no studies have objectively investigated sleepiness in children with behavioral sleep problems, several studies have cited that children with behavioral sleep problems are also sleepy in the day, reporting daytime symptoms of sleepiness, such as problematic behavior [3,57,58].

Circadian disorders

The most common circadian sleep disorder in children is delayed sleep phase syndrome, a very common cause of sleepiness [24,26,34], particularly in adolescents [59]. The natural sleep cycle develops a physiologic tendency for delayed sleep onset. This is coupled with lifestyle factors and early wake times for school. Wake times may occur before the natural conclusion of the circadian sleep cycle. Consequently, adolescents accrue significant sleep debt, which is often repaid by sleeping later and later on weekends further aggravating the potential to delay the sleep phase. When severe, this pattern can develop into delayed sleep phase syndrome.

Sleepiness secondary to other disorders or illnesses

Children with chronic illness and diverse syndromes have reported sleep problems [60,61]. These result not only from disturbances to sleep from physiologic causes but also because disturbed sleep is a strong indicator of both physiologic and psychologic stress [60]. Children and adolescents with special needs, such as developmental disorders (eg, autism), attention-deficit hyperactivity disorder (ADHD), mood disorders, and chronic physical illness (eg, cerebral palsy, epilepsy, rheumatoid arthritis), are at risk of sleepiness because of secondary sleep disruption related to their condition [61].

Sleepiness in children with developmental disabilities

Sleep problems in this population are higher than in comparable groups without developmental disabilities [61]. Studies evaluating daytime sleepiness in these groups, however, are underrepresented in the literature. In addition, generally recognized symptoms of daytime sleepiness seen in normal populations (eg, behavioral and mood disorders and cognitive deficits) may not be reliable indicators of sleepiness in children with special needs because these behaviors are often associated with their conditions.

Attention-deficit hyperactivity disorder

Studies have reported that up to 50% to 60% of children with ADHD present with sleep problems [62,63] including both behavioral sleep disorders

[62,64,65] and physiologic sleep disorders [39,42, 66,67]. Reduced sleep duration in children with ADHD compared with controls has been reported [38,62,65]. Two studies report that children with ADHD have greater physiologic sleepiness than matched controls [8,67], even after three consecutive nights of optimal sleep [8]. Given that the core symptoms of ADHD closely match the daytime symptoms of excessively sleepy children, could children with ADHD be excessively sleepy? If so, this may explain why stimulants improve rather than exacerbate disruptive behavior in these children [63].

Objectively measured sleep of ADHD children, however, seems relatively intact [66,68,69]. Children with ADHD may have sleep disruption that is not detected by current methods of analysis. For example, in pediatric studies, there is a need to develop criteria that include definitions of arousal and sleep disruption that could be based on alternative parameters to visual scoring, because, as the definition of an arousal becomes increasingly subtle, the reliability for visual scoring of that event decreases. Sleep disruption may be more easily detected when criteria are expanded to include changes in autonomic function (blood pressure, heart rate), pulse transit time [70], subcortical arousals, or microarousals as defined by spectral analysis of electroencephalogram [71,72] or by combining measures of electromyogram with electroencephalogram arousal [73]. Recent data suggest that in children with suspected SDB, respiratory cycle-related electroencephalogram changes, detected by computer, may explain sleepiness and inattention better than do standard rates of apnea and hypopnea [74].

Although children with ADHD have sleep problems, the reverse has also been reported. Many daytime symptoms associated with sleep disorders, such as sleep apnea and restless legs syndrome, are similar to the behavioral clusters of ADHD [38,39,66,75]. For example, the excess frequency of hyperactive behavior among habitually snoring children suggests that if SDB contributes to the behavior, then as many as 25% of children with high hyperactivity scores may benefit from the diagnosis and treatment of snoring and any SDB that underlies it [75]. If sleep disturbances cause sleepiness, then sleepy children may try to stay alert by engaging in stimulating, even hyperactive motor behaviors [44]. This is supported by reports of hyperactive symptoms in children whose sleep loss derives from non–disease-related sleep disruption [62].

Mood disorders

Anxiety and depression are the mood disorders most commonly related to sleep disturbances.

Dahl and coworkers [76] suggest that the relationship between the systems that regulate sleep and affect may be bidirectional; however, whether there is a causal association remains unclear. Sleep disturbances present as a symptom for both disorders, yet sleep disturbance and sleepiness may exacerbate mood disorders. Children diagnosed with anxiety disorders complain of more sleep disturbance than do children with any other psychiatric disorders; sleep disturbance that can potentially contribute to daytime sleepiness [61]. Sleep disturbances are also common in children and adolescents with major depressive disorder, with insomnia being the most common complaint [77]. Depressed children and adolescents tend to be sleepier during the day. Whether this is caused by daytime sleepiness from disturbed or insufficient sleep or a behavioral or social withdrawal related to the mood disorder has not been extensively researched.

Other syndromes and illnesses

If it is true that insufficient sleep results in daytime sleepiness, then it follows that any illness, disorder, or syndrome that results in insufficient sleep has the potential to cause daytime sleepiness. A review of all the relevant childhood syndromes and illnesses is beyond the scope of this article, but the contribution of sleepiness to the daytime behavioral symptoms in medically ill children is likely to be significant and underrecognized.

The effects of sleepiness in children

The data that address the specific effects of insufficient sleep and sleepiness in children on daytime function is sparse. They can be categorized into two main areas. First, sleep loss from experimental sleep restriction or deprivation. By experimentally restricting sleep, it is possible to quantify sleep loss and subsequent sleepiness and monitor the consequences. Second, sleep loss from insufficient or impaired sleep. Clinical observations and descriptions of children with insufficient or impaired sleep, most commonly investigated by parental report, describe the range of specific sleep problems (including physiologic and behavioral sleep disorders) that result in sleep loss.

Measurement of the effects of sleepiness on daytime function is accomplished mostly through standardized neuropsychological and neurobehavioral assessment tools. Although these are valuable methods of assessing daytime function in sleepy children, studies using these tests are few. Next, evidence is presented to suggest that sleep loss from either experimental sleep restriction or from insufficient or impaired sleep results in daytime sequelae. Although individual differences to sleep loss exist, studies report problematic behavior, mood disturbances, and deficits in certain cognitive functions.

Behavior

Data collected by parental report [40,58,75,78] and objective methods (polysomnography, actigraphy) [79–82] suggest that behavioral problems are common in children with insufficient or impaired sleep. These clusters of behaviors include a lower frustration threshold leading to irritability, emotional lability and aggression, concentration difficulties, or hyperactive type behaviors [64].

Behavioral inhibition: aggression, impulsivity, risk-taking behavior mood disturbances, hyperactivity

The most common daytime behavioral sequelae in sleepy children are emotional lability [64]. The premise is that children who are sleepy are less able to regulate emotion, have a reduced frustration tolerance, and are more likely to present as aggressive and emotionally volatile [64].

For example, children with SDB [41,52,79,81–83], restless legs syndrome [53], and behavioral sleep disorders [64,57,58] show increased aggression and conduct problems compared with non–sleep-disordered children. Greater levels of sleepiness have been associated with more severe social and conduct problems [78]. These findings have been confirmed in children who have been experimentally sleep deprived. Children restricted to 7 nights of 6.5 hours per night reported increased physiologic sleepiness coupled with an increase in parentally reported oppositional behavior [18].

Children who are sleepy may have difficulty with behavioral inhibition and be more impulsive. They are more likely to engage in risk-taking behaviors when they are less well slept, which could place them at greater risk of injury [84]. Inadequate sleep duration has been shown to increase the risk of injury among children where children who slept less than 10 hours per night were more likely to suffer unintentional injury compared with longer sleepers [85]. Indeed, gross motor tasks seem to be sensitive to sleepiness. In an early study [86] there was a significant reduction in reaction time in gross motor tasks after 18 hours of experimental wakefulness, with balance and agility decreasing after 42 hours of wakefulness.

Evidence suggests that sleepy children have diminished control in various emotional domains [64] including the regulation of mood [87]. Depressed children and adolescents are more sleepy, but whether sleepy children have increased depression remains unclear. Studies of children with SDB [79,83] have reported increased levels of depression and anxiety, but whether this is directly related to sleepiness or another disease-related factor remains unclear.

Another aspect of diminished behavioral control reported in children with sleep loss is hyperactive symptoms. Stores [48] suggests that "sleepiness can take the form of an increase rather than a reduction of activity." Children with sleep problems, particularly before puberty, often show daytime symptoms that resemble those reported in hyperactive children [11].

Neurocognitive function

The effects of sleepiness on daytime neuropsychologic functioning in children have been studied mainly in children with sleep disorders, such as SDB, restless legs, and behavioral sleep problems, with some data available from sleep restriction studies.

Inattention

Sleepy children show impaired attentional capacity on both parental report and standardized tests. Robust findings on attentional deficits in sleepy children have emerged from the literature in children with SDB [44,75,79,81,83] and restless leg syndrome or periodic limb movement disorder [39,49,66]. In addition, children with decreased attentional capacity unselected for sleep complaints show a high frequency of snoring [39,75] and restless legs [88]. Whether inattention results directly from sleepiness in these children or is secondary to a factor intrinsic to disease remains unclear.

Attentional deficits have been detected in children with other sleep problems [65,78]. Sleep loss from behaviorally based sleep disorders has been related to objectively measured ADHD symptoms [76], attentional problems [58], difficulty in focused attention and concentration [89], and poorer performance on sustained attention tasks [58]. Are these attention deficits caused by sleepiness on the premise that sleepy children have difficulty focusing attention? For example, Stein and coworkers [78] reported a negative correlation between sleepiness and parental-reported attentional problems. By contrast, in sleep restriction studies [6,16,17] where MSLT results documented increased sleep tendency, no impairment was noted in auditory [16,17] or sustained attention tasks [6].

The argument for an association between sleepiness and attention deficits is nonetheless strengthened by evidence that treatment of sleep disorders can improve attention. Walters [50] reports that three of six children treated for restless legs reverted to normal scores on a test of variable attention. Furthermore, two studies report withdrawal of stimulant medication in children when sleep disorders were treated [44,50]. Treatment of behavioral sleep disorders [2] and insomnia [64] has similarly resulted in a significant improvement in attentional capacity and impulsivity. These findings, from a variety of sleep disorders, are consistent with a hypothesis that the increased and improved sleep results in greater alertness and improved attentional capacity.

Learning, memory, and academic performance

If sleep disorders result in sleepiness, several studies report reduced neurocognitive functioning in children with sleep disorders. Both standardized tests and anecdotal reports suggest that children with SDB present with lower intelligence quotient, impaired memory and problem solving [79,90–92], and poorer school performance [38,41,42,93]. It has been proposed that these deficits are not solely caused by sleepiness but also by the pathogenesis of the disease itself (hypoxia) [92]. Blunden and coworkers [58], however, report that whereas children with SDB showed reduced memory performance on a working nonverbal memory task, children with behavioral sleep disorders performed worse. Walters [50] reports that children treated for restless legs syndrome and periodic limb movement disorder had a parallel improvement in sleep quality (decreased arousals) and visual memory on standardized tests. These two latter findings suggest factors other than hypoxia contribute to these deficits, potentially sleepiness.

Sleep deprivation studies in children have shown that higher-order function (eg, abstract thinking, verbal fluency, concept formation, creativity) [16] and motor computational speed [16,17] were impaired in experimental sleep restriction studies. In these studies, no memory deficits were reported until sleep restriction was extended from 1 night to 3 nights. Perhaps different cognitive functions require different levels of sleepiness before daytime effects are noted.

Other daytime sequelae of sleepiness in children

Sleep loss is usually associated with stress, increased locomotive activity, changes in hormonal activity, and body temperature [94]. Each of these is known to affect immune function and sleep loss has been associated with changes in cytokines and tumor necrosis factor [94].

Reduced sleep duration produces decreased levels of leptin, an appetite-suppressing hormone, and increased ghrelin, an appetite stimulant [95,96]. Moreover, sleep disturbance increases the preference for lipid-rich, high-calorie foods [95,97]. It remains to be further investigated whether disordered sleep impacts neuroendocrine function enough to make a substantial contribution to childhood obesity. Sleep loss and subsequent sleepiness seem to affect psychosocial, physiologic, and cognitive function.

How does sleepiness impair daytime function?

The sleepiness as direct contributor

Daytime sleepiness and reduced daytime alertness possibly limit the ability to focus and attend to

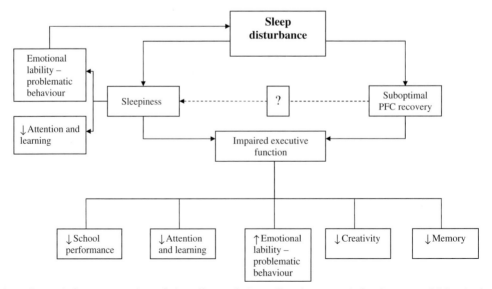

Fig. 1. A theoretical representation of the effects of sleep disturbance and sleepiness on children's daytime function. PFC, prefrontal cortex.

salient information. Reduced attentional capacity may slow leaning and decrease overall knowledge levels. Behavioral problems may be a direct result of emotional volatility caused by sleepiness [Fig. 1]. Indeed, behavioral lability may in turn contribute to sleepiness. A causal relationship between sleep loss and daytime dysfunction is strengthened by studies in which treatment of nonmedical sleep disorders has resulted in amelioration of daytime impairment [2].

Disruption to the development of the prefrontal cortex

Does sleepiness result when significant sections of the brain receive suboptimal recovery? The prefrontal cortex regulates executive function, which includes behavioral regulation (eg, hyperactivity, impulsivity); goal-directed behavior; attentional capacity; and higher-order functions, such as verbal fluency and creativity [98,99], functions reportedly impaired with sleep loss. The prefrontal cortex is among parts of the brain most sensitive to sleep deprivation or sleep disruption [99]. During normal sleep, the prefrontal cortex displays reduced activity across all sleep stages, appearing functionally disconnected from regions with which it interacts during the day [99]. This may reflect a requirement for the prefrontal cortex to rest without interference from other brain activity. Horne [98] maintains that the prefrontal cortex is the hardest working section of the brain, requiring the greatest recovery. This may be the reason that the prefrontal cortex is sensitive to sleep deprivation. If so, it follows that sleep disturbance results in suboptimal recovery and sleepiness, and potentially functional changes to the prefrontal regions of the cerebral cortex, which regulates executive function [see Fig. 1] [99].

Physiologic markers of sleepiness

In recent years, several biologic markers associated with narcolepsy have been identified, including certain HLA haplotypes and the absence of hypocretin in the cerebrospinal fluid [19]. Whether or not these two markers reflect processes that cause sleepiness remains to be further investigated.

Sleep continuity hypothesis

Is it lack of sleep continuity that creates sleepiness? Sleep may be distributed in a manner that is critical to the restorative process, as suggested in the sleep continuity hypothesis [100]. The assumption underlying this theory is that sleep quality is compromised more by positioning of arousals during sleep stages rather than by the length and frequency of the arousals themselves. Bonnet [100] suggests that consolidation of sleep is crucial to optimal

functioning. For example, 6 hours of sleep undisturbed is better than 7 hours with multiple arousals. This may explain the individual differences in sleepiness and why it may not be detected by current methods.

Treatment options

Alleviation of sleepiness through treatment of the underlying sleep loss and disturbance results in improved daytime functioning and reduced cognitive deficits [2,27,64]. Treatment options are usually either pharmacologic or behavioral [Table 2]. Behavioral treatments are usually effective for sleep disorders with an extrinsic cause and are largely based on psychologic techniques that are beyond the scope of this article but are well reviewed elsewhere [27].

In general, determining the use of drug treatment of daytime somnolence is considered only when daytime sleepiness is significant in severity or frequency, when duration of nighttime sleep is sufficient, and when any disturbances of nighttime sleep have been treated to the extent possible. There have been no controlled clinical trials regarding use of stimulants and other wake-promoting medications in children. The medicines most commonly used for these purposes include methylphenidate, amphetamine salts, and modafinil. Dosing for these medications is not well established for the purpose of treating sleepiness in children, but for treatment of ADHD, methylphenidate doses ranging from 0.3 to 1 mg/kg have been reported to be clinically effective [101]. In a small series of children aged 2 to 18 years with narcolepsy and idiopathic hypersomnia treated with modafinil, treatment was reported to be effective and well-tolerated at a mean daily dosage of 346 ± 119 mg/d [102]. Treatment using these agents should be started at relatively low doses with subsequent titration based on tolerance and clinical effect. Optimal timing of doses may differ substantially between children, and even with long-acting agents some children do better with split-day dosing. Side effects of stimulants may include insomnia, weight loss, headache, tachycardia, behavioral changes, and potential for abuse. Modafinil has a good safety profile in most respects, but can cause nausea, poor sleep, excessive perspiration, and other constitutional symptoms.

Challenges for the primary care health professional

The diagnosis and assessment of sleepiness in children can be challenging and the condition is most likely severely underreported. Evidence exists to

Table 2: Examples of common pharmacologic and behavioral treatments for sleep problems that can cause sleepiness

Sleep disturbance	Medical and pharmacologic	Behavioral and psychologic	Possible referral to
Snoring or sleep apnea	Adenotonsillectomy, continuous positive airways pressure	Behavioral treatment for frequently comorbid behavioral sleep disorders	Ear, nose, and throat specialist; overnight sleep unit
Narcolepsy	Stimulants (methylphenidate, pemoline) or REM suppressant (protriptyline) medication	Education, good sleep hygiene, scheduled naps	Overnight sleep unit and daytime sleepiness measures (MSLT)
Insomnia	Zolpidem, benzodiazepines, cough medicines, natural medicines	Relaxation techniques, imagery, cognitive restructuring	Psychologist
Idiopathic hypersomnolence	Stimulant medication		
Periodic limb movement disorder or restless legs syndrome	Dopamine agonists, levodopa, increased iron intake	Massage, heat application	Overnight sleep unit
Sleep association disorder or limit setting disorder		Behavioral reinforcement of desired behaviors, extinction	Sleep psychologist
Frequent night wakings		Behavioral reinforcement of desired behaviors, extinction	Sleep psychologist
Delayed phase syndrome		Chronotherapy, circadian readjustment	Sleep specialist or sleep psychologist

Abbreviations: MSLT, Multiple Sleep Latency Test; REM, rapid eye movement.

confirm that common causes of sleepiness are underreported by parents [3,78,103] and under-diagnosed by clinicians [3,103]. Reasons for under-reporting of sleep problems may be multifactorial including limited parental awareness of the importance and sequelae of sleep problems in children and misattribution of symptoms to other causes.

Summary

Considerable evidence suggests that sleepiness in children is manifested in ways that are less obvious than those seen in sleepy adults. The impact of sleepiness on a range of functional domains is still likely to be substantial, especially in view of unique vulnerabilities during childhood development. A considerable amount of research remains to be undertaken to clarify better the age-dependent manifestations of sleepiness, the extent to which sleepiness causes disruptive behavior and impaired cognition, and the methods for effective interventions in children with sleep disorders.

Sleepiness represents a common but often under-diagnosed problem in children. Sleepiness may accompany a variety of intrinsic (eg, obstructive sleep apnea, restless legs syndrome, narcolepsy) and extrinsic sleep disorders (behavioral sleep disorders) from either primary or secondary sources of sleep disturbance. EDS is likely to have diverse manifestations ranging from overt sleepiness to hyperactive behaviors. Data presented here show that the impact of sleepiness can include reduced attentional and memory capacity; increased emotional volatility and problematic behaviors (eg, aggression and hyperactivity); and poorer executive function. Pathways to these daytime deficits may be multifactorial and treatment needs to encompass a multidisciplinary approach.

References

[1] Brown LW, Billiard M. Narcolepsy, Kleine-Levin syndrome, and other causes of sleepiness in children. In: Ferber R, Kryger M, editors. Principles and practices of sleep medicine in the child. Philadelphia: WB Saunders; 1995. p. 125–34.

[2] Mindell JA, Durand VM. Treatment of childhood sleep disorders: generalization across disorders and effects on family members. J Pediatr Psychol 1993;18:731–50.

[3] Blunden S, Lushington K, Lorenzen B, et al. Are sleep problems under-recognised in general practice? Arch Dis Child 2003;89:708–12.

[4] Saarenpaa OS, Laippala P, Koivikko M. Subjective sleepiness in children. Fam Pract 2000;17:129–33.

[5] Dement WC. Sleepiness. In: Carskadon M, editor. Encyclopedia of sleep and dreaming. New York: Macmillan Publishing Company; 1993. p. 554–67.

[6] Fallone GP, Acebo C, Arendt TA, et al. Effects of acute sleep restriction on behaviour, sustained attention and response inhibition in children. Percept Mot Skills 2001;93:213–29.

[7] Hoban TF, Chervin R. Assessment of sleepiness in children. Semin Pediatr Neurol 2001;8:216–28.

[8] Lecendreux M, Knofl E, Bouvard NM, et al. Sleep and alertness in children with ADHD. J Child Psychol Psychiatry 2000;41:803–12.

[9] Hoddes E, Dement WC, Zarcone V. The development and use of the Stanford Sleepiness Scale (SSS). Psychophysiology 1972;9:150–6.

[10] Johns MW. Daytime sleepiness, snoring, and obstructive sleep apnea: the Epworth Sleepiness Scale. Chest 1993;103:30–6.

[11] Melendres MC, Lutz JM, Rubin ED, et al. Daytime sleepiness and hyperactivity in children with suspected sleep disordered breathing. Pediatrics 2004;14:768–75.

[12] Chervin RD, Archbold KH, Dillon JE, et al. Pediatric Sleep Questionnaire (PSQ): validity and reliability of scales for sleep disordered breathing, snoring, sleepiness and behavioural problems. Sleep Med 2000;1:21–32.

[13] Owens JA, Spirito A, McGuinn M. The children's sleep habits questionnaire (CSHQ): psychometric properties of a survey instrument for school-aged children. Sleep 2000;23:1043–51.

[14] Bruni O, Ottaviano S, Guidetti MR, et al. The sleep disturbance scale for children: construction and validation of an instrument to evaluate sleep disturbance in childhood and adolescence. J Sleep Res 1996;5:251–61.

[15] Drake C, Nickel C, Burduvali E, et al. The pediatric daytime sleepiness scale (PDSS): sleep habits and school outcomes in middle-school children. Sleep 2003;26:455–8.

[16] Randazzo AC, Schweitzer PK, Walsh JK. Cognitive function following acute sleep restriction in children ages 10–14. Sleep 1998;21:861–8.

[17] Carskadon MA, Harvey K, Dement WC. Acute restriction of nocturnal sleep in children. Percept Mot Skills 1981;53:103–14.

[18] Fallone GP, Seifer R, Acebo C, et al. Prolonged sleep restriction in 11 and 12 year old children: effects on behaviour, sleepiness and mood. Sleep 2000;23:A28.

[19] Guilleminault C, Pelayo R. Narcolepsy in prepubertal children. Ann Neurol 1998;43:135–42.

[20] Gozal D, Wang M, Pope DW, et al. Objective sleepiness measures in pediatric obstructive sleep apnea. Pediatrics 2001;108:693–7.

[21] Kotagol S, Gouldin PM. The laboratory assessment of daytime sleepiness in childhood. J Clin Neurophysiol 1996;13:208–18.

[22] Carskadon MA. The second decade. In: Guilleminault C, editor. Sleeping and waking: indica-

tions and techniques. Menlo Park (CA): Addison Wesley; 1982. p. 99–125.

[23] Helbrugge T. The development of circadian rhythms in infants. Cold Spring Harb Symp Quant Biol 1960;25:311–5.

[24] Carskadon MA, Vieira C, Acebo C. Association between puberty and delayed phase preference. Sleep 1993;16:258–62.

[25] Ferber R. Introduction: pediatric sleep disorders medicine. In: Ferber R, Kryger M, editors. Principles and practice of sleep medicine in the child. Philadelphia: WB Saunders; 1995.

[26] Carskadon MA, Wolfson AR, Acebo C, et al. Adolescent sleep patterns, circadian timing, sleepiness at a transition to early school days. Sleep 1998;21:871–81.

[27] Owens J, Palermo TM, Rosen C. Overview of current management of sleep disturbances in children II: Behavioural interventions. Current Therapeutic Research 2001;63:B38–52.

[28] Sadeh A, Raviv A, Gruber R. Sleep patterns and sleep disruptions in school age children. Dev Psychol 2000;36:291–301.

[29] Rona RJ, Leah L, Gulliford MC, et al. Disturbed sleep: effects of socio-cultural factors and illness. Arch Dis Child 1998;78:20–5.

[30] Moore PJ, Adler NE, Williams DR, et al. Socioeconomic status and health: the role of sleep. Psychosom Med 2002;64:337–44.

[31] Richman N. Depression in mothers of preschool children. J Child Psychol Psychiatry 1975; 17:75–8.

[32] Hiscock H, Wake M. Infant sleep problems and post-natal depression: a community based study. Pediatrics 2001;107:1317–22.

[33] Glaze DG, Rosen C, Owens J. Toward a practical definition of pediatric insomnia. Current Therapeutic Research 2002;63:B4–17.

[34] Carskadon MA, Harvey K, Dement WC. Pubertal changes in daytime sleepiness. Sleep 1980;2: 453–9.

[35] Tanner JM. Growth at adolescence. 2nd edition. Oxford: Blackwell; 1962.

[36] Bonnet MH. Cognitive effects of sleep and sleep fragmentation. Sleep 1993;16:S65–7.

[37] Berry D. Hypoxia and neuropsychological functioning. J Sleep Res 1986;3:254–67.

[38] Guilleminault C, Elridge F, Simmons FB, et al. Sleep apnea in eight children. Paediatrics 1976; 58:23–30.

[39] Chervin RD, Dillon JE, Bassetti C, et al. Symptoms of sleep disorders, inattention, and hyperactivity in children. Sleep 1997;20:1185–92.

[40] Ali NJ, Pitson D, Stradling JR. Natural history of snoring and related behaviours problems between the ages of 4 and 7 years. Arch Dis Child 1994;71:74–6.

[41] Guilleminault C, Pelayo R, Leger D, et al. Recognition of sleep disordered breathing in children. Pediatrics 1996;98:871–82.

[42] Richards W, Ferdman R. Prolonged morbidity due to delays in the diagnosis and treatment of obstructive sleep apnea syndrome in children. Clin Pediatr (Phila) 2000;39:103–8.

[43] Carroll JL, McColley SA, Marcus CL, et al. Inability of clinical history to distinguish primary snoring from obstructive sleep apnea. Chest 1995;108:610–8.

[44] Guilleminault C, Winkle R, Korbkin R, et al. Children and nocturnal snoring: evaluation of the effects of sleep related respiratory resistive load and daytime functioning. J Pediatr 1982; 139:165–71.

[45] Dahl RE, Hohum J, Trubnick L. A clinical picture of childhood and adolescent narcolepsy. J Am Acad Child Adolesc Psychiatry 1994; 33:834.

[46] Kotagol S, Haarste KM, Walsh JK. Characteristics of narcolepsy in preteenaged children. Pediatrics 1990;85:205.

[47] Young D, Zorick F, Witting R, et al. Narcolepsy in a paediatric population. Am J Dis Child 1988; 142:210–3.

[48] Stores G. Recognition and management of narcolepsy. Arch Dis Child 1999;81:519–24.

[49] Kotagol S, Silber M. Childhood-onset restless legs syndrome. Ann Neurol 2004;56:803–7.

[50] Walters AS. Is there a subpopulation of children with growing pains who have restless legs syndrome? A review of the literature. Sleep Med 2002;3:93–8.

[51] Allen RP, Pichietti D, Hening WA, et al. Restless legs syndrome: diagnostic criteria, special considerations and epidemiology. A report from the restless legs syndrome diagnosis and epidemiology workshop at the National Institutes of Health. Sleep Med 2003;4:101–19.

[52] Chervin R, Dillon J, Archbold K, et al. Conduct problems and symptoms of sleep disorders in children. J Am Acad Child Adolesc Psychiatry 2003;42:201–8.

[53] Rajaram S, Walters AS, England SJ, et al. Some children with growing pains may actually have restless legs syndrome. Sleep 2004;27:767–73.

[54] Mahowald MW, Rosen G. Parasomnias in children. Paediatrician 1990;17:21–31.

[55] Masand P, Popli AP, Weilburg JB. Sleepwalking. Am Fam Physician 1995;5:649–54.

[56] Guilleminault C, Palombini K, Pelayo R, et al. Sleep walking and sleep terrors in prepubertal children: what triggers them? Pediatrics 2003; 111:e17–25.

[57] Owens J, Opipari L, Nobile C, et al. Sleep and behaviour in children with obstructive sleep apnea and behavioural sleep disorders. Pediatrics 1998;102:1178–84.

[58] Blunden SL, Lushington K, Lorenzen B, et al. Neuropsychological and psychosocial function in children with a history of either snoring or disorders of initiating and maintaining sleep. J Pediatr 2005;146(6):780–6.

[59] Dahl RE, Carskadon M. Sleep and its disorders in adolescence. In: Ferber R, Kryger M, editors. Principles and practices of sleep medi-

cine in the child. Philadelphia: WB Saunders; 1995. p. 19–27.

[60] Glaze DG, Rosen C, Owens J. Toward a practical definition of pediatric insomnia. Current Therapeutic Research 2002;63:B4–17.

[61] Ivanenko A, Crabtree VM, Gozal D. Sleep in children with psychiatric disorders. Pediatr Clin North Am 2004;51:51–68.

[62] Owens J, Maxim R, Nobile C, et al. Parental and self report of sleep in children with attention deficit/hyperactivity disorder. Arch Pediatr Adolesc Med 2000;154:549–55.

[63] Golan N, Shahar E, Ravid S, et al. Sleep disorders and daytime sleepiness in children with attention deficit hyperactive disorder. Sleep 2004;27:261–6.

[64] Dahl R. The impact of inadequate sleep on children's daytime cognitive function. Semin Pediatr Neurol 1996;3:44–50.

[65] Marcotte AC, Thacher PV, Butters M, et al. Parental report of sleep problems in children with attentional and learning disorders. Dev Behav Ped 1998;19:178–86.

[66] Picchetti DL, England SJ, Walters AS, et al. Periodic limb movement disorder and restless legs syndrome in children with attention deficit hyperactivity disorder. J Child Neurol 1998;13: 588–94.

[67] Lebourgeois MK, Avis K, Mixon M, et al. Snoring, sleep quality and sleepiness across attention-deficit hyperactivity disorder subtypes. Sleep 2004; 27:520–5.

[68] Corkum P, Tannock R, Moldofsky H. Sleep disturbance in children with attention-deficit hyperactivity disorder. J Am Acad Child Adolesc Psychiatry 1998;37:637–46.

[69] Gruber R, Sadeh A. Sleep and neurobehavioural functioning in boys with attention deficit hyperactivity disorder ano reported breathing problems. Sleep 2004;27:267–73.

[70] Argod J, Pepin J-L, Smith R, et al. Comparison of oesophageal pressure with pulse transit time as a measure of respiratory effort for scoring obstructive nonapneic respiratory events. Am J Respir Crit Care Med 2000;162:87–93.

[71] Scholle S, Zwacka G. Arousals and obstructive sleep apnea syndrome in children. Clin Neurophysiol 2001;112:984–99.

[72] Bandla HP, Gozal D. Dynamic changes to EEG spectra during obstructive apnea in children. Pediatr Pulmonol 2000;29:359–65.

[73] Brouillette RT, Lavernge J, Leimanis A, et al. Differences in pulse oximetry technology can affect detection of sleep disordered breathing in children. Anaesthetic Anal 2002;94:S47–53.

[74] Chervin RD, Burns JW, Subotic NS, et al. Correlates of respiratory cycle related EEG changes in children with sleep disordered breathing. Sleep 2004;27:116–21.

[75] Chervin RD, Archbold KH, Dillon JE, et al. Inattention, hyperactivity and symptoms of sleep disordered breathing. Pediatrics 2002;109:449–56.

[76] Dahl RE, Pelham WB, Wierson MC. The role of sleep disturbance in attention deficit disorders symptomology: a case study. J Pediatr Psychol 1991;16:229–39.

[77] Frederiksen K, Rhodes J, Reddy R, et al. Sleepless in Chicago: tracking the effects of adolescent sleep loss during middle school years. Child Dev 2004;75:84–95.

[78] Stein MA, Mendelsohn J, Obermeyer WH, et al. Sleep and behaviour problems in school-aged children. Pediatrics 2001;107:e60–74.

[79] Blunden SL, Lushington K, Kennedy D, et al. Behaviour and neurocognitive performance in children aged 5–10 years who snore compared to controls. J Clin Exp Neuropsychol 2000;22: 554–68.

[80] Chervin RD, Archbold KH. Hyperactivity and polysomnographic findings in children evaluated for sleep-disordered breathing. Sleep 2001; 24:313–20.

[81] Lewin DS, Rosen RC, England SJ, et al. Preliminary evidence of behavioural and cognitive sequelae of obstructive sleep apnea in children. Sleep Med 2002;3:5–13.

[82] Ali NJ, Pitson D, Stradling JR. Sleep disordered breathing: effects of adenotonsillectomy on behaviour and psychological functioning. Eur J Pediatr 1996;155:56–62.

[83] Goldstein NA, Post JC, Rosenfeld RM, et al. Impact of tonsillectomy and adenoidectomy on child behaviour. Arch Otolaryngol Head Neck Surg 2000;126:494–9.

[84] Giannotti F, Cortesi F. Sleep patterns and daytime function in adolescents: an epidemiological survey of Italian high school student population. In: Carskadon MA, editor. Adolescent sleep patterns: biological, social, and psychosocial influences. New York: Cambridge University Press; 1998. p. 132–47.

[85] Valent F, Brusaferro S, Barboe F. A case crossover study of sleep and childhood injury. Pediatrics 2001;107:E23–35.

[86] Copes K, Rosentweig J. The effects of sleep deprivation on motor performance of ninth grade student. J Sports Med 1972;12:47–53.

[87] Young W, Knowles J, Maclean A, et al. The sleep of childhood depressives: comparison with age matched controls. Biol Psychiatry 1982;17: 1163–8.

[88] Chervin RD, Archbold KH, Dillon JE, et al. Associations between symptoms of inattention, hyperactivity, restless legs and periodic leg movements. Sleep 2002;25:213–8.

[89] Epstein R, Chillag N, Lavie P. Starting times of school: effects on daytime functioning of fifth grade children in Israel. Sleep 1998;21:47–53.

[90] Rhodes SK, Shimoda KC, Waid LR, et al. Neurocognitive deficits in morbidly obese children with obstructive sleep apnea. J Pediatr 1995; 127:741–4.

[91] Owens J, Spirito A, Marcotte A, et al. Neuropsychological and behavioural correlates of

obstructive sleep apnea syndrome in children: a preliminary study. Sleep Breath 2000; 4:67–78.

[92] Beebe DW, Groesz L, Jerrfies J, et al. Executive dysfunction in children referred for obstructive sleep apnea evaluation. Sleep 2002;25:A225.

[93] Gozal D. Sleep disordered breathing in school aged children: impact on school performance. Pediatrics 1998;102:616–20.

[94] Kryger MH, Roth T, Dement WC, editors. Principles and practices of sleep medicine. 2nd edition. Philadelphia: WB Saunders; 1994.

[95] Spiegel K, Leproult R, Van Cauter E. Impact of sleep debt on metabolic and endocrine function. Lancet 1999;354:1435–9.

[96] Taheri S, Ling L, Austin D, et al. Short sleep duration is associated with reduced leptin, increased ghrelin and increased body mass index. PLoS Medicine 2004;1:e62.

[97] Dinges D, Chigh DK. Physiologic correlates of sleep deprivation. In: Kinney JM, Ticker JB, editors. Physiology, stress and malnutrition: functional correlates, nutritional intervention. New York: Lippincott Raven; 1997. p. 1–27.

[98] Horne JA. Sleep loss and divergent thinking ability. Sleep 1988;11:528–36.

[99] Beebe DW, Gozal D. Obstructive sleep apnea and the prefrontal cortex: towards a comprehensive model linking nocturnal upper airway obstruction to daytime cognitive and behavioural deficits. J Sleep Res 2002;11:1–16.

[100] Bonnet MH. Performance and sleepiness as a function of frequency and placement of sleep disruption. Psychophysiology 1986;23:263–71.

[101] Leonard BE, McCartan D, White J, et al. Methylphenidate: a review of its neuropharmacological, neuropsychological and adverse clinical effects. Hum Psychopharmacol 2004;19:151–80.

[102] Ivanenko AR, Tauman R, Gozal D. Modafinil in the treatment of excessive daytime sleepiness in children. Sleep Med 2003;4:579–82.

[103] Chervin RD, Hedger K, Archbold RH, et al. Sleep problems seldom addressed at two general pediatric clinics. Pediatrics 2001;107:1375–85.

SLEEP
MEDICINE
CLINICS

Sleep Med Clin 1 (2006) 119–125

ELSEVIER
SAUNDERS

Neuromuscular Disorders and Sleepiness

Stephen N. Brooks, MD

- Differential diagnosis of sleepiness in neuromuscular disorders
- Disrupted or insufficient nocturnal sleep
  Sleep-disordered breathing
  Other factors contributing to sleep disruption
- Central nervous system dysfunction
- Other factors related to excessive daytime sleepiness in neuromuscular disorders

- Evaluation of excessive daytime sleepiness in neuromuscular disorders
- Treatment of excessive daytime sleepiness in neuromuscular disorders
- Summary
- References

The medical care of patients with neuromuscular disorders (NMD) is often complicated and challenging. It is easy for the health care provider to become focused on the defining features of the disease, such as muscle weakness or sensory loss, while paying less attention to less primary or obvious symptoms.

Excessive daytime sleepiness (EDS) may be defined as the inability to stay awake and alert during the major waking periods of the day, resulting in unintended lapses into drowsiness or sleep [1]. EDS occurs commonly in the general population. According to the National Sleep Foundation 2005 Sleep in America Poll [2], 27% of males and 31% of females reported daytime sleepiness on at least 3 days per week; 47% of males and 53% of females reported the problem on at least 1 day per week. The symptom may cause or contribute to loss of productivity, cognitive dysfunction, mood disturbance, accidents, and reduced quality of life. In some cases, EDS may be debilitating. Although prevalence estimates of EDS in patients with NMD are not well defined (because of great clinical and pathophysiologic disparity among this group of disorders and the small numbers of subjects in most

clinical studies), the problem is common in this population [3].

EDS is often unidentified in patients with NMD. There are several possible reasons for this. The patient may not complain about it during interactions with health care professionals, because of time constraints of the clinic visit, and the need to focus on other problems believed to be more important; the patient might not recognize that EDS is present; and the patient may believe that the symptom is an intrinsic feature of the primary disease and not amenable to specific treatment. Likewise, the health care provider may not think to inquire about EDS (perhaps because of time limitations); or the symptom may not be distinguished from the physical fatigue that so often accompanies NMD. Patients may use words like "tiredness" or "fatigue" in place of more specific identifiers, such as "sleepiness" or "drowsiness." Input from family members or caregivers can be most valuable in identifying EDS.

Symptoms providing clues to EDS include changes in sleep patterns (eg, insomnia, prolonged sleep time, or difficulty awakening in the morning) or changes in daytime behavior (eg, napping, spending

Stanford Sleep Disorders Clinic, 401 Quarry Road, Suite 3301, Stanford, CA 94305, USA
E-mail address: snbrooks@stanford.edu

1556-407X/06/$ – see front matter © 2006 Elsevier Inc. All rights reserved.
sleep.theclinics.com

doi:10.1016/j.jsmc.2005.11.002

more time in bed, mood alterations, or even cognitive decline). Other signs and symptoms may suggest the presence of processes associated with EDS (eg, sleep-disordered breathing [SDB]), including snoring, gasping or choking, witnessed pauses in breathing during sleep, morning headaches, nocturnal restlessness, peripheral edema or other findings of congestive heart failure, orthopnea, or unexplained polycythemia.

Differential diagnosis of sleepiness in neuromuscular disorders

The causes of EDS in patients with NMD can be grouped into three general categories: (1) disrupted or insufficient nocturnal sleep, (2) central nervous system (CNS) dysfunction, and (3) other factors. The first category is, by far, the most important and is the main focus of this article.

Disrupted or insufficient nocturnal sleep

Numerous factors may cause or contribute to disruption of nocturnal sleep in patients with NMD, including SDB, insomnia, pain, restricted mobility, and secretion clearance problems.

Sleep-disordered breathing

SDB encompasses several clinical entities, including obstructive sleep apnea-hypopnea (OSA), central sleep apnea (CSA), upper airway resistance syndrome, and sleep-related hypoventilation. SDB may occur in more than 42% of patients with NMD [4,5]. To understand why SDB is so prevalent in this population, it is first useful to review some aspects of normal sleep physiology.

Respiration during wakefulness is controlled by metabolic and voluntary systems; during sleep, only the metabolic control of respiration remains functional. At sleep onset, mild hypoventilation occurs because of the subtraction of voluntary control; increased upper airway resistance (decreased activity of upper airway dilator muscles and reduced output from medullary respiratory neurons); and changes in chemoresponsiveness of respiratory neurons [6]. During non–rapid eye movement (REM) sleep, upper airway dilators and accessory muscles of respiration are mildly hypotonic compared with wakefulness. These muscles become significantly hypotonic or atonic during REM sleep, such that the peripheral muscular mechanics of breathing are solely dependant on the diaphragm. Ventilatory responses to hypoxia and hypercapnia are mildly reduced in non-REM sleep and markedly reduced during REM sleep. In normal individuals, these sleep-related changes in ventilation have no important consequences. In patients with NMD,

however, these physiologic events may be significantly magnified, assuming pathologic or even life-threatening proportions. This is especially likely during REM sleep in patients with weakness of the diaphragm [7–9].

Obstructive sleep apnea-hypopnea

OSA generally occurs because of the interaction of sleep-related changes in physiology (neural control of respiration and upper airway musculature) and anatomic compromise of the upper airway. Upper airway muscles become hypotonic during sleep, causing the walls of the airway to become more collapsible. If the caliber of the airway is reduced because of anatomic factors, the air pressure within the lumen of the airway is likewise reduced during airflow. If the intraluminal pressure becomes sufficiently low, the airway may collapse. Complete collapse leads to apnea; partial collapse leads to hypopnea. Other factors are involved, such as state-dependent neural control of respiration. For a more thorough discussion of OSA see the article by Schwab and coworkers [10]. Predisposing anatomic features may include crowding of the upper airway by adipose or soft tissue, adenotonsillar hypertrophy, macroglossia, or craniofacial abnormalities. OSA is common in the general population, with prevalence estimates as high as 24% of men and 9% of women [11]. Many individuals with OSA suffer from EDS as a consequence of sleep fragmentation associated with cortical arousals (related to respiratory effort, hypoxemia, or hypercapnia). Patients with NMD may be further disposed to OSA, because upper airway anatomy may be compromised by adiposity from inactivity; pharyngeal muscle weakness; macroglossia; or craniofacial abnormalities (as in myotonic dystrophy).

Central sleep apnea

CSA during sleep occurs when ventilatory effort is absent or reduced for at least 10 seconds. Events are generally related to ventilatory responsiveness to carbon dioxide and may occur with a decrease in carbon dioxide level below the apneic threshold or a change in the set-point itself (eg, at sleep onset). With conventional polysomnographic recording techniques, obstructive events may seem to be central in situations where inspiratory pressure is limited by muscle weakness. Central hypopnea may be especially difficult to distinguish from obstructive events. In both cases, a sensitive measure of respiratory effort (eg, esophageal pressure) is needed for accurate assessment. Several forms of CSA have been described and may be divided into those associated with hypercapnia and those associated with hypocapnia or normocapnia [1,12]. Central apnea in the latter category may be seen in normal individuals during certain conditions (high altitude, at sleep onset, immediately following cortical arousals, or during REM sleep). An idiopathic form of CSA occurs uncommonly. CSA may also be associated with congestive heart failure (usually with the Cheyne-Stokes pattern) or various disorders of the CNS. Patients with NMD are commonly found to have CSA associated with hypercapnia. The mechanisms responsible for CSA in patients with NMD are not completely understood and may differ among the various disorders. Respiratory control may be affected by direct involvement of the brainstem in some NMD, such as postpolio syndrome [13] and motor neuron disease [14]. Although patients with CSA often complain of insomnia with frequent awakenings, EDS may also be an important consequence of the sleep disruption.

Sleep-related hypoventilation

Hypoventilation occurs during sleep in normal individuals. Patients with NMD often suffer from more severe sleep-related hypoventilation. In severe or advanced cases, hypoventilation during wakefulness may also ensue. The changes during sleep usually occur first, however, and their detection may provide an early indication of disease progression. Weakness of the diaphragm is the most important factor in the development of ventilatory compromise in patients with NMD. Diaphragm muscle weakness may occur in myasthenia gravis, muscular dystrophy, or acid maltase deficiency. Phrenic nerve dysfunction may occur in motor neuron disease, Guillain-Barré syndrome, Charcot-Marie-Tooth disease, and other conditions [14]. Unilateral phrenic nerve involvement is usually asymptomatic, but bilateral involvement produces ventilatory impairment that may be severe and life-threatening. Diaphragmatic weakness is especially important during REM sleep, because other respiratory muscles are hypotonic or atonic during this time. Ventilatory function in patients with NMD may be impaired by additional factors, including scoliosis, chest wall muscle weakness, aspiration of secretions, and pulmonary atelectasis. The significance of sleep-related hypoventilation is also magnified if the patient also suffers from OSA or CSA or in the event of superimposed respiratory infection. Patients with sleep-related hypoventilation may experience arousals from sleep even without episodes of apnea or hypopnea, and symptoms of insomnia or EDS may develop. Over time, nocturnal hypoventilation may lead to blunting of central and peripheral chemoreceptor responses to oxygen and carbon dioxide, worsening the degree of hypoventilation [15,16]. For more detailed discussion about sleep and breathing in specific NMD,

see the reviews by Oztura and Guilleminault [17], Bourke and Gibson [18], and Culebras [14].

Other factors contributing to sleep disruption

In addition to SDB, patients with NMD may suffer from disrupted sleep for several reasons. Chronic pain caused by stiffness, spasticity, muscle cramps, joint contractures, spinal deformity, or pressure sores may disturb sleep. Difficulty with clearance of oral secretions may induce cough or pulmonary aspiration. Lack of mobility caused by muscle weakness or skeletal abnormalities may interfere with normal changes in body position during sleep, causing significant physical discomfort and frustration. Periodic limb movement of sleep may occur in some NMD [19], such as motor neuron disease and postpolio syndrome, causing arousals and sleep fragmentation. Some patients even find muscle fasciculations to be disruptive to sleep. As a consequence of any ongoing problem causing poor sleep, a secondary pattern of insomnia may emerge, further reducing nocturnal sleep time and contributing to daytime symptoms, such as EDS.

Central nervous system dysfunction

Although the clinical and pathologic features of NMD primarily reflect abnormalities of the peripheral nervous system, CNS involvement may also occur in some disorders. Brainstem pathology is known to occur in some cases of motor neuron disease, poliomyelitis, postpolio syndrome, and the Miller Fisher variant of Guillain-Barré syndrome. CNS involvement has also been suggested in myasthenia gravis [20]. With the exception of myotonic dystrophy (discussed later), it is unclear to what extent CNS pathology in NMD might cause EDS (apart from effects on ventilatory control, which might lead to EDS through SDB). There have been reports of decreased cerebrospinal fluid levels of hypocretin (orexin) in patients with Guillain-Barré syndrome [21–23]. At least some of these patients suffered from EDS. Decreased cerebrospinal fluid hypocretin has also been reported in myotonic dystrophy [24]. Hypocretin is believed to play a key role in the orchestration of sleep and wakefulness, and cerebrospinal fluid levels are decreased or undetectable in most patients with narcolepsy-cataplexy [25,26], but the significance of the neuropeptide in NMD remains to be determined.

EDS is common in patients with myotonic dystrophy. In a series of consecutive patients with myotonic dystrophy, Giubilei and coworkers [27] found that 23 of 70 complained of EDS (higher prevalence rates have been reported by others but may reflect referral bias). In many patients with myotonic dystrophy, EDS cannot be explained entirely by SDB [28,29], because it is often present in patients without SDB or persists after SDB is adequately treated. Multiple Sleep Latency Test results, in patients with myotonic dystrophy, may reflect profound sleepiness and even sleep-onset REM periods. CNS abnormalities have been reported in MRI studies of patients with myotonic dystrophy, including diffuse cerebral atrophy, subcortical white matter lesions, and focal involvement of anterior temporal lobes and corpus callosum [30,31]. Autopsy studies by Ono and coworkers [32] revealed loss of serotonin (5-HT) containing neurons in the dorsal raphe and superior central nuclei in patients with myotonic dystrophy; 5-HT neuron density was significantly lower in myotonic dystrophy patients with EDS compared with controls or myotonic dystrophy patients without EDS (although the series was small). Martinez-Rodriguez and colleagues [24] found reduced hypocretin levels compared with controls in the cerebrospinal fluid of six patients with myotonic dystrophy and EDS. Although precise mechanisms have not been determined, the multiple lines of evidence suggest that EDS is a primary feature of myotonic dystrophy and is related to CNS pathology and pathophysiology.

Other factors related to excessive daytime sleepiness in neuromuscular disorders

Aside from nocturnal sleep disruption and CNS pathology, other factors may cause or contribute to EDS in patients with NMD. Although many patients with NMD may experience respiratory instability only during sleep, patients with severe or long-lasting disease may suffer from hypoventilation during wakefulness, leading to hypoxemia, hypercapnia, and consequent daytime somnolence. Depression is common in patients with chronic illness of any nature. Insomnia is the most commonly reported sleep disturbance in depressed patients, but EDS may occur in a significant portion. Patients with NMD may take multiple medications for symptomatic relief of somatic or psychic complaints. Many of these medications, including opioid analgesics, benzodiazepines, muscle relaxants, baclofen, and some antidepressants, may produce daytime sedation.

Evaluation of excessive daytime sleepiness in neuromuscular disorders

EDS must first be identified in affected patients. There should be a high index of suspicion for EDS in patients with NMD, and questions about daytime sleepiness and nocturnal sleep quality should be asked routinely. Additional tools are available to identify and measure sleepiness [33]. Sub-

jective scales query the individual's perception of alertness and sleepiness. One problem with this approach is that patients must have insight into the problem and be able to distinguish sleepiness from other symptoms, such as physical fatigue. The Stanford Sleepiness Scale [34] and the Karolinska Sleepiness Scale [35] assess the momentary degree of alertness and sleepiness. These scales are useful in tracking symptoms during a given time epoch; they are less helpful in identifying a more pervasive state of sleepiness. The Epworth Sleepiness Scale [36] offers a more appropriate method for assessing overall sleepiness. It consists of eight questions, each scored with a degree of severity ranging from 0 to 3. One limitation of this scale is that it asks subjects to imagine themselves in situations that they may rarely or never experience. Semantic issues also may lead to confusion. There may also be individual variation of scores over time. Visual analog scales, on which the subject indicates a response along a linear 100-mm line, are also useful. It is often helpful to ask other individuals who are close to the subject (spouse, bedpartner, caregiver) to complete scales, such as the Epworth Sleepiness Scale or visual analog scales; this adds information, which is not entirely subjective to the individual.

More objective tests, such as the Multiple Sleep Latency Test, rely on measurement of physiologic parameters. The test is performed the day after an overnight polysomnogram (to ensure adequate sleep during the prior night and to exclude obvious causes of nocturnal sleep disruption, which would explain the daytime symptoms). The test consists of four or five opportunities to nap, spaced across the day at 2-hour intervals. Standardized conditions are used; the subject is placed in a quiet, dark, comfortable room and asked not to resist sleep. Outcome measures are mean sleep latency (time from lights-out to unequivocal sleep onset) and presence or absence of sleep-onset REM periods [37].

Once EDS has been identified, a search for causative factors should begin. The patient or caregiver should be asked about total sleep time. Sleep diaries completed over a couple of weeks may be useful in this regard. The patient's medication list should be screened for sedating agents. Questions about or screening tools for depression should also be included in the evaluation of EDS. Overnight polysomnography is essential to look for physiologic disruptions of nocturnal sleep, particularly SDB. In addition to conventional parameters, measurement of carbon dioxide (transcutaneous or end-tidal) is useful in identifying sleep-related hypoventilation in patients with NMD [38]. Esophageal manometry also adds useful information and is especially helpful in distinguishing central from obstructive breathing events and in identifying respiratory effort–related cortical arousals [39]. Polysomnography may also identify abnormal movements during sleep, such as periodic limb movement of sleep.

Treatment of excessive daytime sleepiness in neuromuscular disorders

Basic sleep hygiene should be emphasized in all patients with complaints about sleep or EDS. Sleep-wake schedules should be regular, and as much as possible prolonged time in bed should be avoided when the patient is not asleep. Attention should be given to the physical comfort of the sleeping environment and to the choice of pillows and mattresses. Adjustable beds are helpful for patients with limited mobility. Additional factors disrupting sleep, such as pain or abnormal movements, may require treatment with specific medications. If insomnia is part of the clinical picture, treatment with cognitive-behavioral therapy or pharmacologic agents (drugs that suppress respiration should be used with great caution or not at all) should be considered.

Several treatment modalities are available for SDB. Continuous positive airway pressure is useful for treating OSA. Patients with OSA and mild hypoventilation may derive more benefit from bilevel positive airway pressure (pressure differential between inspiration and expiration), because a degree of ventilatory support is achieved with bilevel positive airway pressure in addition to ensuring upper airway patency. If significant hypoventilation is present (with or without OSA), intermittent positive pressure ventilation is usually needed [40–42]. The use of invasive ventilation with tracheostomy and the use of negative pressure ventilation (iron lung) have become much less frequent but may be appropriate in selected cases. Nocturnal supplemental oxygen may be a useful addition to treatment with ventilatory support in patients with SDB and NMD, but as a sole treatment modality may be ineffective or even deleterious (exacerbating carbon dioxide retention) [43,44].

Patients with CSA may or may not respond to treatment with continuous positive airway pressure. Bilevel positive airway pressure (in spontaneous or timed-cycle mode) or intermittent positive pressure ventilation is often more useful for treating CSA. Supplemental nocturnal oxygen has also been used to treat CSA, but should be used with caution in patients with carbon dioxide retention. Diaphragmatic pacing has been used successfully in selected patients with NMD and respiratory failure [45].

If EDS persists despite treatment of identifiable contributory factors, treatment with modafinil may be beneficial. MacDonald and coworkers [46] reported improvement in EDS and quality of life in patients with myotonic dystrophy treated with modafinil.

Summary

EDS occurs commonly in patients with NMD but is often unrecognized. The causes of EDS may be multifactorial, but SDB is the major contributing factor in many cases. OSA and CSA may occur, but sleep-related hypoventilation is the most important form of SDB in patients with NMD. Abnormalities in respiratory function during sleep may occur without (or before) measurable changes during wakefulness and may herald disease progression. Overnight polysomnography is essential in the evaluation of EDS in patients with NMD. The use of noninvasive ventilatory support during sleep may significantly improve health and quality of life in many of these individuals.

References

[1] National Sleep Foundation 2005 Sleep in America Poll. Washington: National Sleep Foundation; 2005.

[2] Sateia MJ, editor. International Classification of Sleep Disorders – Diagnostic and Coding Manual. 2nd edition. Westchester (IL): American Academy of Sleep Medicine; 2005.

[3] Happe S. Excessive daytime sleepiness and sleep disturbances in patients with neurological diseases: epidemiology and management. Drugs 2003; 63:2725–37.

[4] Labanowski M, Schmidt-Nowara W, Guilleminault C. Sleep and neuromuscular disease: frequency of sleep-disordered breathing in a neuromuscular disease clinic population. Neurology 1996;47:1173–80.

[5] Mellies U, Ragette R, Schwake C, et al. Daytime predictors of sleep disordered breathing in children and adolescents with neuromuscular disorders. Neuromuscul Disord 2003;13:123–8.

[6] Chokroverty S. Physiologic changes in sleep. In: Chokroverty S, editor. Sleep disorders medicine: basic science, technical considerations, and clinical aspects. 2nd edition. Boston: Butterworth-Heinemann; 1999. p. 95–126.

[7] Culebras A. Diaphragmatic insufficiency in REM sleep. Sleep Med 2004;5:337–8.

[8] Arnulf I, Similowski T, Salachas F, et al. Sleep disorders and diaphragmatic function in patients with amyotrophic lateral sclerosis. Am J Respir Crit Care Med 2000;161:849–56.

[9] Mellies U, Ragette R, Schwake C, et al. Sleep-disordered breathing and respiratory failure in acid maltase deficiency. Neurology 2001;57:1290–5.

[10] Schwab RJ, Kuna ST, Remmers JE. Anatomy and physiology of upper airway obstruction. In: Kryger MH, Roth T, Dement WC, editors. Principles and practice of sleep medicine. 4th edition. Philadelphia: WB Saunders; 2005. p. 983–1000.

[11] Young TB, Palta M, Dempsey J, et al. The occurrence of sleep-disordered breathing among middle-aged adults. N Engl J Med 1993;328:1230–5.

[12] Guilleminault C, Robinson A. Central sleep apnea. Neurol Clin 1996;14:611–28.

[13] Dean AC, Graham BA, Dalakas M, et al. Sleep apnea in patients with postpolio syndrome. Ann Neurol 1998;43:661–4.

[14] Culebras A. Sleep disorders and neuromuscular disease. Semin Neurol 2005;25:33–8.

[15] Chokroverty S. Sleep-disordered breathing in neuromuscular disorders: a condition in search of recognition. Muscle Nerve 2001;24:451–5.

[16] Silber MH. Sleep-disordered breathing. In: Bolton CF, Chen R, Wijdicks EFM, editors. Neurology of breathing. Philadelphia: Butterworth Heinemann; 2004. p. 109–35.

[17] Oztura I, Guilleminault C. Neuromuscular disorders and sleep. Sleep 2005;5:147–52.

[18] Bourke SC, Gibson GJ. Sleep and breathing in neuromuscular disease. Eur Respir J 2002;19:1194–201.

[19] George CFP, Guilleminault C. Sleep and neuromuscular disorders. In: Kryger MH, Roth T, Dement WC, editors. Principles and practice of sleep medicine. 4th edition. Philadelphia: WB Saunders; 2005. p. 831–8.

[20] Keesey JC. Does myasthenia gravis affect the brain? J Neurol Sci 1999;170:77–89.

[21] Kanbayashi T, Ishiguro H, Aizawa R, et al. Hypocretin-1 (orexin-A) concentrations in cerebrospinal fluid are low in patients with Guillain Barré syndrome. Psychiatry Clin Neurosci 2002;56:273–4.

[22] Nishino S, Kanbayashi T, Fujiki N, et al. CSF hypocretin levels in Guillain Barré syndrome and other inflammatory neuropathies. Neurology 2003;61:823–5.

[23] Ripley B, Overeem S, Fujiki N, et al. CSF hypocretin/orexin levels in narcolepsy and other neurological conditions. Neurology 2001;57:2253–8.

[24] Martinez-Rodriguez JE, Lin L, Iranzo A, et al. Decreased hypocretin-1 (orexin-A) levels in the cerebrospinal fluid of patients with myotonic dystrophy and excessive daytime sleepiness. Sleep 2003;36:287–90.

[25] Peyron C, Faraco J, Rogers W, et al. A mutation in a case of early narcolepsy and a generalized absence of hypocretin peptides in human narcoleptic brains. Nat Med 2000;6:991–7.

[26] Nishino S, Ripley B, Overeem S, et al. Hypocretin (orexin) deficiency in human narcolepsy [letter]. Lancet 2000;355:39–40.

[27] Giubilei F, Antonini G, Bastianello S, et al. Excessive daytime sleepiness in myotonic dystrophy. J Neurol Sci 1999;164:60–3.

[28] Van der Meche FGA, Bogaard JM, van der Sluys JCM, et al. Daytime sleep in myotonic dystrophy is not caused by sleep apnoea. J Neurol Neurosurg Psychiatry 1994;57:626–8.

[29] Gibbs JW, Ciafaloni E, Radtke RA. Excessive daytime somnolence and increased rapid eye movement pressure in myotonic dystrophy. Sleep 2002;25:662–5.

[30] Bachmann G, Damian MS, Koch M, et al. The clinical and genetic correlates of MRI findings in myotonic dystrophy. Neuroradiology 1996;38:629–35.

[31] Miaux Y, Chiras J, Eymard B, et al. Cranial MRI findings in myotonic dystrophy. Neuroradiology 1997;39:166–70.

[32] Ono S, Takahashi K, Jinnai K, et al. Loss of serotonin-containing neurons in the raphe of patients with myotonic dystrophy: a quantitative immunohistochemical study and relation to hypersomnia. Neurology 1998;51:1121–4.

[33] Guilleminault C, Brooks SN. Excessive daytime sleepiness: a challenge for the practicing neurologist. Brain 2001;124:1482–91.

[34] Hoddes E, Dement W, Zarcone V. The development and use of the Stanford sleepiness scale. Psychophysiology 1972;9:150.

[35] Akerstedt T. Wide awake at odd hours. Swedish council for work life research. Stockholm, Sweden: Fritzes Kundtjanst; 1996.

[36] Johns M. A new method for measuring daytime sleepiness: the Epworth sleepiness scale. Sleep 1991;14:540–5.

[37] Carskadon MA, Dement WC, Mitler MM, et al. Guidelines for the multiple sleep latency test (MSLT): a standard measure of sleepiness. Sleep 1986;9:519–24.

[38] Kotterba S, Patzold T, Malin JP, et al. Respiratory monitoring in neuromuscular disease - capnography as an additional tool? Clin Neurol Neurosurg 2001;103:87–91.

[39] Mikami A, Watanabe T, Motonishi M, et al. Alteration of esophageal pressure in sleep-disordered breathing. Psychiatry Clin Neurosci 1998;52:216–7.

[40] Metha S, Hill NS. Noninvasive ventilation. Am J Respir Crit Care Med 2001;163:540–77.

[41] Schonhoper B, Kohler D. Effect of non-invasive mechanical ventilation on sleep and nocturnal ventilation in patients with chronic respiratory failure. Thorax 2000;55:308–13.

[42] Guilleminault C, Philip P, Robinson A. Sleep and neuromuscular disease: bilevel positive airway pressure by nasal mask as a treatment for sleep disordered breathing in patients with neuromuscular disease. J Neurol Neurosurg Psychiatry 1998;65:225–32.

[43] Buyse B, Meersseman W, Demedts M. Treatment of chronic respiratory failure in kyphoscoliosis: oxygen or ventilation? Eur Respir J 2002;22:525–8.

[44] Masa JF, Celli BR, Riesco JA, et al. Non-invasive positive pressure ventilation and not oxygen may prevent overt ventilatory failure in patients with chest wall diseases. Chest 1997; 112:207–13.

[45] Chervin RD, Guilleminault C. Diaphragmatic pacing for respiratory insufficiency. J Clin Neurophysiol 1997;14:369–77.

[46] MacDonald JR, Hill JD, Tarnopolsky MA. Modafinil reduces excessive somnolence and enhances mood in patients with myotonic dystrophy. Neurology 2002;59:1876–80.

ELSEVIER
SAUNDERS

SLEEP
MEDICINE
CLINICS

Sleep Med Clin 1 (2006) 127–137

Parkinson's Disease and Sleepiness

Alex Iranzo, MD

- Epidemiology and characteristics of
  sleepiness in Parkinson's disease
  Excessive daytime sleepiness
  Sudden onset of sleep episodes
- Etiology of sleepiness in Parkinson's disease
  Excessive daytime sleepiness
  Sudden onset of sleep episodes

- Management of sleepiness in Parkinson's
  disease
- Summary
- Acknowledgments
- References

Parkinson's disease (PD) is the most frequent progressive neurodegenerative movement disorder with a prevalence of 1% to 2% in people over 55 years of age. The cause of PD is unknown, although damage to the dopaminergic central nervous system is implicated in its pathophysiology. The cardinal clinical signs of PD are tremor, rigidity, bradykinesia, and postural and gait abnormalities. In addition, PD patients frequently present with different nonmotor manifestations including mood disorders, anxiety, cognitive impairment, autonomic failure, and sleep disorders.

Sleep complaints in PD are frequent and in some cases they are the initial manifestation of the disease [1]. As many as 60% of parkinsonian patients are affected by sleep disturbances that may have a negative impact on their quality of life. Complaints among PD patients include initial insomnia, frequent awakenings during the night, early awakening, nocturnal akathisia, nocturia, back pain, stiffness, difficulties in turning over in bed, painful cramps, leg jerks, nightmares, vigorous motor and vocal dream-enacting behaviors, visual hallucinations, confusional awakenings, restless legs interfering with sleep initiation and maintenance, loud snoring, wit-

nessed apnea by the bed partner, painful early morning dystonia, and daytime sleepiness. Nocturnal polysomnography (PSG) may detect poor and reduced sleep architecture; decreased amounts of slow wave sleep and rapid eye movement (REM) sleep stages; reduction or loss of spindles and K complexes; periodic leg movements during sleep (repetitive stereotyped jerks of the legs and feet that may disrupt sleep continuity); obstructive or central sleep apnea; and REM sleep behavior disorder (a parasomnia consisting of potentially harmful dream-enacting behaviors associated with nightmares, such as being attacked or chased by unknown people and lack of REM sleep muscle atonia). All these sleep complaints and PSG abnormalities have been related to several conditions, such as damage of the brain structures and mechanisms involved in sleep origin and maintenance; the effects of antiparkinsonian drugs; poor control of parkinsonism; comorbid conditions, such as anxiety, depression, and dementia; aging; and individual genetic susceptibility. In general, sleep disturbances gradually worsen with the invariable progression of the disease. This article briefly reviews the epidemiology, characteristics, etiology, and management of sleepiness in PD.

Neurology Service, Hospital Clínic de Barcelona and Institut D'Investigació Biomèdiques August Pi i Sunyer (IDIBAPS), C/Villarroel 170, Barcelona 08036, Spain
E-mail address: airanzo@clinic.ub.es

doi:10.1016/j.jsmc.2005.11.003

Epidemiology and characteristics of sleepiness in Parkinson's disease

The occurrence of sleepiness in PD has long been recognized [2] but little attention was paid by neurologists until 1999 when Frucht and coworkers [3] described the presence of sudden-onset sleep (SOS) episodes in eight PD subjects, several months after starting therapy with the new dopaminergic agonists pramipexole and ropinirole. These episodes occurred while the subjects were driving and caused road crashes. Five subjects experienced no warning of sleepiness before falling asleep at the wheel and the episodes resolved after the medications were stopped or reduced. The authors termed these episodes "sleep attacks." The controversy and debate generated by this report [4,5] renewed the interest in sleep disorders in PD. As a consequence, a number of studies have been published the last few years showing that the prevalence of sleepiness in subjects treated with dopaminergic agents (levodopa and dopaminergic agonists) is high when compared with controls [6–15]. The high prevalence of sleepiness in PD may have been previously overlooked probably because neurologists paid less attention to sleep symptoms than to the disabling motor problems occurring during wakefulness, such as parkinsonism, dyskinesias, and motor fluctuations, and also because patients and bed partners usually do not spontaneously complain about sleep disturbances. It is common that in PD and other neurodegenerative diseases, such as dementia with Lewy bodies, multiple system atrophy, and progressive supranuclear palsy, a history consistent with daytime sleepiness (and other sleep disorders including REM sleep behavior disorder) is detected only on specific questioning.

There are two possible clinical presentations of sleepiness in the setting of PD. One is a state of excessive daytime sleepiness (EDS), which is perceived by the patient allowing him or her to fight against it but leading to unavoidable napping. The other is the occurrence of SOS episodes (sleep attacks) [1,16]. Both types of sleepiness may impact on the patient's quality of life causing social, professional, and familial problems. In addition, EDS and SOS are both strongly associated with an increased risk of automobile accidents in subjects with PD [17].

In PD, detection of sleepiness is crucial. Clinical history is the most important tool to evaluate the occurrence and characteristics of sleepiness. Several instruments, however, may be necessary to identify and characterize sleepiness better. Subjective methods like the Epworth Sleepiness Scale (ESS) and objective methods, such as the Multiple Sleep Latency Test (MSLT) and the Maintenance of Wakefulness Test (MWT), have been used to measure sleepiness in PD [18–20]. Most of the authors have used the ESS because is a simple self-administered questionnaire that can be completed by the patient, spouse, or caregiver in less than 5 minutes. The ESS is a useful scale in identifying subjects with EDS, assessing the propensity to fall asleep in eight everyday situations (eg, watching television, sitting, and reading). The ESS mainly measures passive sleepiness but active situations like driving a car, working, or eating are not considered. The ESS is not capable of differentiating EDS from SOS. To identify and characterize sleepiness in PD better, new scales have been developed assessing the tendency to fall asleep in active situations like driving, and trying to identify the occurrence of SOS [8,21]. MSLT is considered the gold standard objective method for assessment of EDS and measures the ability to fall asleep when the subject is instructed to sleep in a soporific situation. The MSLT may also identify sleep-onset REM periods (SOREMPs), a characteristic feature in narcolepsy, which may also be observed in some sleepy PD subjects [22–26]. Alternatively, the MWT measures the ability to stay awake when a subject is instructed not to sleep under soporific conditions. The MWT is useful in detecting changes in sleepiness after the administration of a medication. Both MSLT and MWT have only been used in few studies evaluating sleepiness in PD, however, mainly because they are expensive and require a day in the sleep laboratory following overnight PSG. PSG helps to characterize the patient's nocturnal sleep architecture (eg, sleep efficiency, distribution of sleep stages) and to detect primary sleep disorders, such as obstructive sleep apnea that may cause sleepiness in PD and any other condition. Overall, despite their limitations, the ESS, MSLT, and MWT are valid instruments in evaluating the occurrence of sleepiness in PD subjects. The correlation between ESS and MSLT, however, is not particularly strong [27]. Studies evaluating sleepiness in PD showed that MSLT scores correlated with MWT scores but not with the ESS scores [28,29]. This is probably because subjective and objective methods evaluate different aspects of sleepiness.

Excessive daytime sleepiness

The prevalence of EDS in PD ranges from 15.5% to 74% [6–15]. Differences in prevalence among these studies may be explained by different study designs (eg, clinic versus community-based); subject population bias (eg, nondemented versus unselected patients, white versus Asian patients, medicated versus unmedicated patients); the use of different methodologies of ascertainment (eg, subjective scales, such as the ESS, versus objective tools, such as the MSLT); and different definitions of EDS (eg, ESS greater than 7 versus greater than 10).

PD subjects with EDS experience a constant pressure for falling asleep and difficulty with remaining awake. They perceive that they are sleepy and fight against this undesirable sensation. Patients fall asleep and take frequent long naps at inappropriate times or settings, however, especially when situations are not stimulating, such as watching television, listening to music, reading, or driving. This condition may be severe in disabled and in depressed subjects who spend most of the day sitting at home. In severe cases, patients are unable even to stay awake in active situations like eating a meal or having a conversation. This type of sleepiness is not specific to PD, because it is the main feature of other conditions where hypersomnia is common, such as obstructive sleep apnea, idiopathic hypersomnia, depression, sleep deprivation, and idiopathic narcolepsy.

The use of MSLT has demonstrated the existence of a subgroup of sleepy PD subjects with a narcolepsy-like phenotype consisting of short mean sleep latency and the presence of SOREMPs [22,24–26]. When compared with PD patients with nonnarcoleptic features, those in the narcoleptic-like group exhibit shorter mean sleep latency in MSLT (they are sleepier); have longer disease duration; and more frequently experience daytime hallucinations [22,24]. They are significantly sleepier despite exhibiting longer total sleep time and shorter sleep latency in nocturnal PSG [22]. This narcolepsy-like phenotype has also been described in a single de novo untreated juvenile PD subject [30] and in an experimental animal model of PD [31]. In contrast to narcolepsy, sleepy PD subjects with SOREMPs take long and unrefreshing naps, do not report episodes of cataplexy or sleep paralysis, and do not show tight linkage to HLA DQB1*0602 [22,24]. Given that most patients with idiopathic narcolepsy lack hypocretin in the cerebrospinal fluid and because hypocretin neurons project to midbrain dopaminergic cells, it would be interesting to measure hypocretin levels in those PD subjects exhibiting the "full" narcolepsy-without-cataplexy-like phenotype (subjective complaint of severe daytime sleepiness, shortened mean sleep latency and more than one SOREMPs in MSLT, hallucinations, and REM sleep behavior disorder).

Sudden onset of sleep episodes

In PD, SOS episodes are much less common than EDS, if they really exist as an isolated true phenomenon. In PD subjects treated with dopaminergic agents, the prevalence of SOS is estimated to range from 0% to 32% [7,8,10,13,15,17,28,32–40]. The considerable variation of prevalence in SOS can be explained by several factors including lack of a standardized definition of the condition (events occurring without warning of falling asleep versus events occurring with warning of falling asleep); different study designs (retrospective versus prospective, mailed questionnaires or telephone interviews versus face-to-face interviews); and type of selected population (consecutive unselected PD patients versus patients complaining of sleepiness).

It is unclear whether in PD these SOS episodes, termed "sleep attacks," constitute a unique entity or are merely an extreme manifestation of EDS. The initial description of SOS in PD was reported in 1999 by Frucht and colleagues [3]. The authors described these events as a novel condition in PD triggered by two dopaminergic agents and appearing acutely and without warning. This article led to an interesting controversy and debate when several authors questioned the concept of "sleep attack" indicating that it is very well known that PD patients fall asleep because of medication-induced drowsiness on a background of EDS. These authors indicated that PD subjects with SOS are not aware that they are sleepy simply because of the amnesia associated with falling asleep or because they have habituated to the sensation of chronic EDS and are not aware that they are sleepy during the day [4,41,42]. In fact, one study showed that 38% of sleepy PD patients undergoing MSLT do not perceive they had been sleeping during the naps [43]. Subsequently, Frucht and coworkers [5] provided an additional definition of sleep attack as an event of overwhelming sleepiness that occurs without warning, or that occurs with a prodrome that is sufficiently short or overpowering to prevent the patient from taking appropriate protective measures. Interestingly, Möller and coworkers [35] classified EDS in their PD patients in three groups: (1) SOS without previous daytime sleepiness, (2) unusually fast onset of sleep with previous daytime sleepiness, and (3) increased daytime sleepiness without unintended sleep episodes.

Besides occurring with warning, SOS episodes in PD are abrupt, brief, and similar to those originally described in subjects with narcolepsy. In PD, they have been reported to occur while driving and during active situations like eating, drinking, talking, being on the telephone, and writing. Between 1% and 28% of patients with SOS have experienced these abrupt and unexpected events while driving [37,38,44]. An ESS score greater than 10 is found in 71% to 75% of the PD patients reporting SOS episodes [7,37]. In most of the PD patients, SOS episodes occur at least once per week and at any time of the day [37,38]. Some authors, however, have described that SOS events occur after each dose of a dopaminergic agent [42,45] or within the time of peak dose levels [46]. SOS episodes have been reported to be more frequent in men and occurring at any age or stage of the disease [36].

To the best of the present author's knowledge, SOS have not been reported in de novo untreated subjects with PD. It has been documented to be associated with the use of virtually all dopaminergic agents with monotherapy or combined with other drugs, including levodopa [45,47], ropinirole [3], pramipexole [3,32], bromocriptine [33,42], pergolide [33,41,48], lisuride [42], piribedil [42], subcutaneous apomorphine [46], amantadine [33], the monoamine oxidase inhibitor selegiline [33], and the catechol-0-methyl-transferase inhibitor entacapone [49–51]. SOS events occur several days or months after the introduction of the offending agent and they usually resolve or decrease after its withdrawal, reduction, or replacement. The available data indicate that SOS episodes in the setting of PD are considered to be the result of a dopaminergic class effect. It is unclear if SOS only appear with doses above a certain threshold or if some PD patients have a special susceptibility. To date, there is no evidence of a strong association between any particular dopaminergic drug class and the risk for SOS, although dopaminergic agonists alone or in combination with levodopa have been associated more frequently than with levodopa monotherapy. One study showed that levodopa monotherapy was associated with the lowest risk of SOS, followed by dopamine agonist monotherapy and then by the combination of levodopa with a dopamine agonist [37]. This is in line with a recent study showing that those receiving a dopaminergic agonist (pramipexole, ropinirole, or pergolide) were nearly three times more likely to experience SOS when compared with subjects treated with levodopa monotherapy [40]. SOS episodes have been reported to occur in similar fashion with piribedil (50%); ropinirole (41%); bromocriptine (36%); and levodopa (30%) [33]. Moreover, there is no significant difference in the risk for SOS among the different dopamine agonists [37]. Overall, the available data indicate that SOS occurs in a small subset of PD patients; is associated with the introduction of any dopaminomimetic; and is not strongly related to the specific class of dopaminergic agent (eg, levodopa versus ergot and non–ergot-derived D2-D3 receptor-like agonists).

When compared with PD patients without SOS, those with SOS do not exhibit more reduced and fragmented nocturnal sleep architecture and MSLT does not reveal more shortened mean sleep latency [25]. In subjects with SOS, nocturnal PSG does not show a shortened REM sleep latency, which is a characteristic feature in narcolepsy. MSLT in PD patients with SOS shows short [32,45,48,51] or normal [35,52] mean sleep latency. SOREMPs may appear both in subjects with and without SOS [25].

SOS episodes have been recorded by continuous 24-hour PSG monitoring in a few PD subjects treated with dopaminergic agents. Polygraphic recordings showed that most of the SOS events were characterized by rapid transitions from wakefulness to stage II sleep with no intrusions of REM sleep, and lasted between 2 and 16 minutes [39,51–54]. In one PD patient who was taking levodopa and pergolide, SOREMPs were identified in three of the four SOS episodes. In this subject, SOREMPs were still present after pergolide withdrawal [55]. The rapid transitions from wakefulness to sleep seen in PD are indicative of abrupt sleep onset episodes but are probably not very different from those detected by daytime PSG in other diseases associated with severe EDS, such as narcolepsy and dementia with Lewy bodies (personal observation). Rapid transitions from wakefulness to stage II sleep are commonly recorded by MSLT in subjects with any condition associated with severe EDS, such as narcolepsy, obstructive sleep apnea, or idiopathic hypersomnia.

Etiology of sleepiness in Parkinson's disease

The origin and pathophysiology of sleepiness in PD remains ill-defined mainly because of its intrinsic complexity and because most studies have used different methodology. These studies, for example, have used different definitions of EDS (eg, an ESS cutoff score of 7, 10, or 16) or have used different instruments (eg, MSLT, subjective scales, or questionnaires). Moreover, most of the studies assessing sleepiness have not performed nocturnal PSG and the occurrence of primary sleep disorders that may cause sleepiness, such as obstructive sleep apnea, are underestimated. In addition, most studies have excluded patients with dementia to allow completion of questionnaires or the ESS appropriately, or have not taken into account the presence of depression, two well known predisposing factors for sleepiness. The conclusions reported on the origin of sleepiness in PD, both on EDS and SOS, must be interpreted with caution.

The nature of EDS and SOS in PD probably involves multiple factors with the intrinsic effect of the dopaminergic medication and the disease itself being the most relevant [1]. Other predisposing factors for developing sleepiness in PD include disease severity; disease duration; circadian sleep-wake cycle disruption; nocturnal sleep quantity and quality; the occurrence of primary sleep disorders, such as obstructive sleep apnea; coexisting depression and dementia; and individual or genetic susceptibility [1,16]. Male gender, age, use of benzodiazepines, loud snoring (a marker of obstructive sleep apnea), autonomic failure, and hallucinations have also been correlated with sleepiness. The contribution of each of these factors has not yet been elucidated. REM sleep behavior disorder, periodic leg movements in sleep, and restless legs syndrome, although common in PD and impairing sleep architecture to some extent, may not be considered major risk factors for sleepiness in PD [1].

Excessive daytime sleepiness

The main factors contributing to EDS are the sedative effects of the dopaminergic agents and the intrinsic pathology of PD itself.

Effects of dopaminergic agents

Levodopa and dopamine agonists influence sleep mainly through their effects on the mesothalamocortical dopaminergic projections. Experimental studies in animals have shown that the effects of these drugs on sleep are dose dependent in a biphasic fashion. Low doses of levodopa and dopaminergic agonists promote sleep through stimulation of presynaptic D2-like inhibitory autoreceptors in the midbrain ventral tegmental area, thereby inhibiting dopaminergic activity and increasing REM sleep amount. Local applications of D2-like autoreceptor antagonists into the ventral tegmental area reduce REM sleep amount and induce wakefulness. Higher dopaminergic doses induce wakefulness suppressing REM sleep and slow wave sleep through stimulation of D1 postsynaptic receptors. Blockade of D2 autoreceptors and D1 receptors with classical or atypical neuroleptics induces sedation [56,57].

In humans, however, the clinical picture of the effects of dopaminomimetics on sleep is different from animals. This suggests that experiments in animals may not always reflect a complex progressive neurodegenerative disorder, such as PD. In humans, the appearance of somnolence caused by the introduction of a dopaminergic agent may be mediated by several independent factors including the underlying brain disease that affects the dopaminergic systems (eg, PD or restless legs syndrome); different dopaminergic receptor sensitivities; and individual-genetic susceptibility. In restless legs syndrome, for example, the low doses of dopaminergic agents needed to control the symptoms do not induce SOS or EDS. In contrast, in patients with PD, the development of EDS is related to total amount of levodopa dose equivalent rather than with the use of levodopa or any particular agonist [8,9,11,28,29,34,44,58]. In one study, ESS scores were not significantly different between PD patients taking levodopa monotherapy, combination of levodopa and dopamine ago-nist therapy, and dopamine agonist monotherapy [12]. In another study, patients treated with pramipexole, ropinirole, and bromocriptine on polytherapy combinations did not differ in MSLT scores [28]. Two different studies [11,58] found that EDS in PD was associated with the use of any dopamine agonist.

One study found an association between the catechol-0-methyl-transferase low-activity allele and EDS in subjects with PD. The authors of this study speculated that the low activity allele increases the availability of dopamine at the ventral tegmental area thereby promoting sleep [59]. Also, the severity of EDS in PD has been associated with longer duration of dopaminergic treatment [6,34]. Taken together, total amount of dopaminergic dose rather than levodopa or a specific dopamine agonist predicts the occurrence of continuous daytime somnolence in PD. Subjects with higher doses of dopaminomimetics are at higher risk of developing hypersomnia.

Effects of the Parkinson's disease pathology itself

In PD, the development of EDS may be related to the progressive cell loss in the dopaminergic and nondopaminergic brain structures and circuits that modulate the sleep-waking mechanisms. Impairment of both systems may explain some aspects of EDS in the setting of PD [1,56,57].

Two different studies using nocturnal PSG followed by MSLT showed that severity of EDS as measured by MSLT was not correlated with age, parkinsonian motor disability, use and dose of dopamine agonist therapy, cognitive impairment, or poor reduced nocturnal sleep architecture. These observations led to the assumption that EDS in PD may be a primary symptom of the neurodegenerative process itself [22,24].

This is in line with the finding in other studies of the association between EDS and advanced stage of parkinsonism [6,8,9,15,34,58] and also with longer duration of the disease [8,34,58], suggesting that more severe brain damage leads to more severe hypersomnia. Longitudinal studies have shown that the prevalence of EDS in PD increases over time in parallel with disease progression [60–62]. A recent longitudinal study showed that PD patients develop EDS at a rate of 6% a year and that this development is associated with more advanced parkinsonism and dementia. The study also showed that EDS persisted during the 4 years of follow-up in all subjects [61]. The findings of two other studies showed that EDS in PD is linked to advanced stage of disease, dementia, and hallucinations, suggesting an association with a more severe and widespread brain pathology [6,62].

Several findings indicate that integrity of the central dopamine system is crucial for maintaining sleep-wake control and that dopamine cell loss occurring in PD predisposes to EDS. First, non-human primates [31] experimentally depleted of dopamine exhibit reduced mean sleep latency and SOREMPs in MSLT, both of which are reversed with levodopa and bupropion. Second, a single young unmedicated de novo PD patient with EDS showed reduced mean sleep latency and SOREMPs in MSLT [30]. Third, severity of sleepiness and occurrence of SOREMPs in treated PD adults is associated with less reduced and fragmented nocturnal sleep architecture and not with demographic or clinical variables. This indicates that PD itself probably accounts for impairments in the expression of waking and REM sleep [22]. Taken together, these observations suggest that dopamine deficit probably at the level of mesocorticolimbic circuits impairs the thalamocortical arousal state resulting in EDS and inappropriate intrusion of REM sleep into daytime naps [63].

Alternatively, sleepiness and SOREMPs may reflect monoaminergic, GABAergic, or cholinergic dysfunction in other brain regions both known to degenerate in PD and modulate sleep, such as the dorsal raphe, sublocus coeruleus region, locus coeruleus, and pedunculopontine tegmental nucleus [64]. Given the narcolepsy-like phenotype seen in some PD subjects with EDS it is tempting to speculate that damage of the hypothalamic hypocretinergic neurons contributes to the occurrence of hypersomnia and SOREMPs. Some studies in PD brains have shown cell loss in the hypothalamus, although the hypocretin cell population has never been evaluated. Studies evaluating hypocretin levels in PD subjects have presented conflicting results. Two studies showed normal hypocretin-1 values in the lumbar cerebrospinal fluid of eight subjects with sleepiness and no advanced parkinsonism, one of them reporting SOS and the other showing more than one SOREMP in MSLT [65,66]. In contrast, one study showed undetectable or low hypocretin-1 ventricular cerebrospinal fluid levels in 19 PD subjects with advanced disease undergoing deep brain surgery [67]. Methodologic issues (lumbar puncture versus brain surgery to obtain cerebrospinal fluid) or sample bias selection (early versus advanced disease) might account for differences between these studies.

Other contributing factors
Other possible causes of EDS should be considered before determining that it is caused by the disease itself or by the effects of dopaminomimetics. These other causes include poor nocturnal sleep, obstructive sleep apnea, circadian dysrhythmias, depression, dementia, and the use of other sedative drugs.

Reduced and fragmented nocturnal sleep is traditionally associated with the development of EDS. In PD, however, there are conflicting data on the effects of sleep quality and quantity on the development of daytime sleepiness. Most studies using PSG and MSLT have shown that there is no relation between degree of nocturnal sleep disturbance and severity of daytime sleepiness [22,24,25,28]. Two of these studies, contrary to what one would expect, found that the severity of daytime sleepiness inversely correlated with sleep efficiency and total sleep time, and positively correlated with sleep-onset latency [22,25]. These findings indicate that PD subjects with severe EDS are those with the less reduced and fragmented nocturnal sleep [22,25]. In contrast, one recent study involving 20 unselected consecutive PD patients showed that percentage of stage 1 sleep correlated with the MSLT, whereas pergolide equivalents correlated with the MWT scores, suggesting that poor nocturnal sleep, in conjunction with the somnogenic effect of the dopaminergic drugs, is responsible for the development of EDS [29].

Obstructive sleep apnea is one of the most common causes of EDS in the general population. One study in PD subjects showed motor abnormalities of the upper airway muscles and lung function impairment [68]. This could predispose to sleep apnea and thereby the development of EDS. Indeed, two studies found that loud snoring, a marker of obstructive sleep apnea, is associated with the development of EDS in PD [12,69]. Obstructive sleep apnea might be expected to be common in PD. As a result of decreased upper airway caliber with age [70], however, sleep-disordered breathing is very prevalent in older adults, and as many as 62% of subjects older than 65 years demonstrate an apnea-hypopnea index greater than 10 events per hour [71]. Few PSG data, however, are available on the prevalence of obstructive sleep apnea in PD. Several studies have shown that sleep-disordered breathing is common in PD, especially in those subjects complaining of EDS, but it is not significantly more prevalent than in age-matched population [24,26,29,72–74]. It seems that PD itself does not confer increased risk for obstructive sleep apnea and that the frequent presence of this condition in PD is a reflection of aging. Nevertheless, PD patients with EDS should undergo routine PSG to exclude the occurrence of obstructive sleep apnea because correct treatment of this condition with continuous positive airway pressure can be of great help.

Circadian sleep-wake cycle disruption is another cause of EDS in subjects with PD. These patients have an exaggerated tendency toward an advancement of phase, thereby developing an irregular sleep-wake pattern characterized by early morning awakening and evening sleepiness. In PD, this situation is frequently associated with advanced disease; depression; and dementia (personal observations).

Depression and cognitive impairment are two other conditions that may cause EDS in PD and in other neurodegenerative disorders, such as Alzheimer disease and dementia with Lewy bodies. Because most of the studies in PD have not taken into account these two variables, their real impact on sleepiness is unknown.

In addition to dopaminergic agents, other medications frequently prescribed may induce EDS, such as neuroleptics, antidepressants, anxiolytics, and hypnotics. Clonazepam, the treatment of choice in REM sleep behavior disorder, and other long-acting benzodiazepines may also induce EDS as a side effect.

In PD, periodic leg movements in sleep may not be a main cause of sleepiness because most of these movements are not associated with arousals (personal observations). Also, REM sleep behavior disorder per se is not considered another cause of EDS because sleep disruption caused by this parasomnia is not significant (personal observations).

Sudden onset of sleep episodes

There are few systematically collected data evaluating the origin and risk factors for SOS in PD. Many reported cases are retrospective and may miss clinically relevant data. Nocturnal PSG and MSLT data in SOS are scarce. One study compared PD subjects with SOS (defined by the authors as unintended sleep episodes) and sleepy PD subjects without SOS. The study did not find any difference between the groups in demographic variables, severity of parkinsonism, therapy with dopaminergic agents, cognitive status, degree of daytime sleepiness, presence of SOREMPs in the MSLT, and nocturnal sleep architecture. The authors of this study concluded that unintended sleep episodes occur on a background of EDS, they are not the result of poor nocturnal sleep, and that they are probably primary to the disease itself [25].

Other studies evaluating risk factors for SOS in PD, however, disclosed associations between these episodes and several variables. SOS has been reported to occur with almost all dopaminergic drugs and it seems that patients taking dopamine agonists are at a higher risk than subjects on levodopa. The most common variables associated with SOS are therapy with dopamine agonists [33,37,38], duration of parkinsonism [7,37,38], higher ESS scores [7,37–39], higher age [37,38], and male gen-

der [37,38]. Other variables that have been associated with SOS are autonomic failure [33], better subjective sleep quality [38], heavy snoring [39], REM sleep behavior disorder [39], and higher nocturnal total sleep time on PSG [33]. Despite being considered as main risk factors for EDS in PD, total dopaminergic equivalent dose and advanced disease are two variables that do not seem to be predictive for SOS.

Episodes of irresistible onset of sleepiness occurring 30 to 60 minutes after meals and after drug dose intake have been thought to be linked to the hypotensive effect of levodopa and dopamine agonists [75]. Interestingly, one study found a strong association between autonomic failure and SOS [33].

A study evaluating dopamine receptors polymorphisms found that the dopamine D4 receptor DRD4*Short/Short variant was more frequent in PD patients with SOS than in those without SOS. The authors of this study found no associations with the other genes coding for dopamine receptors 2 and 3 [76]. In contrast, a recent study documented the association of SOS with the dopamine D2 receptor allele A2. Given the fact that D2 autoreceptors are prominent in the midbrain ventral tegmental area, it can be speculated that impairment in the mesocorticolimbic dopamine system may be associated with the occurrence of SOS [77]. Another recent study from the same group has found that the allele T of the preproohypocretin polymorphism is associated with SOS [78]. Because dopaminergic neurons in the ventral tegmental area are excited by hypocretinergic projections, it is tempting to speculate that genetic factors in the dopaminergic and hypocretinergic systems may play a role in the pathogenesis of SOS in subjects with PD. It would be very interesting to measure cerebrospinal fluid hypocretin-1 levels in PD subjects reporting SOS, especially in those exhibiting SOREMPs in MSLT.

Management of sleepiness in Parkinson's disease

Subjects with PD need comprehensive and individualized treatment of their sleep complaints, including sleepiness. Management of sleepiness is challenging because it is a multifactorial complex phenomenon [1,79]. In general, EDS and SOS may be treated similarly.

Sleep hygiene measures should be advised to all subjects and particularly to those with disruption of the circadian sleep-wake cycle and depression. These measures include schedule of regular bed time and waking time, consolidation of sleep during the night, not spending time in bed awake, avoiding long daytime naps, and promoting daytime activities. Short-acting sleeping aids and other sedating medications may be useful only in a few selected cases because it has been shown that the sleepier PD subjects are those with better nocturnal sleep [22].

Physicians must also consider that an underlying comorbidity, such as depression, may be the main cause of EDS in some subjects. In these cases, adequate treatment of the underlying cause may resolve the associated sleepiness.

Before determining that EDS is caused by the disease itself or by the effects of dopaminomimetics, routine PSG should be performed to exclude obstructive sleep apnea, especially in snorers. If this sleep disorder is detected, treatment with continuous positive airway pressure should be considered. Patients and relatives need instruction, support, and encouragement for the correct use of the nasal continuous positive airway pressure mask.

Patients taking dopaminergic drugs should be warned of the occurrence of EDS and SOS as an adverse effect of these medications. They should be informed about the risk of road accidents. These patients should be advised to stop driving if they experience any sign of somnolence while driving. If EDS or SOS are thought to be related to the introduction or dose increase of a dopaminergic medication, dose reduction, drug discontinuation, or switching to a different dopaminomimetic may be useful [80]. Other sedating drugs (hypnotics; benzodiazepines, such as clonazepam; sedating antidepressants, such as trazodone; antipsychotics; and antihistaminics) should be avoided. In subjects taking dopaminergic agents, treatment of sleepiness with waking-promoting agents, such as modafinil, is only moderately effective [81–84].

Summary

In PD, sleepiness is a common feature that in some cases may lead to automobile accidents and professional, social, and familial problems. Sleepiness manifests in PD as a state of EDS with difficulty to remain awake leading to frequent naps, and less frequently as SOS episodes, which have been termed "sleep attacks." EDS is associated with advanced parkinsonism and higher doses of dopaminomimetics, although it may occur in unmedicated subjects at earlier stages of the disease. The main factors contributing to EDS are the intrinsic pathology of PD and the sedative effects of the dopaminergic agents. Depression, cognitive impairment, and obstructive sleep apnea may also predispose to sleepiness. Poor nocturnal sleep, REM sleep behavior disorder, periodic leg movements in sleep,

and restless legs syndrome, although frequent in PD, are not considered major risk factors for sleepiness. Treatment strategies include sleep hygiene; reduction or discontinuance of sedative medications; treatment of an underlying condition (eg, obstructive sleep apnea); and using stimulant medications, such as modafinil. The common occurrence of sleepiness and documentation of REM sleep intrusions into daytime naps in PD subjects and animal models of parkinsonism indicate that central dopaminergic transmission participates in the sleep-wake control.

Acknowledgments

I thank Dr. J. Santamaria for his comments while reviewing this manuscript.

References

[1] Rye D, Iranzo A. The nocturnal manifestations of waking movement disorders: focus on Parkinson's disease. In: Guilleminault C, editor. Handbook of clinical neurophysiology, vol. 6. Sleep and its disorders. Philadelphia: Elsevier; 2005. p. 263–72.

[2] Nausieda PA. Sleep in Parkinson's disease. In: Koller WC, editor. Handbook of Parkinson's disease. 2nd edition. New York: Marcel Dekker; 1992. p. 451–67.

[3] Frucht S, Rogers MD, Greene PE, et al. Falling asleep at the wheel: motor vehicle mishaps in persons taking pramipexole and ropinirole. Neurology 1999;52:1908–10.

[4] Olanow CW, Schapira AHV, Roth T. Waking up to sleep episodes in Parkinson's disease. Mov Disord 2000;15:212–5.

[5] Frucht SJ, Greene PE, Fahn S. Sleep episodes in Parkinson's disease: a wake-up call. Mov Disord 2000;15:601–3.

[6] Tandberg E, Larsen JP, Karlsen K. Excessive daytime sleepiness and sleep benefit in Parkinson's disease: a community-based study. Mov Disord 1999;14:922–7.

[7] Tan EK, Lum SY, Fook-Chong SMC, et al. Evaluation of somnolence in Parkinson's disease: comparison with age and sex-matched controls. Neurology 2002;58:465–8.

[8] Hobson DE, Lang AE, Martin WWR, et al. Excessive daytime sleepiness and sudden-onset sleep in Parkinson disease: a survey by the Canadian movement disorder group. JAMA 2002;287:455–63.

[9] Kumar S, Bhatia M, Behari M. Sleep disorders in Parkinson's disease. Mov Disord 2002;17:775–81.

[10] Fabbrini G, Barbanti P, Aurilia C, et al. Excessive daytime sleepiness in de novo and treated Parkinson's disease. Mov Disord 2002;17:1026–30.

[11] O'Suilleabhain PE, Dewey RB. Contributions of dopaminergic drugs and disease severity to day-

time sleepiness in Parkinson disease. Arch Neurol 2002;59:986–9.

[12] Högl B, Seppi K, Brandauer E, et al. Increased daytime sleepiness in Parkinson's disease: a questionnaire survey. Mov Disord 2003;18:319–23.

[13] Brodsky MA, Godbold J, Roth T, et al. Sleepiness in Parkinson's disease: a controlled study. Mov Disord 2003;18:668–72.

[14] Kumar S, Bhatia M, Behari M. Excessive daytime sleepiness in Parkinson's disease as assessed by Epworth Sleepiness Scale (ESS). Sleep Med 2003; 4:339–42.

[15] Furumoto H. Excessive daytime somnolence in Japanese patients with Parkinson's disease. Eur J Neurol 2004;11:535–40.

[16] Arnulf I. Excessive daytime sleepiness in parkinsonism. Sleep Med Rev 2005;9:180–200.

[17] Meindorfner C, Körner Y, Möller JC, et al. Driving in Parkinson's disease: mobility, accidents, and sudden onset of sleep at the wheel. Mov Disord 2005;20:832–42.

[18] Santamaria J. How to evaluate excessive daytime sleepiness in Parkinson's disease. Neurology 2004; 63(Suppl 3):S21–3.

[19] Johns MW. A new method for measuring daytime sleepiness: the Epworth sleepiness scale. Sleep 1991;14:540–5.

[20] Arand D, Bonnet M, Hurwitz T, et al. The clinical use of the MSLT and MWT. Sleep 2005;28:123–44.

[21] Marinus J, Visser M, van Hilten JJ, et al. Assessment of sleep and sleepiness in Parkinson disease. Sleep 2003;26:1049–54.

[22] Rye DB, Bliwise DL, Dihenia B, et al. FAST TRACK. Daytime sleepiness in Parkinson's disease. J Sleep Res 2000;9:63–9.

[23] Arnulf I, Bonnet AM, Damier P, et al. Hallucinations, REM sleep, and Parkinson's disease: a medical hypothesis. Neurology 2000;55:281–8.

[24] Arnulf I, Konofal E, Merino-Andreu M, et al. Parkinson's disease and sleepiness: an integral part of PD. Neurology 2002;58:1019–24.

[25] Roth T, Rye DB, Borcher LD, et al. Assessment of sleepiness and unintended sleep in Parkinson's disease patients taking dopamine agonists. Sleep Med 2003;4:275–80.

[26] Kaynak D, Kiziltan G, Kaynak H, et al. Sleep and sleepiness in patients with Parkinson's disease before and after dopaminergic treatment. Eur J Neurol 2005;12:199–207.

[27] Chervin RD, Aldrich MS. The Epworth Sleepiness Scale may not reflect objective measures of sleepiness or sleep apnea. Neurology 1999;52:125–31.

[28] Razmy A, Lang AE, Shapiro CM. Predictors of impaired daytime sleep and wakefulness in patients with Parkinson disease treated with older (ergot) vs newer (nonergot) dopamine agonists. Arch Neurol 2004;61:97–102.

[29] Stevens S, Comella CL, Stepanski EJ. Daytime sleepiness and alertness in patients with Parkinson disease. Sleep 2004;27:967–72.

[30] Rye DB, Johnston LH, Watts RL, et al. Juvenile Parkinson's disease with REM sleep behavior disorder, sleepiness, and daytime REM onset. Neurology 1999;53:1868–70.

[31] Daley J, Turner R, Bliwise D, et al. Nocturnal sleep and daytime alertness in the MPTP-treated primate. Sleep 1999;22(Suppl):S218–9.

[32] Hauser RA, Gauger L, McDowell-Anderson W, et al. Pramipexole-induced somnolence and episodes of daytime sleep. Mov Disord 2000;15:658–63.

[33] Montastruc JL, Brefel-Courbon C, Senard JM, et al. Sleep attacks and antiparkinsonian drugs: a pilot prospective pharamacoepidemiologic study. Clin Neurol 2001;24:181–3.

[34] Pal S, Bhattacharya KF, Agapito C, et al. A study of excessive daytime sleepiness and its clinical significance in three groups of Parkinson's disease patients taking pramipexole, cabergoline and levodopa mono and combination therapy. J Neural Transm 2001;108:71–7.

[35] Möller JC, Stiasny K, Hargutt V, et al. Evaluation of sleep and driving performance in six patients with Parkinson's disease reporting sudden onset of sleep under dopaminergic medication: a pilot study. Mov Disord 2002;17:474–81.

[36] Homann CN, Wenzel K, Suppan K, et al. Sleep attacks in patients taking dopamine agonists: review. BMJ 2002;324:1483–7.

[37] Paus S, Brecht HM, Köster J, et al. Sleep attacks, daytime sleepiness, and dopamine agonists in Parkinson's disease. Mov Disord 2003;18:659–67.

[38] Körner Y, Meindorfner C, Möller JC, et al. Predictors of sudden onset of sleep in Parkinson's disease. Mov Disord 2004;19:1298–305.

[39] Manni R, Terzaghi M, Sartori I, et al. Dopamine agonist and sleepiness in PD: review of the literature and personal findings. Sleep Med 2004;5:189–93.

[40] Avorn J, Scneeweiss S, Sudarsky LR, et al. Sudden uncontrollable somnolence and medication use in Parkinson disease. Arch Neurol 2005;62:1242–8.

[41] Schapira AHV. Sleep attacks (sleep episodes) with pergolide. Lancet 2000;355:1332–3.

[42] Ferreira JJ, Galitzky M, Montastruc JL, et al. Sleep attacks and Parkinson's disease treatment. Lancet 2000;355:1333–4.

[43] Merino-Andreu M, Arnulf I, Konofal E, et al. Unawareness of naps in Parkinson's disease and in disorders with excessive daytime sleepiness. Neurology 2003;60:1553–4.

[44] Schlesinger I, Ravin PD. Dopamine agonists induce episodes of irresistible daytime sleepiness. Eur Neurol 2003;49:30–3.

[45] Garcia-Borreguero D, Schwarz C, Larrosa O, et al. L-DOPA-induce excessive daytime sleepiness in PD: a placebo-controlled case with MSLT assessment. Neurology 2003;61:1008–10.

[46] Homann CN, Homann B, Ott E, et al. Sleep attacks may not be a side-effect dopaminergic medication. Mov Disord 2003;18:1569–71.

[47] Ferreira JJ, Thalamas C, Montastruc JL, et al.

Levodopa monotherapy can induce "sleep attacks" in Parkinson's disease patients. J Neurol 2001;248:426–7.

[48] Jimenez-Jimenez FJ, Velasco I, Toledo M, et al. Multiple latency test in a patient with episodes of sleep induced by pergolide. Rev Neurol (Barc) 2002;34:1140–1.

[49] Bares M, Kanovsky P, Rektor I. Excessive daytime sleepiness and "sleep attacks" induced by entacapone. Fundam Clin Pharmacol 2003;17:113–6.

[50] Santens P. Sleep attacks in Parkinson's disease induced by entacapone, a COMT-inhibitor. Fundam Clin Pharmacol 2003;17:121–3.

[51] Tracik F, Ebersbach G. Sudden daytime sleep onset in Parkinson's disease: polysomnographic recordings. Mov Disord 2001;16:500–6.

[52] Ebersbach G, Norden J, Tracik F. Sleep attacks in Parkinson's disease: polysomnographic recordings. Mov Disord 2000;15(Suppl 3):89.

[53] Schäfer D, Greulich W. Effects of parkinsonian medication on sleep. J Neurol 2000;247(Suppl 4): 24–7.

[54] Romigi A, Brusa L, Marciani MG, et al. Sleep episodes and daytime somnolence as a result of individual susceptibility to different dopaminergic drugs in a PD patient: a polysomnographic study. J Neurol Sci 2005;228:7–10.

[55] Ulivelli M, Rossi S, Lombardi C, et al. Polysomnographic characterization of pergolide-induced sleep attacks in idiopathic PD. Neurology 2002;58:462–5.

[56] Rye DB, Jankovic J. Emerging views of dopamine in modulating sleep/wake state from an unlikely source: PD. Neurology 2002;58:341–6.

[57] Rye DB. The two faces of Eve: dopamine's modulation of wakefulness and sleep. Neurology 2004; 63(Suppl 3):S2–7.

[58] Ondo WG, Dat Vuong K, Khan H, et al. Daytime sleepiness and other sleep disorders in Parkinson's disease. Neurology 2001;57:1392–6.

[59] Frauscher B, Höghl B, Maret S, et al. Association of daytime sleepiness with COMT polymorphism in patients with Parkinson disease: a pilot study. Sleep 2004;27:733–6.

[60] Happe S, Berguer K on behalf of the FAQT study investigators. The association of dopamine agonists with daytime sleepiness, sleep problems and quality of life in patients with Parkinson's disease: a prospective study. J Neurol 2001;248: 1062–7.

[61] Gjerstad MD, Aarsland D, Larsen JP. Development of daytime somnolence over time in Parkinson's disease. Neurology 2002;58:1544–6.

[62] Fabbrini G, Barbanti P, Aurilia C, et al. Excessive daytime somnolence in Parkinson's disease: follow-up after 1 year of treatment. Neurol Sci 2003;24: 178–9.

[63] Freeman A, Ciliax B, Bakay R, et al. Nigrostriatal collaterals to thalamus degenerate in parkinsonian animal models. Ann Neurol 2001;50:321–9.

[64] Jellinger KA. Post mortem studies in Parkinson's disease: is it possible to detect brain areas for specific symptoms? J Neural Transm Suppl 1999;56: 1–29.

[65] Overeem S, van Hilten JJ, Ripley B, et al. Normal hypocretin-1 levels in Parkinson's disease with excessive daytime sleepiness. Neurology 2002; 58:498–9.

[66] Baumann C, Ferini-Strambi L, Waldvogel D, et al. Parkinsonism with excessive daytime sleepiness: a narcolepsy-like disorder? J Neurol 2005;252: 139–45.

[67] Drouot X, Moutereau S, Nguyen JP, et al. Low levels of ventricular CSF orexin/hypocretin in advanced PD. Neurology 2003;61:540–3.

[68] Vincken WG, Gauthier SG, Dollfuss RE, et al. Involvement of upper-airway muscles in extrapyramidal disorders. N Engl J Med 1984;311: 438–42.

[69] Braga-Neto P, Pereira da Sila-Junior F, Sueli Monte F, et al. Snoring and excessive daytime sleepiness in Parkinson's disease. J Neurol Sci 2004; 217:41–5.

[70] Martin SE, Mathur R, Marshall I, et al. The effect of age, sex, obesity and posture on upper airway size. Eur Respir J 1997;10:2087–90.

[71] Anconi-Israel S, Kripke DF, Klauber MR, et al. Sleep-disordered breathing in community-dwelling elderly. Sleep 1991;14:486–95.

[72] Bittinger LJ, McNear KK, Khan F, et al. Obstructive sleep apnea on polysomnography in patients with parkinsonism. Sleep 2005;28:A283.

[73] Hitchcock SE, Greer SA, Pour Ansari F, et al. Sleep disordered breathing (SDB) in Parkinsons disease (PD). Sleep 2005;28:A286–7.

[74] Diederich NJ, Vaillant M, Leischen M, et al. Sleep apnea syndrome in Parkinson's disease: a case-control study in 49 patients. Mov Disord 2005; 11:1413–8.

[75] Contin M, Provini F, Martinelli P, et al. Excessive daytime sleepiness and levodopa in Parkinson's disease: polygraphic, placebo-controlled monitoring. Clin Neuropharmacol 2003;26:115–8.

[76] Paus S, Seeger G, Brecht HM, et al. Association study of dopamine D2, D3, D4 receptor and serotonin transporter gene polymorphisms with sleep attacks in Parkinson's disease. Mov Disord 2004;19:705–7.

[77] Rissling I, Geller F, Bandmann O, et al. Dopamine gene receptor gene polymorphisms in Parkinson's disease patients reporting sleep attacks. Mov Disord 2004;19:1279–84.

[78] Rissling I, Köner Y, Geller F, et al. Prehypocretin polymorphysms in Parkinson disease patients reporting sleep attacks. Sleep 2005;28:871–5.

[79] Barone P, Amboni M, Vitale C, et al. Treatment of nocturnal disturbances and excessive daytime sleepiness in Parkinson's disease. Neurology 2004;63(Suppl 3):S35–8.

[80] Del Dotto P, Gambaccini G, Caneparo D, et al. Bedtime cabergoline in Parkinson's disease patients with excessive daytime sleepiness induced by dopamine agonists. Neurol Sci 2003;24:170–1.

[81] Hauser RA, Wahba MN, Zesiewicz TA, et al.

Modafinil treatment of pramipexole-associated somnolence. Mov Disord 2000;15:1269–71.

[82] Högl B, Saletu M, Brandauer E, et al. Modafinil for the treatment of daytime sleepiness in Parkinson's disease: a double-blind, randomized, crossover, placebo-controlled polygraphic trial. Sleep 2002;25:905–9.

[83] Adler CH, Caviness JN, Hentz JG, et al. Random-

ized trial of modafinil for treating subjective daytime sleepiness in patients with Parkinson's disease. Mov Disord 2003;18:287–93.

[84] Nieves AV, Lang AE. Treatment of excessive daytime sleepiness in patients with Parkinson's disease with modafinil. Clin Neuropharmacol 2002;25:111–4.

ELSEVIER
SAUNDERS

SLEEP
MEDICINE
CLINICS

Sleep Med Clin 1 (2006) 139–155

Poststroke Hypersomnia

Claudio L. Bassetti, MD*, Philipp Valko, MD

- Historical remarks
- Neuroanatomy and physiology of
  wakefulness and sleep
- Pathophysiology of poststroke
  hypersomnia
- Epidemiology of poststroke hypersomnia
- Clinical features of poststroke hypersomnia
  *Clinical varieties of poststroke
  hypersomnia*
    Fatigue
    *Stroke topography and poststroke
    hypersomnia*
- Sleep-wake studies in poststroke
  hypersomnia
- Treatment and prognosis of poststroke
  hypersomnia
- References

Poststroke hypersomnia can be defined on clinical grounds as an exaggerated sleep propensity with excessive daytime sleepiness, increased daytime napping, or prolonged nighttime sleep following cerebrovascular event. As a consequence, patients may be difficult to arouse or keep awake once awakened.

The clinician is faced with various problems in dealing with patients suffering from poststroke hypersomnia. First, the clinical presentation of hypersomnia can be very similar despite different underlying pathophysiology. Hypersomnia as a consequence of brain disease may arise from decreased (deficient) arousal or enhanced sleep mechanisms. The former has been named "passive" hypersomnia, somnolence, or dearousal, and the latter "active" hypersomnia or abnormal sleepiness [1]. Somnolence lies in the wakefulness-coma continuum. The somnolent patient usually presents additional neurologic or neuropsychologic deficits. Sleepiness lies in the wakefulness-sleep continuum. The sleepy patient, once aroused, usually does not exhibit neurologic abnormalities. In clinical practice, somnolence and sleepiness may be difficult to separate, evolve into each other, or even coexist (see later). Second, hypersomnia is often underrecognized or underreported by patients. Sleep needs and behavior are highly variable in the normal population and heavily depend on motivation and environment. Milder forms of poststroke hypersomnia may not be noticed by the patient and his or her environment until their return home or to work. Napping in the hospital is less alarming than at work. As a consequence, the diagnosis of poststroke hypersomnia often requires questioning of third parties (nurses, relatives) and knowledge of sleep habits and behavior preceding the onset of stroke. One should also be aware that certain motor deficits, such as bilateral ptosis, tetraparesis, or akinetic mutism (see later) can be mistaken for hypersomnia. Third, sleep behavior and electroencephalogram (EEG) correlates of sleep are regulated by distinct albeit interrelated neuronal systems, which focal brain disease can derange separately. Sleep may occur, at least to some extent, even in the absence of its EEG correlates. Fourth, hypersomnia following focal brain damage is often overshadowed by the additional presence of mental, behavioral, or motor deficits. Finally, the anarchy in the use of terms, such as hypersomnia, sopor, stupor, coma, apathy, akinetic mutism, in part caused by divergent meanings of the same terms in

Department of Neurology, University Hospital of Zurich, Frauenklinikstrasse 26, CH-8091 Zurich, Switzerland
* Corresponding author.
E-mail address: claudio.bassetti@usz.ch (C.L. Bassetti).

1556-407X/06/$ – see front matter © 2006 Elsevier Inc. All rights reserved.
sleep.theclinics.com

doi:10.1016/j.jsmc.2005.11.012

different languages (eg, stupor), makes it sometimes difficult to interpret correctly reports in the literature [2].

Historical remarks

Although hypersomnia following stroke was mentioned by MacNish [3] already in 1830, subsequent reports on the occurrence of sleep-wake disorders in patients with cerebrovascular diseases remained scarce until the beginning of the twentieth century [4,5]. In the classic monographs on sleep by Manasseina [6] and Kleitman [7] there are no remarks on poststroke hypersomnia.

At the end of the nineteenth century the first clinical observations were made that attributed sleep-wake disorders to distinctly localized intracerebral lesions. They concerned mostly patients with inflammatory or tumorous pathologies. In 1881, Wernicke [8] reported several patients in whom autopsy revealed punctate hemorrhages affecting the gray matter around the third and fourth ventricles and the aqueduct of Sylvius. In describing the clinical features of "polioencephalitis hemorrhagica superioris," now referred to as "Wernicke-Korsakoff syndrome," he already reported the occasional occurrence of impaired consciousness. The idea that wakefulness may depend on the integrity of specific areas of the brain was further supported in 1890 by Mauthner [9], who related somnolence and coma in patients with "sleeping sickness" (encephalitis lethargica) to the presence of inflammatory lesions in the periventricular gray (Höhlengrau) of the midbrain. He speculated that sleep might be the (passive) result of a functional break between brainstem and cerebral cortex.

In the 1920s, considering the presence of persistent insomnia in some patients with postencephalitic lesions of the anterior hypothalamus, von Economo [10] first postulated that sleep might represent an active process of the brain, and not just the absence of wakefulness. In other cases of encephalitis lethargica von Economo showed that hypersomnia was associated with lesions in the posterior hypothalamus. In 1949 Moruzzi and Magoun [11] induced abrupt wakefulness in the sleeping cat by electrical stimulation of the mesencephalic ascending reticular activating system (ARAS), thereby experimentally confirming von Economo's clinical observations.

The fundamental role of the thalamus in sleep generation was first demonstrated by Hess' [12] observation of sleep induction in cats following low-frequency stimulation of the medial thalamus. The description in 1986 of fatal familial insomnia, characterized by a complete loss of sleep spindles and slow wave sleep because of a degeneration of the thalamic nuclei, has further advanced the understanding of the thalamic regulation of sleep and wakefulness [13]. Finally, in 1998 the excitatory hypothalamic neurotransmitter hypocretin (orexin) and, subsequently, its diffuse projections to structures involved in the regulation of sleep and wakefulness have been discovered [14].

Neuroanatomy and physiology of wakefulness and sleep

Arousal systems consist of several anatomically and chemically (eg, monoaminergic and cholinergic) distinct neuronal networks that are located in upper pons, midbrain, and posterior hypothalamus and project diffusely to the cortex through synaptic relays in the midline (intralaminar) and dorsomedial thalamic nuclei (thalamic route) and in the basal forebrain (extrathalamic route, [Fig. 1]) [15–17]. The previously mentioned monoaminergic systems include noradrenergic (from the locus coeruleus); serotoninergic (from the dorsal raphae nucleus); dopaminergic (from ventral tegmental area); and histaminergic (from tuberomamillary nucleus) neurons [18]. In addition, excitatory hypocretin neurons in the posterolateral hypothalamus probably play a crucial role in promoting arousal and wakefulness, as is suggested by its widespread projections to the arousal systems in the brainstem, thalamus, and basal forebrain [14]. The main activating cholinergic influences come from neurons in the laterodorsal tegmental and pedunculopontine nuclei of the pons [18–20]. The increased cortex excitability induced by the arousal systems is accompanied by a potentiation and synchronization of fast (30–40 Hz) spontaneous gamma rhythms in intracortical and thalamocorticothalamic networks [21,22].

There is increasing support for the hypothesis that mental, motor, vegetative, and EEG arousal may depend on the action of different subunits of the arousal systems and their specific ascending or descending connections [17,23,24]. For example, the role of thalamostriatocortical and corticostriatothalamic circuits in regulating arousal and more generally sleep-wake functions remains to be determined [16]. This variety of arousal systems may explain how different focal brain lesions may lead to a spectrum of hypersomnolent syndromes with variable impairment of motor, mental, and EEG arousal. Dissociated states characterized by normal mental arousal with insufficient motor arousal (akinetic mutism), or hyperkinesia and mutism [25], or coma with normal (alpha) EEG activity [26], or wakefulness with EEG slowing [27] may then arise.

Corticofugal neuronal systems, such as Nauta's forebrain-midbrain circuit, project back to thalamus, basal ganglia, and brainstem [1,28]. These

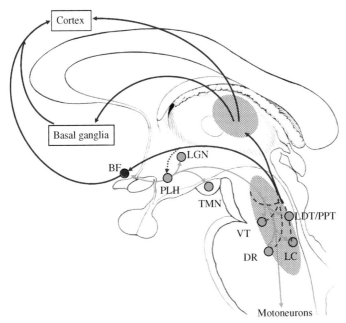

Fig. 1. Arousal systems. The previously called ARAS (*red shaded*) consists of neuronal areas located in upper pons, midbrain, and posterior hypothalamus which project diffusely to the cortex through synaptic relays in the midline (intralaminar) and dorsomedial thalamic nuclei (thalamic route) and in the basal forebrain (extrathalamic route). Corticofugal neuronal systems (not shown) project back to thalamus, basal ganglia, and brainstem and modulate the activity of the ARAS. This regulation of the level of cortical activation subserves the capacity to focus and sustain attention to specific tasks and stimuli. Hypocretin neurons in the posterolateral hypothalamus excite brainstem neurotransmitter systems: serotoninergic cells in the dorsal raphe, norepinephrinergic neurons in the locus coeruleus, cholinergic cells in the basal forebrain and the LDT-PPT, histaminergic cells in the tuberomammillary nucleus, and dopaminergic cells in the substantia nigra and ventral tegmentum. BF, basal forebrain; DR, dorsal raphe; LC, locus coeruleus; LDT, laterodorsal tegmental; LGN, local glutamatergic neurons; PLH, posterolateral hypothalamus; PPT, pedunculopontine tegmental; TMN, tuberomammillary nucleus; VT, ventral tegmentum.

corticothalamic neurons outnumber thalamocortical projections and modulate the activity. This regulation of cortical activation subserves, among others, the capacity to focus and sustain attention to specific tasks and stimuli [28–30]. In addition, corticofugal systems and hypocretinergic projections contribute to the regulation of the motor expression (body sleep) of activated and deactivated states [24].

Generally speaking, supratentorial structures (particularly thalamocortical networks) are crucial for the generation of non–rapid eye movement (NREM) sleep, whereas infratentorial structures (particularly neurons in the dorsolateral upper pons) are essential for the generation of REM sleep. A descending (corticofugal) contribution of the cerebral cortex in regulating wakefulness, NREM, and REM sleep mechanisms has been suggested [28,30–32].

Experimental work in the last four decades has led to the recognition of sleep-promoting neurons in anterior hypothalamus, basal forebrain, thalamus, pons, and medulla. A particularly important group of neurons firing at sleep onset has been recently identified in the ventrolateral preoptic nu-

cleus of the anterior hypothalamus [33]. Moreover, hypocretin neurons, which are supposed to play a pivotal role in the maintenance of a stable waking state [34], have been found to be inhibited during sleep by GABAergic neurons located in the ventrolateral preoptic nucleus and basal forebrain [35]. The inhibition of hypocretin neurons may be crucially involved in the sleep initiation, which in turn is accompanied by a decreased activity of the arousal systems [36,37]. As a result the transfer of sensory information at the level of the thalamic relay nuclei is diminished and thalamocortical neurons become hyperpolarized. Sleep spindles (12–16 Hz beta rhythms) and slow wave sleep (1–4 Hz delta rhythms), the electrophysiologic hallmarks of NREM sleep, arise from the interaction of increasingly hyperpolarized thalamocortical neurons with neuronal oscillators in the reticular thalamic nucleus (pacemaker of sleep spindles) and cerebral cortex (pacemaker of <1 Hz rhythms) [38]. The generators of the different REM sleep phenomena (EEG activation, muscle atonia, REM, and so forth) are located in the mediolateral tegmentum of the pontomesencephalic junction and include neurons of the laterodorsal tegmental and pedunculopontine tegmental nuclei [18–20]. Phasic and tonic events of REM sleep may depend on different neuronal populations in the pontine tegmentum [39]. Although in REM sleep brain excitability is as high as during wakefulness, the pattern of activation and the involved transmitter systems differ between the two states [40]. During wakefulness hypocretinergic, cholinergic, and monoaminergic neurons are activated. During REM sleep cholinergic neurons are active while monoaminergic neurons are inhibited (the degree of activation of hypocretin neurons is unclear at this point).

Pathophysiology of poststroke hypersomnia

Environmental disturbances (eg, noise, light, intensive care, and monitoring), cardiorespiratory disorders including sleep-disordered breathing, sedative drugs, and complications of stroke (eg, seizures, infections, fever, emotional stress) represent stroke-associated factors that, often by means of sleep deprivation and sleep fragmentation, can cause transient hypersomnia and changes of the sleep EEG. The importance of such factors is well illustrated by the high frequency of sleep disturbances observed in patients without brain damage treated in intensive care units [41,42].

Because the modulation of wakefulness, NREM sleep, and REM sleep occurs in multiple and overlapping areas of brainstem and cerebral hemispheres, it is no surprise that strokes of different topography can directly affect sleep-wake functions, stroke-dependent factors. The net detrimental effect on both wakefulness promoting and sleep-inducing systems may give rise to poststroke hypersomnia or insomnia. The occasional observation of patients with rapid transition from insomnia to hypersomnia ([43], see also later) emphasizes the dual influence of such brain areas as thalamus, basal forebrain, and pontomesencephalic junction on sleep-wake regulation [1,44].

A reduction in the activity of the arousal systems, often called dearousal, underlies most forms of poststroke hypersomnia. This dearousal, also called cortical deafferentation or disconnection, corresponds to a focal, multifocal, or diffuse cortical brain hypometabolism, which can be demonstrated by positron emission tomography (PET) [45]. The most severe and persisting forms of dearousal are seen in patients with bilateral lesions of the posterior subthalamus (hypothalamus), tegmental midbrain, and upper pons, where fibers of the arousal systems are bundled and can be severely lesioned by a single lesion. The mental arousal seems to be affected more by medial lesions, whereas involvement of lateral portions of the arousal systems may impair the motor arousal preferentially [1,46]. In

paramedian thalamic lesions (even without subthalamic extension) the initial clinical picture may be similar to impairment of consciousness of midbrain origin but recovery is usually better, probably because of the existence of an extrathalamic route of cerebral activation [18]. The core of the lesion in these patients involves the dorsomedial nucleus (particularly its magnocellular part) and intralaminar (midline) nuclei [47,48]. Lesions in lower pons and medulla have usually no or only little effect on arousal. In deep hemispheric lesions sparing the thalamus dearousal is usually mild and transient, probably because of the widespread distribution of arousal systems projections at this level. The occasional observation of significant hypersomnia following anterior caudate and other deep (subcortical) hemispheric stroke (see later) suggests, however, that basal ganglia and more generally subcortical centers may play a more important role in sleep-wake functions than previously thought [16,31,49,50]. A disruption of both ascending (corticopetal) and descending (corticofugal) fibers may be involved in such cases. As for thalamomesencephalic lesions, also in deep hemispheric lesion, cortical hypometabolism can be demonstrated (ipsilateral to the lesion) by PET [51,52]. In large hemispheric strokes dearousal results from disruption of the arousal systems in the upper brainstem secondary to vertical (transtentorial) or horizontal (midline shift) displacement of the brain secondary to brain edema [53]. In (pseudotumoral) cerebellar infarcts similar mechanisms are responsible for dearousal [54]. The rare occurrence (see later) of sleep-wake disturbances following smaller superficial (cortical) hemispheric strokes without mass effect supports the hypothesis of a role of the cerebral cortex in sleep-wake functions [30,32,55]. A few PET studies suggested that hypersomnia may be associated in these patients with a reduced metabolism of the contralateral (unaffected) hemisphere (transhemispheric diaschisis) [56,57].

Sleep-disordered breathing is particularly frequent after stroke and may additionally contribute to poststroke fatigue and excessive daytime sleepiness. Approximately 50% to 70% of stroke patients exhibit sleep-disordered breathing, as defined by an apnea-hypopnea index ≥10 per hour [58]. No major differences have been reported in the frequency of sleep-disordered breathing according to topography and subtype (ischemic versus hemorrhagic) of stroke [59–62].

Epidemiology of poststroke hypersomnia

Focal ischemic brain damage causes sleep-wake disorders in 20% to 40%, most commonly in the

Table 1: Poststroke hypersomnia in 100 consecutive acute stroke patients with no coma or respiratory insufficiency: sleep and stroke characteristics

	Hypersomnia* (N = 22)	No hypersomnia (N = 78)	P value
Age	52.3 ± 13.3	55.2 ± 12.4	
Male:female	3:9	53:25	
Before stroke			
Epworth score	6.2 ± 4.8	5.4 ± 3.8	
Estimated sleep per 24 hours	7.4 ± 0.8	7.3 ± 1.5	
After stroke			
NIHSS	12 ± 5.7	6.2 ± 3.3	P < .0001
Apnea-hypopnea-index[b]	6.4 ± 13.4	16.3 ± 14.4	
Actigraphic findings (within the first week after stroke, in 20 patients)			
Sleep-wake ratio	1.3 ± 0.6[a]	0.5 ± 0.1	P = .0001
Short-term outcome (at hospital discharge, in 100 patients)			
Barthel-Index	67.7 ± 30.5	90.3 ± 15.5	P = .0049
Rankin score	3 ± 1.5	1.7 ± 1.2	P = .0011
Long-term outcome (at 1 year, in 42 patients)			
Epworth score	5.9 ± 4.5	5.8 ± 3.5	
Estimated sleep per 24 hours	8.3 ± 1.6	7.9 ± 1.5	
Rankin score	1.8 ± 1.1	1.5 ± 1.1	

Abbreviation: NIHSS, National Institute of Health Stroke Score.
[a] Excessive daytime sleepiness or increased sleep per 24 hours (as compared with prestroke situation), assessed prospectively within the first week after stroke onset.
[b] As assessed by automatic-CPAP within a mean of 3 days after stroke.
Courtesy of Neurology Department, University of Berne, Berne, Switzerland.

form of increased sleep needs (hypersomnia); excessive daytime sleepiness; or insomnia [63]. Clinical experience has shown that poststroke hypersomnia is frequent in paramedian thalamic and mesencephalic stroke, large hemispheric stroke, and bilateral tegmental pontine stroke. Poststroke hypersomnia is occasionally and usually only transiently seen in caudate and other deep (subcortical) hemispheric strokes, being rare in unilateral pontine, medullary, and small superficial (cortical) hemispheric strokes. The exact frequency of poststroke hypersomnia is unknown. In large series of stroke patients the frequency of disturbed level of consciousness was estimated around 10% to 20% and has been associated with the presence of hemorrhagic strokes, severe deficits, and poor outcome [64,65].

In a prospective (unpublished) study of 100 consecutive patients with acute ischemic stroke not requiring admission to an intensive care unit (no coma or respiratory insufficiency) the authors observed hypersomnia, as defined previously, in 22% of cases during the first week following the onset of symptoms [Table 1]. The presence of hypersomnia was well documented by actigraphy and correlated with a more severe stroke and a worse short-term outcome. Conversely, there were no differences between patients with and without hypersomnia in Epworth Sleepiness Score, and estimated sleep duration preceding the onset of stroke, and severity of sleep-disordered breathing. Poststroke hypersomnia was more common in large (corticosubcortical) and in deep (subcortical) hemispheric strokes [Table 2].

Table 2: Poststroke hypersomnia in 100 consecutive acute stroke patients with no coma or respiratory insufficiency: topography of the lesion

	Hypersomnia (N = 22)	No hypersomnia (N = 78)
Supratentorial strokes (N = 70)		
Superficial	2 (20%)	10
Superficial and deep	12 (43%)	16
Deep	6 (35%)	17
Thalamic (isolated)	1 (17%)	6
Infratentorial strokes (N = 19)	1 (6%)	18
Multiple strokes (N = 11)	0	11

Courtesy of Neurology Department, University of Berne, Berne, Switzerland.

Clinical features of poststroke hypersomnia

Clinical varieties of poststroke hypersomnia

The clinical features of poststroke hypersomnia vary according to stroke topography. In addition to an increased sleep propensity, these patients may present disturbances in circadian distribution of sleep and wakefulness; control of sleep-wake transition (eg, awakening); regulation of tonic and phasic attention; eating; sexual behavior; and mood.

Most patients with poststroke hypersomnia present a continuous hypersomnia with inattention, decreased motor activity, reduced speech production, and mood flattening. Hypersomnia can appear after an initial period of sopor or coma, less commonly of hyperalertness with insomnia. In some patients hypersomnia coexists or evolves to extreme apathy with lack of spontaneity and initiative, slowness and poverty of movement, and catalepsy, a condition for which the term "akinetic mutism" was coined [66,67]. Akinetic mutism, and its less severe form, usually referred to as "abulia" [68], may persist despite normalization of vigilance or even after appearance of insomnia.

Only exceptionally, patients after stroke develop an episodic or periodic hypersomnia. In a 51-year-old man, narcolepsy-like symptoms (excessive daytime sleepiness, hypnagogic hallucinations, sleep paralysis, and cataplexy) appeared following pontine stroke, despite the absence of the HLA-DR2 haplotype [69]. Another case with a narcolepsy-like syndrome developed after bilateral diencephalic stroke following surgical removal of a craniopharyngioma. In this patient, cerebrospinal fluid hypocretin-1 (orexin-A) levels were low, suggesting a link between poststroke hypersomnia and deficient neurotransmission. In two of the authors' patients with hypersomnia following thalamic and pontine stroke, however, cerebrospinal fluid hypocretin-1 levels were normal (unpublished observations). The exact role of the hypocretinergic system in poststroke hypersomnia still remains to be established. Hypersomnia with hyperphagia (incorrectly referred to as Kleine-Levin syndrome) was reported in one patient after multiple cerebral strokes [70].

In patients with thalamic or deep hemispheric strokes hypersomnolent behavior may mimic physiologic sleep with normal postures, regular quiet breathing, and rapid arousability. In patients with large hemispheric or brainstem lesions hypersomnia is usually accompanied by abnormal sleep with altered posturing and breathing. A few patients with deep hemispheric and thalamic stroke may exhibit a so-called "presleep behavior," during which they yawn, stretch, close their eyes, curl up, and assume a normal sleeping posture while complaining of a constant urge to sleep [71]. When stimulated or given explicit tasks to perform these patients are, however, able to control their behavior. For this peculiar dissociation between lack of (loss of) autoactivation in the presence of preserved heteroactivation (arousability from external stimuli) Laplane [72] suggested the term "athymormia" or "pure psychic akinesia" [73]. PET and single-photon emission CT studies in patients with athymormia and bipallidal, paramedian mesencephalodiencephalic, and bilateral genu capsula infarcts point to a frontal cortex deactivation [74]. These cases illustrate the existing overlap between disorders of motor and mental arousal.

In some patients, phases of hypersomnia, mutism, and akinesia alternate with phases of insomnia, psychomotor agitation, confusional state with logorrhea, and hallucinations [68,75–78]. These behavioral shifts can be rapid, similar to paradox kinesia in hypokinetic extrapyramidal syndromes, and associated with an inversion of sleep-wake cycle [75]. At times the transition from wakefulness to sleep and vice versa may be difficult; some patients can be aroused only by repeated, vigorous stimuli; others may present after awakening a dream-reality confusion (oneiric states).

Fatigue

A continuum exists between hypersomnia and fatigue, which is defined as a feeling of physical or mental tiredness and lack of energy which cannot be improved by sleep extension [79]. The patients complain to be rapidly exhausted and have a strong desire for sleep, despite an often normal or (paradoxically) decreased sleep propensity. The Epworth Sleepiness Scale is a useful tool to differentiate fatigue from excessive daytime sleepiness [80]. The high frequency of fatigue, which affects up to 68% of patients 3 to 13 months after stroke, has only recently been recognized [81]; fatigue was not related to time poststroke, stroke severity, or lesion location. Fatigue may develop following stroke in association with sleep-wake disturbances, mood and emotional changes, neurologic deficits, and neuropsychologic sequelae. A significant overlap exists particularly between poststroke fatigue and poststroke depression. Poststroke fatigue may occur in the absence of depression, however, and even persist after recovery from the neurologic deficits [82,83]. A dysfunction of arousal and attentional circuits, as suggested also for some forms of poststroke hypersomnia, has been postulated for poststroke fatigue [84].

Stroke topography and poststroke hypersomnia

Severe and persistent poststroke hypersomnia is suggestive of a bilateral thalamic or mesencephalic stroke. Less severe and only transient hypersomnia is seen with other stroke localizations and associated neurologic deficits often point to the topography of the underlying lesion.

In large hemispheric strokes with brain edema hypersomnia is typically associated with ipsilateral (to the lesion) gaze palsy or gaze preference and head deviation, severe contralateral sensorimotor hemisyndrome, visual field deficits, and variable neuropsychologic deficits. Hypersomnia typically develops between the second and fifth day together with slight pupillary asymmetry; paratonia with Babinski's sign contralateral to the hemiparesis; and periodic (Cheyne-Stokes) breathing secondary to the development of brain edema with mass effect [85]. A more or less severe hypersomnia, which is usually only transient, can be seen also in the absence of significant brain edema in anterior more than posterior strokes, and in left more than right hemispheric strokes [86]. Plum and Posner [87] also refer in their monograph to the existence of patients with unilateral hemispheric stroke and early drowsiness probably unrelated to cerebral swelling.

Case 1: Castaigne and Escourolle [46] reported a 66-year-old patient with bilateral anterior cerebral artery stroke and severe hypersomnia persisting over a few months.

Case 2: The authors observed a 40-year-old patient with left middle-cerebral artery stroke in whom profound hypersomnia was present for the first 4 to 5 days after stroke despite the absence of both mass effect on brain MRI and medical complications.

In patients with frontal (particularly cingulate) stroke akinetic mutism, usually with normal wakefulness (anterior or vigilant variant of akinetic mutism [67]), may be misinterpreted as hypersomnia [88,89]. In a literature review of patients with bilateral infarctions in the territory of the anterior cerebral artery akinetic mutism was found in seven of eight cases [90].

In reports of deep (subcortical) hemispheric strokes involving unilaterally or bilaterally caudate nucleus, putamen, globus pallidus, or capsula interna the presence of apathy, fatigue, athymormia, and akinetic mutism but not hypersomnia is frequently mentioned. These deficits are usually explained by the disruption of basal ganglia-thalamo-frontal circuits modulating motor and behavioral control [77,91–94]. Caplan and coworkers [77] reported abulia in 10 of 18 patients with acute caudate stroke, occasionally alternating with periods of confused hyperactivity with restlessness, insomnia, and hallucinations. Mendez and coworkers [95] reported 12 patients with caudate infarcts, 6 of them being confined to the caudate nucleus and the remainder extending additionally into the adjacent anterior limb of the internal capsule. According to the clinical and neuropsychologic findings the patient were divided into three groups. Group I patients showed apathy and diminished verbal and motor activity, group II patients were disinhibited and impulsive, and group III patients had prominent anxiety or depression. No correlation was found between clinical findings and the side of the lesion, but the presence of depression or anxiety was associated with larger lesions. A few contributions reported on bilateral caudate infarcts, which mostly lead to severe abulia, flattened affect, and inattention [96,97]. In

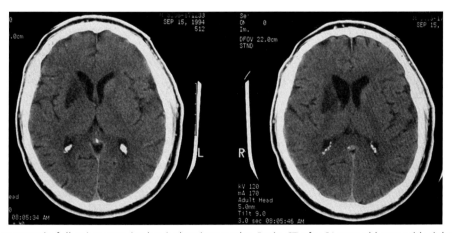

Fig. 2. Hypersomnia following anterior lenticulostriate stroke. Brain CT of a 61-year-old man with right anterior lenticulostriate stroke involving the head of the caudate nucleus and persisting hypersomnia. The patient initially presents with insomnia, agitated confusional state, visual hallucinations, and involuntary crying. During the following days he develops a severe hypersomnia with sleep-like behavior up to 16 hours per day, which is documented by actigraphy. Three months later the patient sleeps 10 to 11 hours per day. At 1 year sleep needs have normalized. The patient has to retire from work, however, because of persisting attentional deficits and affective lability. (Courtesy of G. Schroth, Division of Neuroradiology, University Hospital, Bern, Switzerland.)

the authors' experience, however, hypersomnia, and not only decreased motor arousal (akinesia), is not uncommon in patients with nonlacunar deep (subcortical) hemispheric strokes.

Case 3: A 61-year-old man presents with right anterior caudate stroke with initial insomnia, hallucinations, and agitation, followed after a few hours by hypersomnia with a sleep-like behavior over 13 to 16 hours per day [Fig. 2]. Three months later the patient sleeps only 10 to 11 hours per day and at 1 year his sleep needs have normalized.

Case 4: In a 68-year-old woman with left paraventricular striatocapsular stroke and mild neurologic deficits a profound inversion of sleep-wake cycle is first noted. Two weeks later daytime hypersomnia has almost recovered, whereas nighttime insomnia with estimated 2 to 3 hours of sleep per night is still present. Sleep-wake functions finally normalize 4 weeks after stroke onset. The authors made similar observations in patients with posterior lenticulostrate and capsular infarcts.

In thalamic strokes hypersomnia is seen in paramedian lesions because of occlusion of the thalamoperforating (thalamic-subthalamic) arteries. Severe and persistent hypersomnia is usually seen with bi-

lateral lesions [Fig. 3] but occasionally also after unilateral stroke [5,48,98,99]. Less commonly, the authors observed hypersomnia also in patients with unilateral anterior or ventroposterolateral thalamic stroke. Patients with bilateral paramedian thalamic stroke typically present with the triad hypersomnia; confabulatory (Korsakow-like) amnesia; and vertical gaze palsy [46,47,100]. Additional somatic symptoms include dysarthria, gait instability, skew deviation, Horner's syndrome, hypogeusia, hyposmia, and incontinence. Breathing is usually unaffected. Some patients also present a "frontal lobe syndrome" with anosognosia; hyperphagia (and weight gain); hypersexuality; and altered mood [48,100,101]. Flat or depressed mood is frequently observed and parallel hypersomnia with decreased speech and motor activity. Less commonly patients present with insomnia, hallucinatory confusional state, logorrhea, euphoria with childish behavior [102], and motor restlessness with compulsive-like activity [78]. Hypersomnia usually appears after an initial coma, less commonly with an agitated delirium, which can last for hours to a few days [43]. Sleep-like behavior can be present initially for >20 hours per day and may correspond in some patients to a preparatory

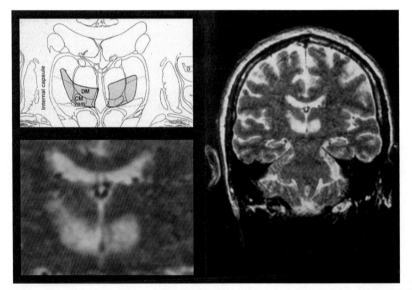

Fig. 3. Hypersomnia following bilateral paramedian thalamic stroke. Coronal T2-weighted brain MRI of a 51-year-old man with bilateral, butterfly-like paramedian thalamic stroke and persisting hypersomnia. The patient initially presents with a short phase of agitation followed by coma. One hour later the patient can be aroused and severe hypersomnia with sleep-like behavior over 15 to 18 hours per day, vertical gaze palsy, dysarthria, and mild memory deficits are noted. A polysomnography at 1 month documents a reduction of sleep spindles, NREM sleep stage 2, and REM sleep and the absence of stage 3 to 4 NREM sleep [see **Fig. 5**]. In the following weeks the patient is asleep, based on actigraphic recordings, over 70% of the time. Four months later sleep needs are still about 12 to 13 hours per day. Multiple Sleep Latency Test documents a moderate sleepiness with a mean sleep latency of 5 minutes. Levodopa brings no improvement. Three years later the patient sleeps 9 to 10 hours per day (compared with 7–8 hours before stroke) and has a decreased attentional span but no other neuropsychologic deficits. He has returned to his old job and works 50% of the time. (Courtesy of G. Schroth, Division of Neuroradiology, University Hospital, Bern, Switzerland.)

behavior for sleep or akinetic mutism rather than true sleep. Twelve patients with combined polar paramedian thalamic infarction have been recently described [103]. With one exception, all patients showed acute impairment of consciousness. Three patients with bilateral lesions had acute coma, eye movement disturbances, and neurobehavioral symptoms; the main findings consisted of severe anterograde amnesia and incomplete recovery requiring institutional or private care. Right-sided infarcts showed a less favorable outcome with respect to recovery from anterograde amnesia.

In mesencephalic strokes hypersomnia is usually seen with tegmental lesions. The presence of a bilateral lesion is usually required but mild and transient hypersomnia is occasionally observed also in unilateral lesions [4]. Isolated infarcts of the midbrain are less common than thalamomesencephalic strokes (see previously) and strokes involving simultaneously midbrain, superior cerebellum, and occipital cortex (so-called "top of the basilar" syndrome [104]). In addition to hypersomnia, the clinical syndrome usually includes a III nerve palsy; a vertical gaze palsy; and contralateral sensory and, occasionally, motor deficits (tremor, hemiparesis, or ataxia). The severity of hypersomnia is variable and even in a single patient fluctuations between coma, hypersomnia, and akinetic mutism are observed [105].

Case 5: Façon and coworkers [75] reported a 78-year-old patient with bilateral tegmental thalamomesencephalic stroke presenting with bilateral III nerve palsy, hallucinations, inversion of sleep-wake cycle, and severe hypersomnia persisting until death 3 years later.

Case 6: Castaigne and coworkers [106] described a 66-year-old patient with similar lesion and initial clinical presentation in whom severe hypersomnia (20 hours sleep per day) persisted for 8 months until death.

Patients with tegmental mesencephalic strokes and, less commonly, with paramedian thalamic strokes, may experience vivid dream-like hallucinations that are complex, colorful, full of motion, and typically occur in the evening and at sleep onset (Lhermitte's peduncular hallucinosis [107–110]). The original patient described by Lhermitte [107] had, in addition to the complex visual hallucinations, an inversion of the sleep-wake cycle with nocturnal insomnia and daytime hypersomnia. Severe and persisting insomnia following a presumed thalamomesencephalic stroke was reported also by Van Bogaert [111].

In pontine strokes hypersomnia is seen in unilateral and particularly bilateral supratrigeminal tegmental lesions, which are suggested by the presence of a IV nerve palsy; internuclear ophthalmoplegia; nystagmus; contralateral (or bilateral) sensorimotor deficits; and irregular breathing [112]. Bilateral upper pontine tegmental lesions are invariably associated with disturbed level of consciousness [87,112]. Not infrequently, these lesions extend to the midbrain and even thalamus [46]. Compared with thalamic and midbrain lesions, pontine strokes lead more commonly to coma than to hypersomnia or akinetic mutism [27,46,112]. In ventromedial pontine infarcts hypersomnia can be observed, but is typically short-lived.

Case 7: Van Bogaert [111] reported a 47-year-old patient with right tegmental pontomesencephalic stroke presenting with right IV and VII nerve palsy; facial myoclonus; right hemiparesis; severe, imperative (narcolepsy-like) hypersomnia; and increased dreaming persisting until death 5 months later.

In medullary strokes a mild hypersomnia is occasionally seen with bilateral but also unilateral medial lesions, which usually present clinically with a motor hemisyndrome and contralateral XII nerve palsy [113]. Less commonly hypersomnia is mentioned also in reports of more lateral, usually hemorrhagic, medullary strokes [114,115].

Sleep-wake studies in poststroke hypersomnia

The diagnosis of poststroke hypersomnia relies primarily on clinical observation and direct questioning of the patient and their relatives. Actigraphy can document the presence of altered sleep-wake cycle with excessive amounts of sleep over several days to weeks. In the authors' experience actigraphic findings correlate quite well with the clinical diagnosis of poststroke hypersomnia [see Table 1].

Case 8: A 60-year-old patient with bilateral paramedian thalamic stroke previously reported presents with abrupt coma followed by sleep behavior over 19 hours per day, complete vertical gaze palsy, frontal behavior, and moderate amnesia [48]. Actigraphy during the first week after stroke onset shows periods of motor inactivity compatible with sleep during 80% of recording time [Fig. 4A]. Two years later hypersomnia has improved and the patient reports sleep over 10 to 12 hours per day. A second actigraphy documents this improvement with "sleep," as assessed by actigraphy, present now only over 45% of the time [Fig. 4B].

On should be aware that in patients with disorder of motor arousal (eg, with akinetic mutism) or depression (with clinophilia) actigraphy may overestimate the severity of hypersomnia.

The wake-EEG of patients with poststroke hypersomnia typically shows focal or lateralized EEG slowing (polymorphic delta activity) in hemispheric and thalamic lesions. In subthalamic, midbrain, and upper pontine lesions a more or less

A

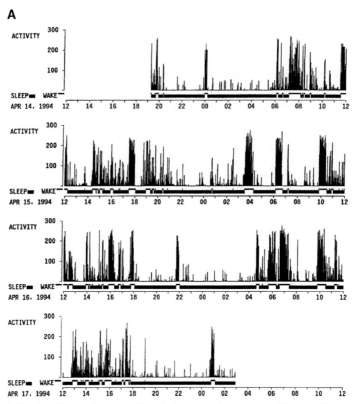

Fig. 4. Hypersomnia following bilateral paramedian thalamic stroke. Actigraphic recordings of a 60-year-old man with bilateral paramedian thalamic stroke and severe hypersomnia. In the acute stage the patient presents with sudden coma, followed by sleep behavior over 19 hours per day, moderate amnesia, complete vertical gaze palsy, hyperphagia, and hypersexuality. (*A*) One week after stroke onset the patient is asleep, by actigraphic criteria, over 80% of the time. Sleep-wake patterns seem greatly disorganized. At 8 months the patient still sleeps 12 hours per day. Methylphenidate (20 mg per day) and mazindol (4 mg per day) do not improve hypersomnia. Because of attentional and amnestic deficits the patient has to retire from work. Two years after stroke onset hypersomnia has clinically improved to 9 to 11 hours sleep per day. (*B*) Actigraphy now shows that the patient is asleep over 45% of the time and that sleep-wake pattern has greatly improved. Four years after stroke the patient's sleep behavior has almost normalized.

symmetric, diffuse EEG slowing in the theta or delta range with paradoxical or absent reactivity to external stimuli is most commonly found [106,112, 116–121]. Patients with disturbed levels of consciousness caused by bilateral thalamic strokes or infratrigeminal pontine lesions often present a low-voltage, fast EEG activity in the alpha-beta range. The correlation between EEG and clinical findings, including lesion topography, is generally poor, particularly with infratentorial strokes [120]. In brainstem lesions the relationship between the EEG (and its reactivity to stimuli) and the level of consciousness becomes worse the lower and the more lateral (in the tegmentum) the localization of stroke [117]. Coma caused by pontine stroke may be associated with fast (alpha) EEG activity [26], whereas diffuse, high-voltage EEG slowing was reported, for example, in an alert patient with unilateral tegmental stroke [112]. Paradoxical improvement of EEG paralleling

clinical worsening has also been reported (case 13 in [46]).

Because of the possible dissociation in focal brain lesions between EEG activity and behavioral arousal [122], the correlation of poststroke hypersomnia with production of sleep by EEG criteria is, as for wake-EEG, relatively poor. Prolonged EEG monitoring and Multiple Sleep Latency Test may fail to demonstrate an increased production of sleep despite the presence of clinically and actigraphically obvious excessive sleep behavior [Fig. 5] [48,123]. Daytime sleep may be associated, particularly in patients with thalamic and thalamomesencephalic stroke, with a variety of EEG patterns including diffuse low-voltage alpha-beta activity, NREM stage 1 sleep, NREM stage 2 to 4 sleep, diffuse slow wave activity, and REM sleep [see Fig. 5] [48,124–126]. In a few patients with paramedian thalamic stroke the authors observed a paradoxical decrease of

B

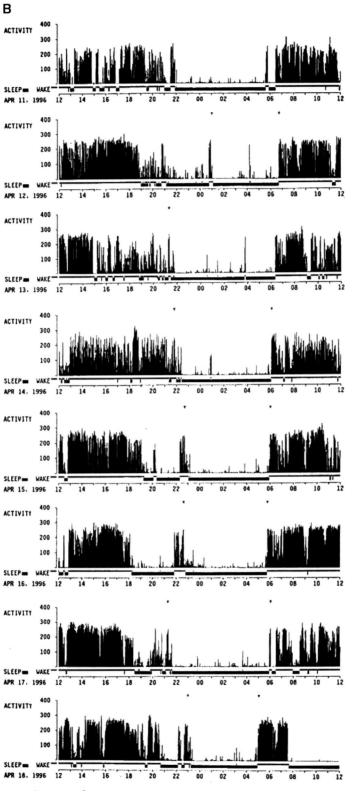

Fig. 4 (continued).

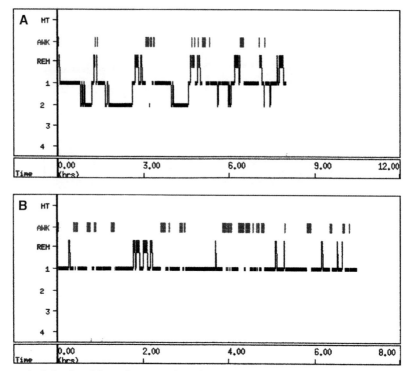

Fig. 5. Hypersomnia following bilateral paramedian thalamic stroke. Hypnogram of a prolonged polysomnographic recording (from 10:30 PM–2:00 PM) of a 51-year-old man with bilateral paramedian thalamic stroke [see Fig. 3] and severe hypersomnia performed 3 weeks after stroke onset. The recording time is of 481 minutes at night and 419 minutes during the day. (*A*) At night there is a good sleep efficiency (91%); an increase in stage 1 sleep (59% of total sleep time [TST]), a decrease in stage 2 sleep (28% TST), spindling (<100 per hour sleep) and REM sleep (13% TST), and the absence of stage 3 to 4 sleep. (*B*) During the day the patient has a good sleep efficiency (80%) related to the presence of stage 1 sleep (92% of time) and REM sleep (8%).

sleep latency in the Multiple Sleep Latency Test paralleling the recovery of hypersomnia, which the authors attributed to an improved electrogenesis [48]. Nighttime sleep is characterized in hemispheric and thalamic stroke by an ipsilateral reduction (or abolition) of sleep spindles, K-complexes, and slow wave sleep [48,125,127–129]. In patients with bilateral paramedian thalamic stroke, Bassetti and coworkers [48] found a correlation between severity of hypersomnia and reductions of sleep spindles. Reduction of sleep spindle was usually, but not invariably, associated with a reduction of slow wave sleep. Bilateral effects on sleep EEG with unilateral supratentorial lesions have also been reported. In a patient with large hemispheric stroke Hachinski and coworkers [128] observed the disappearance of sleep spindles over the infarcted side in the first days following stroke onset. After 9 days sleep spindles began, however, to decrease also over the healthy hemisphere reaching by the fiftieth night 10% to 20% of the baseline values. Similarly, Santamaria and coworkers [130] found a bilateral (but no ipsilateral) reduction of sleep spindles in patients with unilateral, isolated thalamic

stroke. Occasionally, a reduction of REM sleep and sawtooth waves has also been noted with supratentorial strokes [48,128,131]. In subthalamic and midbrain lesions sleep spindles may also be decreased, and upper pontine tegmental strokes are typically associated with a reduction of both NREM and REM sleep [132–134]. On rare occasions, an increased production of sleep by EEG criteria is found in patients with poststroke hypersomnia. Increased slow wave sleep was reported with subthalamic and midbrain lesions, and enhanced REM sleep in bithalamic, mesencephalic, lower pontine, and medullary lesions [132,135,136].

Case 9: Arpa recently reported a 44-year-old man with a right lateral-tegmental pontine hematoma and severe hypersomnia, in whom long-term EEG monitoring showed during the first 3 months after stroke increased amounts of sleep ranging from 10.8 to 14.6 hours per day [137,138]. The relative amounts of slow wave sleep (4%–11% of total sleep time) and REM sleep (8%–10%) were slightly above normal values.

Case 10: Bastuji and coworkers [124] described a patient with severe hypersomnia caused by bilateral thalamomesencephalic stroke with an initial sleep behavior over 18 hours per day. Eight months after stroke hypersomnia had regressed clinically to 12 hours per day. By EEG criteria sleep was similarly present over about 12 hours per day, with an increase in both slow wave sleep (30% of total sleep time) and REM sleep (22%).

Case 11: Popoviciu and coworkers [133] described a patient with akinetic mutism caused by bilateral, ventrotegmental pontine stroke in whom a polygraphic recording demonstrated an increase of REM sleep (317 minutes per 24 hours) and wakefulness (541 minutes per 24 hours).

When considering abnormalities in sleep architecture of acute stroke patients one should always be aware that such changes may only in part be related to acute brain damage. Similar sleep changes also were reported in patients admitted to an intensive care unit after acute myocardial infarction [41].

Treatment and prognosis of poststroke hypersomnia

Treatment of poststroke hypersomnia with stimulants is usually difficult and often ineffective [48,125]. In single patients some improvement was seen in thalamic and mesencephalic stroke with amphetamines (case 14 in [46], modafinil [124]) or methylphenidate [48].

Case 12: Catsman-Berrevoets and Harskamp [71] reported improvement of apathy and presleep behavior with 20 to 40 mg bromocriptine, supporting the hypothesis that dopaminergic neurons may be implicated not only in motor but also mental arousal (and attention) [15,17,137].

Case 13: The authors observed a 57-year-old patient with hypersomnia (12 hours per day compared with 7 before stroke), excessive daytime sleepiness, and loss of dream recall following bilateral paramedian thalamomesencephalic stroke. Moderate improvement of hypersomnia and marked reduction of daytime sleepiness was achieved with levodopa, 250 mg daily (modafinil was also effective, but had to be stopped because of headache); at 14 months after stroke, the patient reported a decrease in sleep needs (10 hours per day) and the return of dreaming experiences.

More generally, treatment of sleep-wake disturbances in acute stroke should include placement of patients in private rooms at night; protection from nocturnal light, noise, and unnecessary arousals; increased mobilization with exposure to light during the day; and, when unavoidable, temporary use of hypnotics that are relatively free of cognitive side effects, such as zolpidem. Some hypersomnolent patients with apathy and depression may also profit from the prescription of stimulant antidepressants and light therapy.

The pattern of recovery of poststroke hypersomnia is highly variable. In most cases hypersomnia improves within a few days to weeks. Hypersomnia within the first week after stroke does not seem to preclude a good long-term outcome [see Table 1]. Conversely, persistent hypersomnia over weeks or months, which is usually expression of a thalamic or thalamomesencephalic strokes, often heralds long-term disability. In the most severely affected patients significant hypersomnia can persists over years. In other patients hypersomnia evolves to akinetic mutism with normal wakefulness but apathy; amnesia; attentional deficits; diminished psychomotor drive; and depressed mood (thalamic dementia) [46,139]. Finally, in less severe cases patients may report at follow-up only a mildly prolonged nighttime sleep and daytime napping. Associated disturbances of attention and short-term memory, indifference, lack of initiative, and mood flattening may dominate the clinical picture.

References

[1] Passouant P, Cadilhac J, Baldy-Moulinier M. Physio-pathologie des hypersomnies. Rev Neurol 1967;116:585–629.

[2] Bassetti C. Disturbances of consciousness and sleep-wake functions. In: Caplan L, Bogousslavsky J, editors. Stroke syndromes. Cambridge: Cambridge University Press; 2001. p. 108–17.

[3] MacNish R. The philosophy of sleep. New York: D Appleton; 1834.

[4] Claude H, Loyez M. Ramollissement du noyau rouge. Rey Neurologique 1912;23:40–51.

[5] Freund SC. Zur klinik und anatomie der vertikalen blicklähmung. Neurol Zentralbl 1913; 32:1215–29.

[6] Manasseina M. (de Manacéïne M). Sleep: its physiology, pathology, hygiene and psychology. St. Petersburg (Russia): Walter Scott, Ltd, Paternoster Square; 1892.

[7] Kleitman N. Sleep and wakefulness. Chicago: Midway Reprint edition, The University of Chicago Press; 1963.

[8] Wernicke C. Lehrbuch der gehirnkrankheiten. Kassel und Berlin: Theodor Fischer; 1881.

[9] Mauthner L. Zur pathologie und physiologie des schlafes nebst bemerkungen über die Nona. Wien Med Wochenschr 1890;23:961.

[10] Von Economo C. Encephalitis lethargica. Wien Med Wochenschr 1923;73:777–82.

[11] Moruzzi G, Magoun HW. Brainstem reticular formation and activation of the EEG. Electroencephal Clin Neurophysiol 1949;1:455–73.

[12] Hess WR. Hirnreizversuche über den mechanismus des schlafes. Arch Psychiatrie 1929;86: 287–92.

[13] Lugaresi E, Medori R, Montagna P, et al. Fatal familial insomnia and dysautonomia with selective degeneration of thalamic nuclei. N Engl J Med 1986;315:997–1003.

[14] Baumann CR, Bassetti CL. Hypocretins (orexin) and sleep-wake disorders. Lancet Neurol 2005; 4:673–82.

[15] Jouvet M. Les mécanismes de l'éveil: du système réticulée mésencéphalique aux réseaux multiples. Arch Physiol Biochem 1996;104: 762–9.

[16] Groenewegen HJ, Berendse HW. The specificity of the nonspecific midline and intralaminar thalamic nuclei. Trends Neurosci 1994;17:52–7.

[17] Berlucchi G. One or many arousal systems? Reflections on some of Giuesppe Moruzzi's foresights and insights about the intrinsic regulation of brain activity. Arch Ital Biol 1997;135: 5–14.

[18] Jones BE. Basic mechanisms of sleep-wake states. In: Kryger MH, Roth T, Dement WC, editors. Principles and practice of sleep medicine. 3rd edition. Philadelphia: WB Saunders; 2000. p. 134–54.

[19] Siegel JM. Brainstem mechanisms generating REM sleep. In: Kryger MH, Roth T, Dement WC, editors. Principles and practice of sleep medicine. 3rd edition. Philadelphia: WB Saunders; 2000. p. 112–33.

[20] Rye DB. Contributions of the pedunculopontine region to normal and altered REM sleep. Sleep 1997;20:757–88.

[21] Munk MHJ, Roelfema PR, König P, et al. Role of reticular activation in the modulation of intracortical synchronization. Science 1996; 272:271–4.

[22] Sillito AM, Jones HE, Gerstein GL, et al. Feature-linked synchronization of thalamic relay cell firing induced by feedback from the visual cortex. Nature 1994;369:479–82.

[23] Koella WP. Die physiologie des schlafes. Stuttgart: Gustav Fischer Verlag; 1988.

[24] Chammas DZ, Magana O, Krilowicz BL. The posterior basal diencephalon of rats enhances expression of an activated state. Sleep 1999; 22:284–92.

[25] Inbody S, Jankovic J. Hyperkinetic mutism: bilateral ballism and basal ganglia calcification. Neurology 1986;36:825–7.

[26] Loeb C, Poggio G. Electroencephalogram in a case with ponto-mesencephalic haemorrhage. Electroencephal Clin Neurophysiol 1953;5: 295–6.

[27] Cravioto H, Silberman J, Feigin I. A clinical and pathologic study of akinetic mutism. Neurology 1960;10:10–21.

[28] Contreras D, Destexhe A, Sejnowski TJ, et al. Control of spatiotemporal coherence of a thalamic oscillation by corticothalamic feedback. Science 1996;274:771–4.

[29] Villablanca J, Salinas-Zeballos ME. Sleep-wakefulness, EEG, and behavioural studies of chronic cats without the thalamus: the athalamic cat. Arch Ital Biol 1972;110:348–82.

[30] Villablanca JR, Marcus RJ, Olmstead CE. Effect of caudate nuclei or frontal cortex ablations in cats. II. Sleep-wakefulness, EEG, and motor activity. Exp Neurol 1976;53:31–50.

[31] Villablanca J, Marcus R. Sleep-wakefulness, EEG and behavioural studies of chronic cats without neocortex and striatum: the diencephalic cat. Arch Ital Biol 1972;110:383.

[32] Penaloza-Rojas JH, Elterman M, Olmos N. Sleep induced by cortical stimulation. Exp Neurol 1964;10:140–7.

[33] Gallopin T, Fort P, Eggermann E, et al. Identification of sleep-promoting neurons in vitro. Nature 2000;404:992–5.

[34] Eggermann E, Bayer L, Serafin M, et al. The wake-promoting hypocretin-orexin neurons are in an intrinsic state of membrane depolarization. J Neurosci 2003;23:1557–62.

[35] Estabrooke IV, McCarthy MT, Ko E, et al. Fos expression in orexin neurons varies with behavioral state. J Neurosci 2001;21:1656–62.

[36] Szymusiak R. Magnocellular nuclei of the basal forebrain: substrates of sleep and arousal regulation. Sleep 1995;18:478–500.

[37] Sherin JE, Shiromani PJ, McCarley RW, et al. Activation of ventrolateral preoptic neurons during sleep. Science 1996;271:216–9.

[38] Amzica F, Steriade M. Electrophysiological correlates of sleep delta waves. Electroencephal Clin Neurophysiol 1998;107:69–83.

[39] Shouse MN, Siegel JM. Pontine regulation of REM sleep components in cats: integrity of the pedunculopontine tegmentum (PPT) is important for phasic events but unnecessary for atonia during REM sleep. Brain Res 1992;571:50–63.

[40] Kahn D, Pace-Schott EF, Hobson JA. Consciousness in waking and dreaming: the roles of neuronal oscillation and neuromodulation in determining similarities and differences. Neuroscience 1997;78:13–38.

[41] Broughton R, Baron R. Sleep patterns in the intensive care unit and on the ward after acute myocardial infarction. Electroencephal Clin Neurophysiol 1978;45:348–60.

[42] Krachmann SL, D'Alonzo GE, Criner GJ. Sleep in the intensive care unit. Chest 1995;107: 1713–20.

[43] Walther H. Ueber einen dämmerzustand mit triebhafter erregung nach thalamusschädigung. Bern (Switzerland): Universität Bern; 1945.

[44] Hösli L. Dämpfende und fördernde systeme im medialen thalamus und im retikularapparat (nachweis der funktionellen dualität durch selektive reizungen und ausschaltungen). Inauguraldissertation. Basel: Buchdruckerei Birkhäuser; 1962.

[45] Levasseur M, Baron JC, Sette G, et al. Brain energy metabolism in bilateral paramedian thalamic infarcts: a PET study. Brain 1992;115: 795–807.

[46] Castaigne P, Escourolle R. Etude topographique des lésions anatomiques dans les hypersomnies. Rev Neurol 1967;116:547–84.

[47] Castaigne P, Lhermitte F, Buge A, et al. Paramedian thalamic and midbrain infarcts: clinical and neuropathological study. Ann Neurol 1981;10:127–48.

[48] Bassetti C, Mathis J, Gugger M, et al. Hypersomnia following thalamic stroke. Ann Neurol 1996;39:471–80.

[49] Braun AR, Balkin TJ, Wesensten NJ, et al. Regional cerebral blood flow throughout the sleep-wake cycle: an H215O study. Brain 1997; 120:1173–97.

[50] Heuaser G, Buchwald NA, Wyers EJ. The caudate spindle. II. Facilitatory and inhibitory caudate cortical pathways. Electroencephal Clin Neurophysiol 1961;13:519–24.

[51] Vallar G, Perani D, Capra SF, et al. Recovery from aphasia and neglect after subcortical stroke: neuropsychological and cerebral perfusion study. J Neurol Neurosurg Psychiatry 1988; 51:1269–76.

[52] Bogousslavsky J, Miklossy J, Regli F, et al. Subcortical neglect: neuropsychological, SPECT, and neuropathological correlations with anterior choroidal artery territory infarction. Ann Neurol 1988;23:448–52.

[53] Ropper AH. A preliminary MRI study of the geometry of brain displacement and level of consciousness with acute intracranial masses. Neurology 1989;39:622–7.

[54] Amarenco P, Hauw JJ, Caplan LR. Cerebellar infarctions. In: Lechtenberg R, editor. Handbook of cerebellar diseases. New York: Marcel Dekker; 1993. p. 251–90.

[55] Davison C, Demuth EL. Disturbances in sleep mechanism: a clinicopathologic study. V. Anatomic and neurophysiologic considerations. Arch Neurol Psychiatr 1946;55:364–81.

[56] Lenzi GL, Frackowiack RSJ, Jones T. Cerebral oxygen metabolism and blood flow in human cerebral ischemic infarction. J Cereb Blood Flow Metab 1982;2:321–35.

[57] Müller C, Achermann P, Bischof M, et al. Visual and spectral analysis of sleep EEG in acute hemispheric stroke. Eur Neurol 2002;48:164–71.

[58] Turkington PM, Bamford J, Wanklyn P, et al. Prevalence and predictors of upper airway obstruction in the first 24 hours after acute stroke. Stroke 2002;33:2037–42.

[59] Bassetti C, Aldrich M, Chervin R, et al. Sleep apnea in the acute phase of TIA and stroke. Neurology 1996;47:1167–73.

[60] Wessendorf TE, Teschler H, Wang YM, et al. Sleep-disordered breathing among patients with first-ever stroke. J Neurol 2000;247:41–7.

[61] Parra O, Arboix A, Bechich S, et al. Time course of sleep-related breathing disorders in first-ever stroke or transient ischemic attack. Am J Respir Crit Care Med 2000;161:375–80.

[62] Bassetti C, Aldrich M. Sleep apnea in acute cerebrovascular diseases: final report on 128 patients. Sleep 1999;22:217–23.

[63] Hermann D, Bassetti CL. Sleep apnea and other sleep-wake disorders in stroke. Curr Treat Options Neurol 2003;5:241–9.

[64] Bogousslavsky J, Van Melle G, Regli F. The Lausanne stroke registry: analysis of 1000 consecutive patients with first stroke. Stroke 1988; 19:1083–92.

[65] Asplund K, Britton M. Ethics of life support in patients with severe stroke. Stroke 1989;20: 1107–12.

[66] Cairns H, Oldfield RC, Pennybacker JB, et al. Akinetic mutism with an epidermoid cyst of the 3rd. Brain 1941;64:273–90.

[67] Segarra J. Cerebral vascular disease and behaviour. I. The syndrome of the mesencephalic artery. Arch Neurol 1970;22:408–18.

[68] Fisher CM. Abulia minor versus agitated behaviour. Clin Neurosurg 1983;31:9–31.

[69] Rivera VM, Meyer JS, Hata T, et al. Narcolepsy following cerebral hypoxic ischemia. Ann Neurol 1986;19:505–8.

[70] Drake ME. Kleine-Levine syndrome after multiple cerebral infarctions. Psychosomatics 1987; 28:329–30.

[71] Catsman-Berrevoets CE, Harskamp F. Compulsive pre-sleep behaviour and apathy due to bilateral thalamic stroke. Neurology 1988;38: 647–9.

[72] Laplane D, Baulac M, Widlöcher D, et al. Pure psychic akinesia with bilateral lesions of basal ganglia. J Neurol Neurosurg Psychiatry 1984;47: 377–85.

[73] Engelborghs S, Marien P, Pickut BA, et al. Loss of psychic self-activation after paramedian bithalamic infarction. Stroke 2000;31:1762–5.

[74] Carota A, Staub F, Bogousslavsky J. Emotions, behaviours and mood changes in stroke. Curr Opin Neurol 2002;15:57–69.

[75] Façon E, Steriade M, Wertheim N. Hypersomnie prolongée engendrée par des lésions bilatérale du système activateur medial: le syndrome thrombotique de la bifurcation du tronc basilaire. Rev Neurol 1958;98:117–33.

[76] Rondot P, Recondo J, Dvous P, et al. Infarctus thalamique bilatéral avec mouvements abnormaux et amnésie durable. Rev Neurol 1986; 142:389–405.

[77] Caplan LR, Schmahmann JD, Kase CS, et al. Caudate infarcts. Arch Neurol 1990;47:133–43.

[78] Bogousslavsky J, Ferrazzini M, Regli F, et al. Manic delirium and frontal-lobe syndrome with paramedian infarction of the right thalamus. J Neurol Neurosurg Psychiatry 1988;51:116–7.

[79] Hossain JL, Ahmad P, Reinish LW, et al. Subjective fatigue and subjective sleepiness: two independent consequences of sleep disorders? J Sleep Res 2005;14:245–53.

[80] Johns MW. Sleepiness in different situations measured by the Epworth Sleepiness Scale. Sleep 1994;17:703–10.

[81] Ingles JL, Eskes GA, Phillips SJ. Fatigue after stroke. Arch Phys Med Rehabil 1999;80:173–8.

[82] Choi-Kwon S, Han SW, Kwon SU, et al. Poststroke fatigue: characteristics and related factors. Cerebrovasc Dis 2005;19:84–90.

[83] Staub F, Bogousslavsky J. Fatigue after stroke: a major but neglected issue. Cerebrovasc Dis 2001;12:75–81.

[84] Bogousslavsky J. William Feinberg lecture 2002: emotions, mood, and behavior after stroke. Stroke 2003;34:1046–50.

[85] Ropper AH, Shafran B. Brain edema after stroke: clinical syndrome and intracranial pressure. Arch Neurol 1984;41:26–9.

[86] Albert ML, Silverberg R, Reches A, et al. Cerebral dominance for consciousness. Arch Neurol 1976;33:453–4.

[87] Plum F, Posner JB. The diagnosis of stupor and coma. 3rd edition. Philadelphia: FA Davis; 1980.

[88] Barris RW, Schuman HR. Bilateral anterior cingulate gyrus lesions: syndrome of the anterior cingulate gyri. Neurology 1953;3:44–52.

[89] Buge A, Escourolle R, Rancurel R, et al. Mutisme akinétique et ramollissement bicingulaire. Rev Neurol 1975;131:121–37.

[90] Minagar A, David NJ. Bilateral infarction in the territory of the anterior cerebral arteries. Neurology 1999;52:886–8.

[91] Kumral E, Evyapan D, Balkir K. Acute caudate lesions. Stroke 1999;30:100–8.

[92] Helgason C, Wilbur A, Weiss A, et al. Acute pseudobulbar mutism due to discrete bilateral capsular infarction in the territory of the anterior choroidal artery. Brain 1988;111:507–24.

[93] Helgason C, Caplan L. Anterior choroidal artery-territory infarction. Arch Neurol 1986;43: 681–6.

[94] Alexander G. Parallel organization of functionally segregated circuits linking basal ganglia and cortex. Annu Rev Neurosci 1986;9:357–81.

[95] Mendez MF, Adams NL, Lewandowski KS. Neurobehavioral changes associated with caudate lesions. Neurology 1989;39:349–54.

[96] Trillet M, Croisile B, Tourniaire D, et al. Disorders of voluntary motor activity and lesions of caudate nuclei. Rev Neurol (Paris) 1990;146: 338–44.

[97] Richfield EK, Twyman R, Berent S. Neurological syndrome following bilateral damage to the head of the caudate nuclei. Ann Neurol 1987; 22:768–71.

[98] Schuster B. Beiträge zur pathologie des thalamus opticus. Arch Psychiatr Nervenkr 1937; 107:201–33.

[99] Schaltenbrand G. Thalamus und schlaf. Allg Zeitschr Psychiatr Grenzgeb 1949;125:48–62.

[100] Gentilini M, De Renzi E, Crisi G. Bilateral paramedian thalamic artery infarcts. J Neurol Neurosurg Psychiatry 1987;50:900–9.

[101] Guberman A, Stuss D. The syndrome of bilateral paramedian thalamic infarction. Neurology 1983;33:540–6.

[102] Fukatsu R, Fujii T, Yamadori A, et al. Persisting childish behavior after bilateral thalamic infarcts. Eur Neurol 1997;37:230–5.

[103] Perren F, Clarke S, Bogousslavsky J. The syndrome of combined polar and paramedian thalamic infarction. Arch Neurol 2005;62: 1212–6.

[104] Caplan LR. Top of the basilar syndrome. Neurology 1980;30:72–9.

[105] Brage D, Morea R, Copello AR. Syndrome nécrotique tegmento-thalamique avec mutisme akinétique. Rev Neurol 1961;104:126–37.

[106] Castaigne P, Buge A, Escourolle R, et al. Ramollissement pédonculaire médian tegmento-thalamique avec ophtalmoplégie et hypersomnia: etude anatomo-clinique. Rev Neurol 1962;106: 357–61.

[107] Lhermitte MJ. Syndrome de la calotte du pédoncule cerebral: les troubles psycho-sensoriels dans les lésions mésocéphaliques. Rev Neurol 1922;29:1359–65.

[108] Van Bogaert L. Syndrome inférieur du noyau rouge, troubles psycho-sensoriels d'origine mésocéphalique. Rev Neurol 1924;31:417–23.

[109] Feinberg WM, Rapcsack SZ. Peduncular hallucinosis after paramedian thalamic infarction. Ann Neurol 1989;26:125–6.

[110] Garrel S, Fau R, Perret J, et al. Troubles du sommeil dans deux syndromes vasculaires du tronc cérébral dont l'un anatomo-clinique. Rev Neurol 1966;115:575–84.

[111] Van Bogaert M. Syndrome de la calotte protubérantielle avec myoclonie localisée et troubles du sommeil. Rev Neurol 1926;45:977–88.

[112] Chase TN, Moretti L, Prensky AL. Clinical and electroencephalographic manifestations of vascular lesions of the pons. Neurology 1968; 18:357–68.

[113] Bassetti C, Bogousslavsky J, Mattle H, et al. Medial medullary infarction: report of seven patients and review of the literature. Neurology 1997;48:882–90.

[114] Rousseaux M, Caron J, Cattelat C. Hypotension othostatique transitoire sévère et hématome du tegmentum pontin. Rev Neurol 1993;149: 468–75.

[115] Davison C, Demuth EL. Disturbances in sleep mechanism: a clinicopathologic study. IV. Lesions at the mesencephalometencephalic level. Arch Neurol Psychiatry 1946;55:126–33.

[116] Kubik CS, Adams RD. Occlusion of the basilar artery: a clinical and pathological study. Brain 1946;69:73–121.

[117] Ketz E. Die vertebro-basilaris-thrombose im konventionellen EEG. Zeitschr EEG EMG 1970;2: 36–43.

[118] Gloor P, Ball G, Schall N. Brain lesions that produce delta waves in the EEG. Neurology 1977;27:326–33.

[119] Hirose G, Saeki M, Kosoegawa H, et al. Delta waves in the EEGs of patients with intracerebral hemorrhage. Arch Neurol 1981;38:170–5.

[120] Schaul N, Gloor P, Gotman J. The EEG in deep midline lesions. Neurology 1981;31:157–67.

[121] Lhermitte F, Gautier JC, Marteau R, et al. Troubles de la conscience et mutisme akinétique. Rev Neurol 1963;109:115–31.

[122] Feldman SM, Waller HJ. Dissociation of electrocortical activation and behavioural arousal. Nature 1962;4861:1320–2.

[123] Karabelas G, Kalfakis N, Kasvikis I, et al. Unusual features in a case of bilateral paramedian thalamic infarction. J Neurol Neurosurg Psychiatry 1984;47:186.

[124] Bastuji H, Nighoghossian N, Salord F, et al. Mesodiencephalic infarct with hypersomnia: sleep recording in two cases [abstract]. J Sleep Res 1994; 3:16.

[125] Guilleminault C, Quera-Salva MA, Goldberg MP. Pseudo-hypersomnia and pre-sleep behaviour with bilateral paramedian thalamic lesions. Brain 1993;116:1549–63.

[126] Graff-Radford NR, Eslinger PJ, Damasio AR, et al. Nonhemorrhagic infarction of the thalamus: behavioural, anatomic and physiologic correlates. Neurology 1984;34:14–23.

[127] Körner E, Flooh E, Reinhart B, et al. Sleep alterations in ischemic stroke. Eur Neurol 1986; 25:104–10.

[128] Hachinski V, Mamelak M, Norris JW. Clinical recovery and sleep architecture degradation. Can J Neurol Sci 1990;17:332–5.

[129] Bassetti CL, Aldrich MS. Sleep electroencephalogram changes in acute hemispheric stroke. Sleep Med 2001;2:185–94.

[130] Santamaria J, Pujol M, Orteu N, et al. Unilateral thalamic stroke does not decrease ipsilateral sleep spindles. Sleep 2000;23:333–9.

[131] Giubilei F, Iannilli M, Vitale A, et al. Sleep patterns in acute ischemic stroke. Acta Neurol Scand 1992;86:567–71.

[132] Beck U, Kendel K. Polygraphische nachtsschlafuntersuchugnen bei patienten mit hirnstammläsionen. Arch Psychiatr Nervenkr 1971;214: 331–46.

[133] Popoviciu L, Asgian B, Corfarici D, et al. Anatomoclinical and polygraphic features in cerebrovascular diseases with disturbances of vigilance. In: Tirgu-Mures L, Popoviciu L, Asgia B, et al, editors. Sleep 1978: Fourth European congress on sleep research. New York: S. Karger; 1980. p. 165–9.

[134] Autret A, Laffont F, De Toffol B, et al. A syndrome of REM and non-REM sleep reduction and lateral gaze paresis after medial tegmental pontine stroke. Arch Neurol 1988;45: 1236–42.

[135] Vighetto A, Confavreux C, Boisson D, et al. Paralysie de l'abaissement du regard et amnésie globale durables par lésion thalamosousthalamique bilatérale. Rev Neurol 1986;142: 449–55.

[136] Schott B, Maugière F, Laurent B, et al. L'amnésie thalamique. Rev Neurol 1980;136:117–30.

[137] Powell JH, Al-Adawi S, Morgan J, et al. Motivational deficits after brain injury: effects of bromocriptine in 11 patients. J Neurol Neurosurg Psychiatry 1996;60:416–21.

[138] Arpa J, Rodriguez-Albarino R, Izal E, et al. Hypersomnia after tegmental pontine hematoma: case report. Neurologia 1995;10:140–4.

[139] Castaigne P, Buge A, Cambier J, et al. Démence thalamique d'origine vasculaire par ramollissement bilatéral, limité au territoire du pédicule rétro-mamillaire: apropos de deux observation anatomo-cliniques. Rev Neurol 1966;114:89–107.

SLEEP
MEDICINE
CLINICS

Sleep Med Clin 1 (2006) 157–163

Periodic Leg Movements in Sleep and Restless Legs Syndrome Relation to Daytime Alertness and Sleepiness

Richard P. Allen, PhD

- ▪ Periodic leg movements in sleep definition and measurement
- ▪ Periodic leg movements in sleep and sleepiness
- ▪ Restless legs syndrome, periodic leg movements in sleep, and sleepiness
- ▪ References

There had long been an assumption in sleep medicine that the sleep disruption associated with the commonly observed periodic leg movements in sleep (PLMS) produces significant daytime sleepiness, particularly if there are a large number of arousals associated with these leg movements. Fig. 1 provides an example of the profoundly frequent PLM and arousals observed in an all-night physiologic recording (polysomnogram [PSG]) observed in some patients complaining of poor sleep or excessive daytime sleepiness). It seemed intuitively obvious that such pronounced and frequent phenomena disrupt sleep causing the patient's sleep-wake complaint. The sleep field identified a periodic limb movement disorder characterized by these PLMS plus a complaint of insomnia or daytime sleepiness. The appealing implicit assumption of a causal relation between PLMS and simultaneous occurrence of a sleep compliant remained largely unchallenged for the early years of sleep medicine. These peculiar PLMS events held such appeal that apparently few if any appreciated the high probability that two commonly occurring events (PLMS and sleep problems) co-occur by chance, not because of linked biology. This failure contributed to a basic misunderstanding of the biologic significance of PLMS and their relation to

daytime functioning. Two important windows informing clinicians about these issues are explored here: the studies of relationship of PLMS to insomnia and daytime sleepiness; the evaluation of daytime functioning of patients with restless legs syndrome (RLS), a disorder with PLMS as a motor sign. This later also indicates the complexity of daytime alertness suggesting multiple biologic or psychologic dimensions.

Periodic leg movements in sleep definition and measurement

PLMS were described in 1953 by Symonds [1] as a sleep myoclonus. These were later found to be very common in patients with RLS [2]. The recording of these events, as shown in Fig. 1, made it immediately apparent that the electromyographic activation and patterns were not generally myoclonic but rather represented a distinct pattern more appropriately referred to as "periodic leg movements" (PLM). When they occur in sleep they are called PLMS, but they also occur during resting waking, particularly in RLS patients, and then they are referred to as PLM of waking (PLMW) [3]. The movements are predominately but not exclusively flexor and electromyographic recording of the anterior

Neurology and Sleep Medicine, John Hopkins University, Bayview Medical Center, Asthma and Allergy Building, 1B76B, 5501 Hopkins Bayview Circle, Baltimore, MD 21224, USA
E-mail address: richardjhu@aol.com

1556-407X/06/$ – see front matter © 2006 Elsevier Inc. All rights reserved.
sleep.theclinics.com

doi:10.1016/j.jsmc.2005.11.013

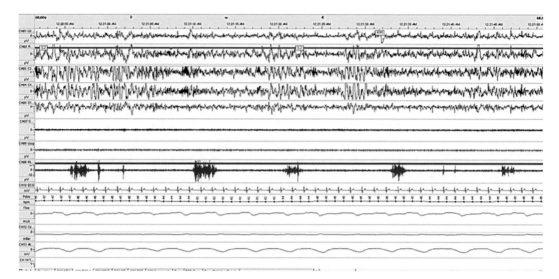

Fig. 1. One-minute polysomnogram recording from stage 2 sleep showing repeated PLM, several followed by brief arousal. The top two lines are the eye movements. The next three are electroencephalogram (EEG) (two central and one occipital). The lines below these in descending order are the submental electromyogram (EMG), left and then right anterior tibialis EMG, ECG, pulse rate, airflow from a nasal cannula, and thoracic and abdominal respiratory efforts.

tibialis from each leg defines the events. The current definition of PLM requires that the anterior-tibialis electromyographic envelope for each event must be 0.5 to 5 seconds long for PLMS and 0.5 to 10 seconds for PLMW. There must be at least four consecutive events occurring with intermovement intervals (time from onset to onset of consecutive movements) of 5 to 90 seconds [4,5]. The PLMW

during all-night physiologic recordings are not common except for RLS patients, where they actually have somewhat more diagnostic value than the PLMS [6]. PLMW and PLMS may be combined in some assessments.

A large night-to-night variation in PLMS per hour significantly complicates the measurement of these events and where possible multiple nights of re-

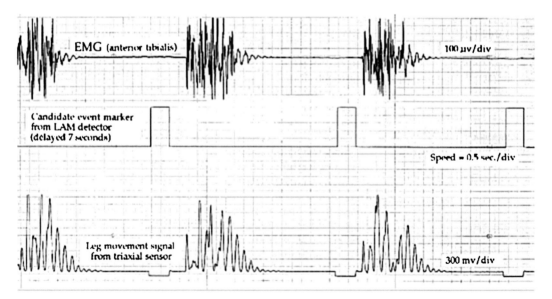

Fig. 2. PLM from a patient with RLS recorded simultaneously with anterior tibialis EMG and PAM-RL (IM Systems, Baltimore, MD) activity meter. Note the similar patterns from the two signals permitting use of the same measures for the activity data that are used for the EMG. The vertical lines represent 0.5-second intervals. The middle line notes when a PLM event is detected (after 7-second delay) by an automatic real-time PLM detector built into the PAM-RL.

cording provide a more stable assessment of the PLMS characteristics for a given individual [3,7]. Because these events generally produce some leg or foot movement they can also be detected by a currently available sophisticated leg activity meter (IM Systems, Baltimore, Maryland) worn at the ankle with a digital sampling rate of 40 Hz. This type of recording can separate the movements by leg position to remove those when not lying in bed and provides an accurate assessment of the combined PLMW and PLMS during the night [8]. Fig. 2 shows the repetitive nature of the leg movements captured by the leg activity meter demonstrating that this recording provides a resolution of each event similar to the envelope of the electromyography. The activity meter has the advantage of reduced cost and providing recording for multiple nights (up to 5 with one meter). It has the disadvantage of not providing information to exclude PLM associated with arousal from a sleep-disordered breathing event as shown in Fig. 3. Any evaluation of PLMS for a patient needs to exclude significant sleep-disordered breathing. The leg monitor also has the disadvantage of not separating PLMW from PLMS, but PLMW rarely occur for conditions other than RLS and for RLS they become important to include for diagnosis. Even for RLS the PLMW are far less common than PLMS and their rate during waking is somewhat similar. The activity meter includes the wake time and the PLMW in its measurement with the wake time generally being much less than the sleep time.

This combination of PLMW and PLMS produces a remarkably accurate assessment of the standard PSG recording of PLMS [8]. The mild loss in accuracy of the recoding is compensated by the multiple nights of recording and the reduced cost.

Periodic leg movements in sleep and sleepiness

The confusion between essential PLMS and the PLMS-like artifacts arising from episodic arousals caused by sleep-disordered breathing complicates evaluation of effects of PLMS. The brief arousals at the end of a sleep-disordered breathing event often occur with a brief leg movement of the same duration as that for PLMS and the periodicity of these events often fall within that defined for PLMS [see Fig. 3]. These PLMS are always considered products of the respiratory events and as a general rule disappear with effective treatment of the sleep-disordered breathing. The exceptional situations in which after effective continuous positive airway pressure treatment the PLMS do not disappear and even in some unusual cases become more severe remain poorly understood [9], but these puzzling cases represent a small minority of sleep-disordered breathing patients and evaluating the significance of PLMS themselves requires some effort to separate out PLMS associated with sleep-disordered breathing.

The common occurrence of PLMS with RLS and also narcolepsy, rapid eye movement behavior dis-

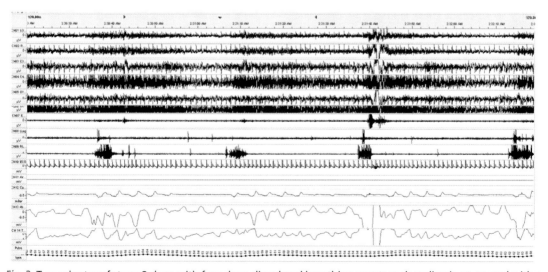

Fig. 3. Two minutes of stage 2 sleep with four sleep-disordered breathing events each ending in an arousal with a leg movement that qualifies as a PLM in sleep. Note the clear periodicity of these leg movements on the sixth line from the bottom of the chart matching that of the sleep-disordered breathing events shown by the airflow decreases on the fourth line from the bottom of the chart. The top two lines are the eye movements, the next three are EEG, and the sixth line is the submental EMG directly above the left leg and right leg anterior tibialis EMG. The EKG is above the airflow from a nasal cannula with thoracic and abdominal movements for respiratory effort. The finger oximetry makes up the last three lines.

order, and synucleinopathies further complicates interpretation of the significance of the PLMS themselves. Like sleep-disordered breathing each of these disorders alters daytime functioning. Unfortunately, many of the studies evaluating effects of PLMS themselves fail to evaluate for sleep-disordered breathing and fail to exclude these other disorders. But even with these problems the early studies attempting to relate PLMS to any sleep complaint including daytime sleepiness produced largely negative results. In a community-based sample of 427 adults 65 or older Ancoli-Israel and coworkers [10], using a home recording system, recorded respiration, and leg-movements combined with an activity record of sleep and wake. They reported higher PLMS per hour related significantly to breathing problems and decreased satisfaction with sleep but also to decreased inadvertent napping. This study failed to control for sleep-disordered breathing events and still, if anything, suggested PLMS were associated with decreased daytime problems with sleep. Mosko and coworkers [11] in a smaller sleep laboratory study of 46 elderly subjects also failed to find any relation between PLMS per hour and subjective reports of sleep-wake complaints including no relation to subjectively reported daytime sleepiness. These initials studies expecting to relate PLMS and its subsequent sleep disruption to daytime sleepiness produced surprising results that should have raised concern about the validity of the implicit assumptions underlying the concept of a periodic limb movement disorder. But there was a strong tendency to discount these studies and even claim the patients had significant disease even though they had no subjective complaints with any indication for any associated health consequence [11].

It should not have come as a surprise that more recent studies failed to find any relation between PLMS per hour and sleep complaints in patients without other sleep disorders. Mendelson [12] reviewed data on 67 patients diagnosed at a university-based sleep disorder center with periodic limb movement disorder and found no relation between PLMS per hour or PLMS with arousal per hour of sleep and either subjective or objective Multiple Sleep Latency Test measures of sleepiness. Nicolas and coworkers [13] in a sleep laboratory study of 34 patients with PLMS without other sleep-related disorders known to cause PLMS found no relation between PLMS per hour and sleep efficiency at night or the Multiple Sleep Latency Test measure of daytime sleepiness. Still, given the sample size of these studies it remained unclear whether or not the PLMS or possibly PLMS associated with arousals is associated with sleep fragmentation and daytime sleepiness. Chervin [14] reviewed data from a larger group of 321 patients evaluated with PSG at a sleep-disorder center and found a surprising relation between PLMS associated with arousals per hour and decreased objective sleepiness and no relation between PLMS without arousal and daytime sleepiness.

In total there seems to be no obvious relation at all between PLMS and sleep-wake complaints except, if anything, in one study the occurrence of PLMS associated with arousals may indicate less daytime sleepiness. The study by Chervin [14], however, failed to exclude patients with RLS and this may have contributed to the unexpected result. This finding must be balanced against recent data showing a clear association between PLMS and both heart rate and EEG changes [15], indicating these events mark a brain process with multiple effects including but not limited to the leg muscle activation. This relation has been best documented for RLS patients [16–18], but aside from disorders associated with altered autonomic function, such as rapid eye movement behavior disorder [19], there is no reason to assume these results do not generalize to most PLMS. The extent to which these processes have health significance either by themselves or in the presence of other biologic factors remains to be established. The paradigm shift is that PLMS and even PLMS associated with arousals do not significantly disrupt sleep causing sleepiness; rather, they mark a biologic process that may in itself be significant. The observations by Montplaisir and colleagues [20] of a link between PLMS and sleep disorders with dopamine impairment support the potential biologic significance of the broader-based PLM process.

Restless legs syndrome, periodic leg movements in sleep, and sleepiness

RLS is a commonly occurring (about 7% prevalence in the United States and Europe [21]) sensory-motor neurologic disorder. The condition presents with a primary symptom of a strong urge to move the leg precipitated by rest or the transition state permitting sleep and relieved by movement or any strongly alerting activity. The urge to move is often associated with other peculiar sensations that patients find hard to describe, but usually have elements of an unpleasant sense of motion deep in the leg (eg, worms crawling in the leg) that are often noxious and sometimes like an ache or even peculiar pain. RLS has a strong circadian pattern with symptoms much worse or sometimes only occurring during the evening or night. There seems to be a protected period around 8 to 10 AM when the symptoms are markedly reduced if they occur at all [22]. **Fig. 4** gives an example of an RLS sleep log

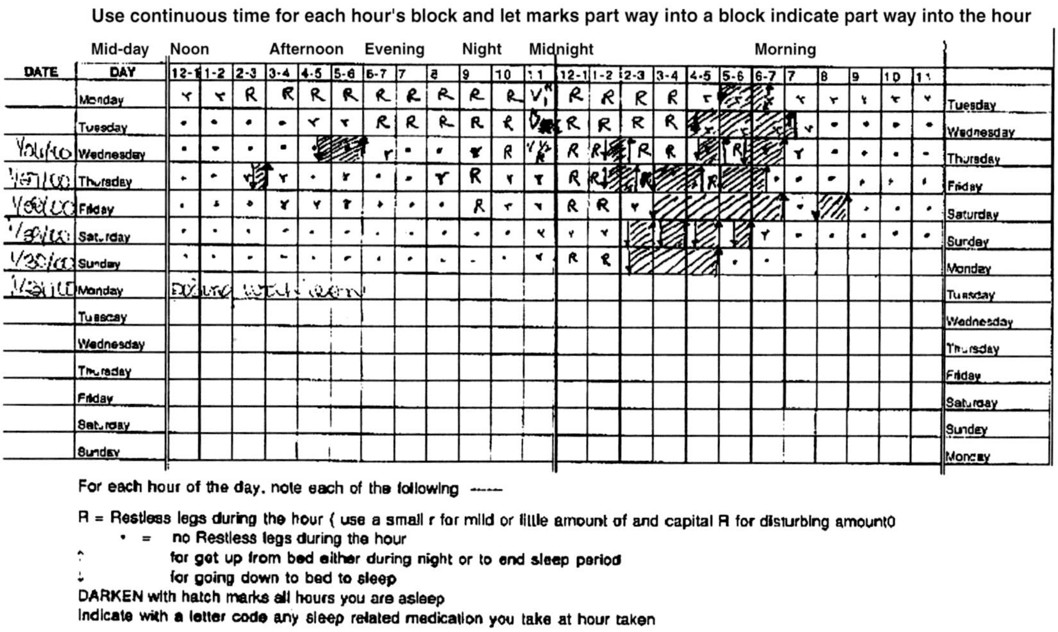

Fig. 4. RLS sleep log for a week in the life of moderately severe untreated RLS patient. Note the markedly reduced bed and sleep times and the circadian pattern of RLS symptoms with no effort to sleep-in late in the morning despite the lack of any symptoms.

completed by one patient showing the hours of each day for a week marked for occurrence of RLS symptoms by either a large "R" for moderate to severe symptoms and small "r" for minimal to mild symptoms. Sleep times are indicated by hatch marks darkening the hourly square. The pattern reported by this patient typifies that of moderately severe RLS patients. Note the very short sleep time for most nights and the circadian pattern with virtually no symptoms in the morning. Also typical of RLS patients is the failure to sleep-in late in the morning despite the absence of symptoms and the lack of sleep the prior night. This failure to use the morning to catch up on sleep seems typical of the disorder and not consistent with the daytime sleepiness expected for the degree of chronic sleep loss observed.

PLMS represent the motor sign of RLS and at this time provide the only objective marker of the disorder. Although nonspecific, PLMS are sensitive, occurring in at least 80% of the RLS patients [23], and significantly linked to the clinical evaluation of symptom severity [24,25]. PLMS support the diagnosis and provide an objective measure of disease severity. Mild RLS has little effect on sleep, but moderate to severe RLS marked by increased PLMS produces significant sleep disruption. PSGs on a case series of 31 moderate to severely affected RLS patients showed sleep efficiency to be significantly reduced to less than 60% with PLMS in-

creased to over 100 per hour [25]. Another PSG case series of 131 RLS patients of similar severity showed similar reduction in sleep efficiency (average ± SD 75% ± 18.9%) [23]. About 85% of these moderate to severe RLS patients reported difficulty falling asleep and 84% reported difficulty staying asleep [23].

There are relatively few studies comparing the PSG sleep of RLS patients with age- and gender-matched controls. Three small studies with samples of 12 to 16 subjects in each of the RLS patient and matched control groups each reported RLS patients had significantly less total sleep time and sleep efficiency. Sleep latency was longer for RLS patients but for these samples this difference from controls was not statistically significant [3,26–28]. One study with a larger sample size (100 RLS patients and 50 matched control subjects) found the same significant differences and with the larger sample size the longer sleep latency was also statistically significant [6]. These objective indications of profoundly disturbed sleep of the more severe RLS patients matches the reported subjective complaints with over 75% of those in a population-based survey with at least moderately severe RLS symptoms reporting significant sleep disruption as a primary compliant [21].

Sleep deprivation even less than that reported for RLS when produced experimentally in normal subjects has been found to cause daytime sleepiness and disruption of cognitive and vigilance performance [29]. Similar effects would be expected for more severe RLS patients with the increased PLMS per hour marking the disease severity. Studies of RLS patients, however, have failed consistently to find the expected daytime sleepiness. The situation is somewhat confused by the failure in many studies to discriminate between frank sleepiness and fatigue or lack of energy. Even those who do not or even could not fall asleep in the daytime may answer affirmatively to a single question on presence of daytime sleepiness. Indeed, in the one larger PSG study comparing RLS with control subjects 34% reported daytime sleepiness [23], significantly less than the 85% reporting sleep disruption, but significantly more than for controls. When the daytime sleepiness is evaluated more carefully a different picture emerges.

In a study of the daytime alertness in 12 RLS patients in sleep clinic compared with 12 matched controls, RLS patients showed increased simple reaction time in response to a visual stimulus but showed no difference from controls on a standard measure of attention and concentration from the Grünberger alphabetic cancellation test (percent errors) [27]. In this small study the RLS patients reported more drowsiness than controls on a visual analog scale, but again this was not clearly defined. The Epworth Sleepiness Scale provides a better assessment of actual sleepiness tendency and one series of 31 untreated RLS patients showed about the same Epworth scores as 33 matched controls (average ± SD of 5.9 ± 4.5 versus 5.1 ± 2.1) [30].

Larger population-based epidemiologic studies have reported increased daytime sleepiness for RLS patients [31,32], but the complaint was more of lack of attention and concentration making it difficult to work [31] than of falling asleep at inappropriate times. The Epworth test when used in population-based studies again fails to show statistically significantly increases for those with RLS symptoms to that of controls [31].

RLS when severe has perhaps the greatest chronic sleep loss of any sleep disorder. It appropriately produces decreased concentration and a subjective sense of some effects of sleep loss but none or at most minimal actual daytime sleepiness. It is tempting to see this as partly an expression of increased arousal associated with increased hypocretin [33–35] that was reported in one study of more severe RLS patients off medication [36], but not in a second study [37]. This discrepancy, regardless of cause, points out at least two dimensions to the concept of daytime sleepiness: one actual tendency to fall asleep as assessed by the Epworth Sleepiness Scale and the Multiple Sleep Latency Test, the other the loss of ability to maintain focused atten-

tion as measured by vigilance-type tests. The well-documented cognitive deficits of one night of sleep deprivation apparently specific to prefrontal lobe function [29] might represent yet another dimension of the subjective complaint of daytime sleepiness. One recent study comparing RLS patients with controls also showed cognitive deficits associated with prefrontal lobe function but otherwise normal cognitive functioning (Pearson and coworkers, unpublished data, 2005). RLS despite not producing actual sleepiness in the day may produce at least two of the features of daytime sleepiness (ie, decreased concentration and impaired frontal lobe function).

References

[1] Symonds CP. Nocturnal myoclonus. J Neurol Neurosurg Psychiatr 1953;16:166–71.

[2] Lugaresi G, Coccagna G, Berti Ceroni G, et al. Restless legs syndrome and nocturnal myoclonus. In: Gastaut H, Lugaresi E, Berti Ceroni G, editors. The abnormalities of sleep in man. Bologna: Aulo Gaggi Editore; 1968. p. 285–94.

[3] Montplaisir J, Boucher S, Nicolas A, et al. Immobilization tests and periodic leg movements in sleep for the diagnosis of restless leg syndrome. Mov Disord 1998;13:324–9.

[4] Michaud M, Poirier G, Lavigne G, et al. Restless legs syndrome: scoring criteria for leg movements recorded during the suggested immobilization test. Sleep Med 2001;2:317–21.

[5] Atlas Task Force of the American Sleep Disorders Association. Recording and scoring leg movements. Sleep 1993;16:748–59.

[6] Michaud M, Paquet J, Lavigne G, et al. Sleep laboratory diagnosis of restless legs syndrome. Eur Neurol 2002;48:108–13.

[7] Mosko SS, Dickel MJ, Ashurst J. Night-to-night variability in sleep apnea and sleep-related periodic leg movements in the elderly. Sleep 1988; 11:340–8.

[8] Sforza E, Johannes M, Bassetti C. The PAM-RL ambulatory device for detection of periodic leg movements: a validation study. Sleep Med 2005; 6:407–13.

[9] Fry JM, DiPhillipo MA, Pressman MR. Periodic leg movements in sleep following treatment of obstructive sleep apnea with nasal continuous positive airway pressure. Chest 1989;96:89–91.

[10] Ancoli-Israel S, Kripke DF, Klauber MR, et al. Periodic limb movements in sleep in community dwelling elderly. Sleep 1991;14:496–500.

[11] Mosko SS, Dickel MJ, Paul T, et al. Sleep apnea and sleep-related periodic leg movements in community resident seniors. J Am Geriatr Soc 1988;36:502–8.

[12] Mendelson WB. Are periodic leg movements associated with clinical sleep disturbance? Sleep 1996;19:219–23.

[13] Nicolas A, Lesperance P, Montplaisir J. Is ex-

cessive daytime sleepiness with periodic leg movements during sleep a specific diagnostic category? Eur Neurol 1998;40:22–6.

[14] Chervin RD. Periodic leg movements and sleepiness in patients evaluated for sleep-disordered breathing. Am J Respir Crit Care Med 2001; 164(8 Pt 1):1454–8.

[15] Sforza E, Nicolas A, Lavigne G, et al. EEG and cardiac activation during periodic leg movements in sleep: support for a hierarchy of arousal responses. Neurology 1999;52:786–91.

[16] Sforza E, Juony C, Ibanez V. Time-dependent variation in cerebral and autonomic activity during periodic leg movements in sleep: implications for arousal mechanisms. Clin Neurophysiol 2002;113:883–91.

[17] Gosselin N, Lanfranchi P, Michaud M, et al. Age and gender effects on heart rate activation associated with periodic leg movements in patients with restless legs syndrome. Clin Neurophysiol 2003;114:2188–95.

[18] Sforza E, Pichot V, Barthelemy JC, et al. Cardiovascular variability during periodic leg movements: a spectral analysis approach. Clin Neurophysiol 2005;116:1096–104.

[19] Fantini ML, Michaud M, Gosselin N, et al. Periodic leg movements in REM sleep behavior disorder and related autonomic and EEG activation. Neurology 2002;59:1889–94.

[20] Montplaisir J, Michaud M, Denesle R, et al. Periodic leg movements are not more prevalent in insomnia or hypersomnia but are specifically associated with sleep disorders involving a dopaminergic impairment. Sleep Med 2000;1: 163–7.

[21] Allen RP, Walters AS, Montplaisir J, et al. Restless legs syndrome prevalence and impact: REST general population study. Arch Intern Med 2005; 165:1286–92.

[22] Allen RP, Picchietti D, Hening WA, et al. Restless legs syndrome: diagnostic criteria, special considerations, and epidemiology. A report from the restless legs syndrome diagnosis and epidemiology workshop at the National Institutes of Health. Sleep Med 2003;4:101–19.

[23] Montplaisir J, Boucher S, Poirier G, et al. Clinical, polysomnographic, and genetic characteristics of restless legs syndrome: a study of 133 patients diagnosed with new standard criteria. Mov Disord 1997;12:61–5.

[24] Garcia-Borreguero D, Larrosa O, de la Llave Y, et al. Correlation between rating scales and sleep laboratory measurements in restless legs syndrome. Sleep Med 2004;5:561–5.

[25] Allen RP, Earley CJ. Validation of the Johns Hopkins Restless Legs Severity Scale (JHRLSS). Sleep Med 2001;2:239–42.

[26] Saletu M, Anderer P, Saletu B, et al. Sleep laboratory studies in restless legs syndrome patients as compared with normals and acute effects of ropinirole. 2. Findings on periodic leg movements, arousals and respiratory variables. Neuropsychobiology 2000;41:190–9.

[27] Saletu B, Gruber G, Saletu M, et al. Sleep laboratory studies in restless legs syndrome patients as compared with normals and acute effects of ropinirole. 1. Findings on objective and subjective sleep and awakening quality. Neuropsychobiology 2000;41:181–9.

[28] Garcia-Borreguero D, Larrosa O, Granizo JJ, et al. Circadian variation in neuroendocrine response to L-dopa in patients with restless legs syndrome. Sleep 2004;27:669–73.

[29] Durmer JS, Dinges DF. Neurocognitive consequences of sleep deprivation. Semin Neurol 2005;25:117–29.

[30] Saletu B, Anderer P, Saletu M, et al. EEG mapping, psychometric, and polysomnographic studies in restless legs syndrome (RLS) and periodic limb movement disorder (PLMD) patients as compared with normal controls. Sleep Med 2002;3:S35–42.

[31] Ulfberg J, Nystrom B, Carter N, et al. Restless legs syndrome among working-aged women. Eur Neurol 2001;46:17–9.

[32] Bjorvatn B, Leissner L, Ulfberg J, et al. Prevalence, severity and risk factors of restless legs syndrome in the general adult population in two Scandinavian countries. Sleep Med 2005;6:307–12.

[33] Kilduff TS, Peyron C. The hypocretin/orexin ligand-receptor system: implications for sleep and sleep disorders. Trends Neurosci 2000;23: 359–65.

[34] Moore RY, Abrahamson EA, Van Den Pol A. The hypocretin neuron system: an arousal system in the human brain. Arch Ital Biol 2001;139: 195–205.

[35] Xi M, Morales FR, Chase MH. Effects on sleep and wakefulness of the injection of hypocretin-1 (orexin-A) into the laterodorsal tegmental nucleus of the cat. Brain Res 2001;901(1–2):259–64.

[36] Allen RP, Mignot E, Ripley B, et al. Increased CSF hypocretin-1 (orexin-A) in restless legs syndrome. Neurology 2002;59:639–41.

[37] Stiasny-Kolster K, Mignot E, Ling L, et al. CSF hypocretin-1 levels in restless legs syndrome. Neurology 2003;61:1426–9.

SLEEP
MEDICINE
CLINICS

Sleep Med Clin 1 (2006) 165–170

Index

Note: Page numbers of article titles are in **boldface** type.

doi:10.1016/S1556-407X(06)00011-7

Changing Your Address?

Make sure your subscription changes too! When you notify us of your new address, you can help make our job easier by including an exact copy of your Clinics label number with your old address (see illustration below.) This number identifies you to our computer system and will speed the processing of your address change. Please be sure this label number accompanies your old address and your corrected address—you can send an old Clinics label with your number on it or just copy it exactly and send it to the address listed below.

We appreciate your help in our attempt to give you continuous coverage. Thank you.

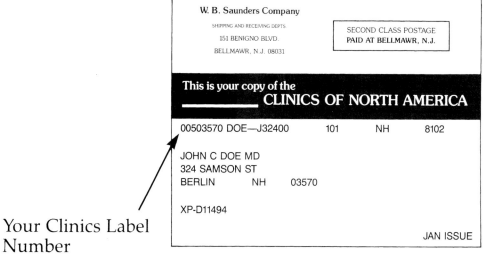

Your Clinics Label Number
Copy it exactly or send your label along with your address to:
W.B. Saunders Company, Customer Service
Orlando, FL 32887-4800
Call Toll Free 1-800-654-2452

Please allow four to six weeks for delivery of new subscriptions and for processing address changes.